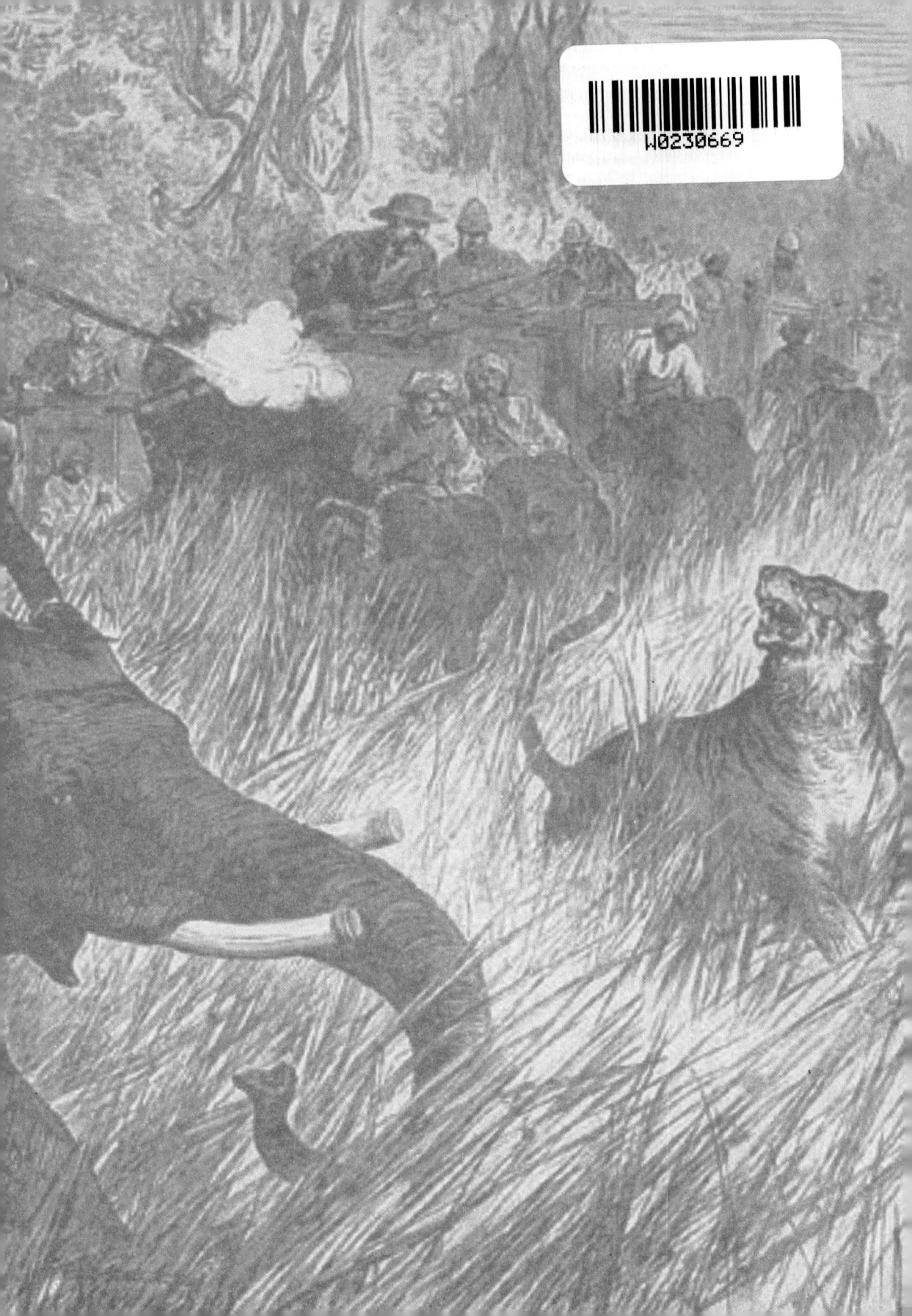

TIGERS

IN THE LONG GRASS

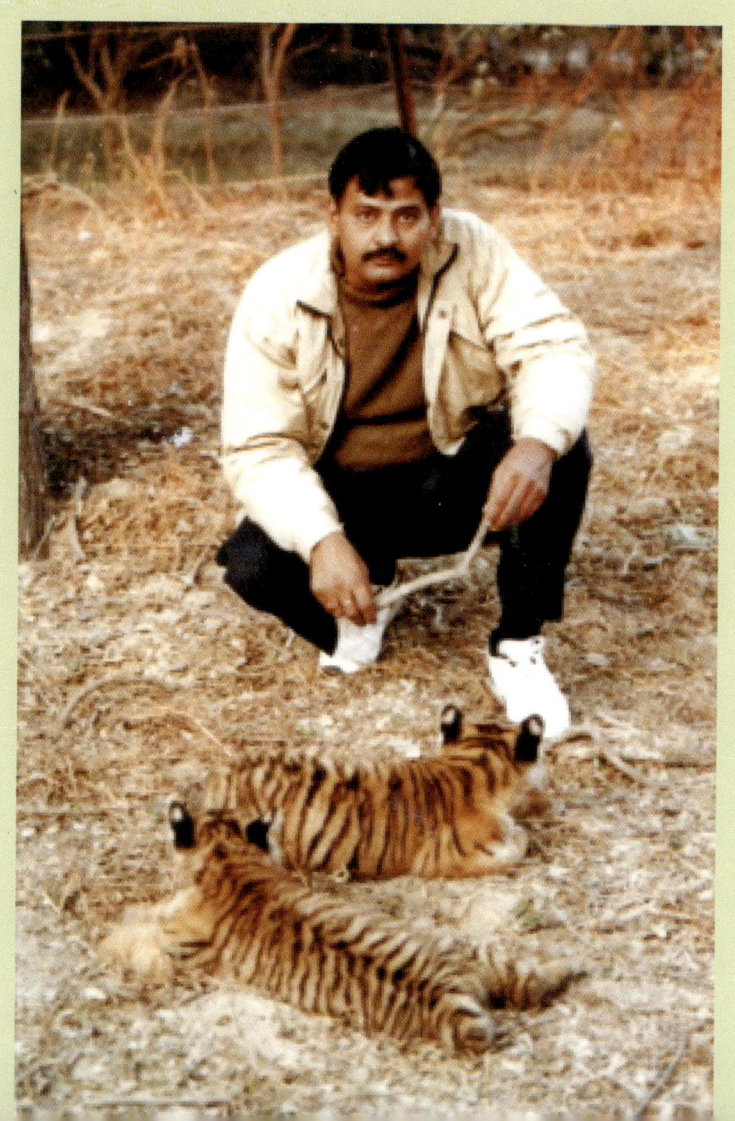

Accolades for Rahul Shukla's Sugarcane Tiger

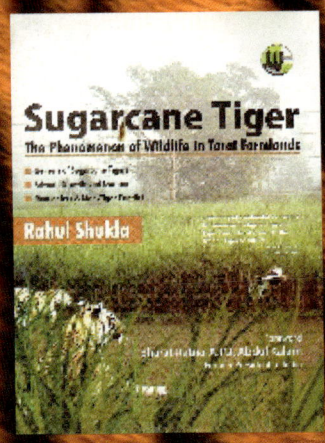

"Rahul Shukla has for many years followed the lives of tigers that live and breed in sugarcane fields of the Terai region of India and Nepal, once home to thousands of tigers and a unique assemblage ungulate prey found nowhere in Asia. Thanks to ravages inflicted by humans, only remnants of the magnificent Terai remains, much of it replaced by a human-dominated ecosystem of extensive sugarcane farms, harboring a simplified prey base consisting of wild pigs, livestock, and Nilgai in some places. Dr. Shukla has with single-minded passion, unearthed their unique adaptations. His natural history accounts add value to our collective knowledge about our national animal".

Dr. K. Ullas Karanth, Director for Science-Asia, Wildlife Conservation Society

In my official capacity as Secretary, Home, to the Government of Uttar Pradesh (1994-98), I got the chance to associate with Dr Rahul Shukla in many of his Tarai visits, admiring his extraordinary endeavour to protect farmland wildlife… I am influenced by his accredited work on Sugarcane Tiger and the narrative of their ruthless decimation which is the history of the greatest theft of tigers in the Tarai farmlands. I endorse that he is the only expert with the right credentials who could have presented this record of farmland wildlife so meticulously.

- N. Ravi Shanker, IAS, Chief Secretary, Uttarakhand

Drawn to dangerous challenges, Rahul Shukla enjoys worldwide repute in the field of tiger studies. His deep and profound understanding of the subject and immense contribution to the cause of conserving tigers makes this chronicle highly appealing for readers.

- Rupak De, IFS, Head of the Forest Department & Principal Chief Conservator of Forests, Uttar Pradesh

This book, written from the heart, is an important one as it lays bare the predicament of half-way tigers living in sugarcane between man and wilderness. The author is one and alone who saw its portents in mid 1970's and brought them forth through a series of articles in the esteemed newspaper of north India "The Pioneer." This book, carrying many old press reports, is a *cri de coeur* that crosses an emotional threshold to protect farmland wildlife.

- Abhilash Khandekar, Environmentalist & National Editor, *Bhaskar Group*

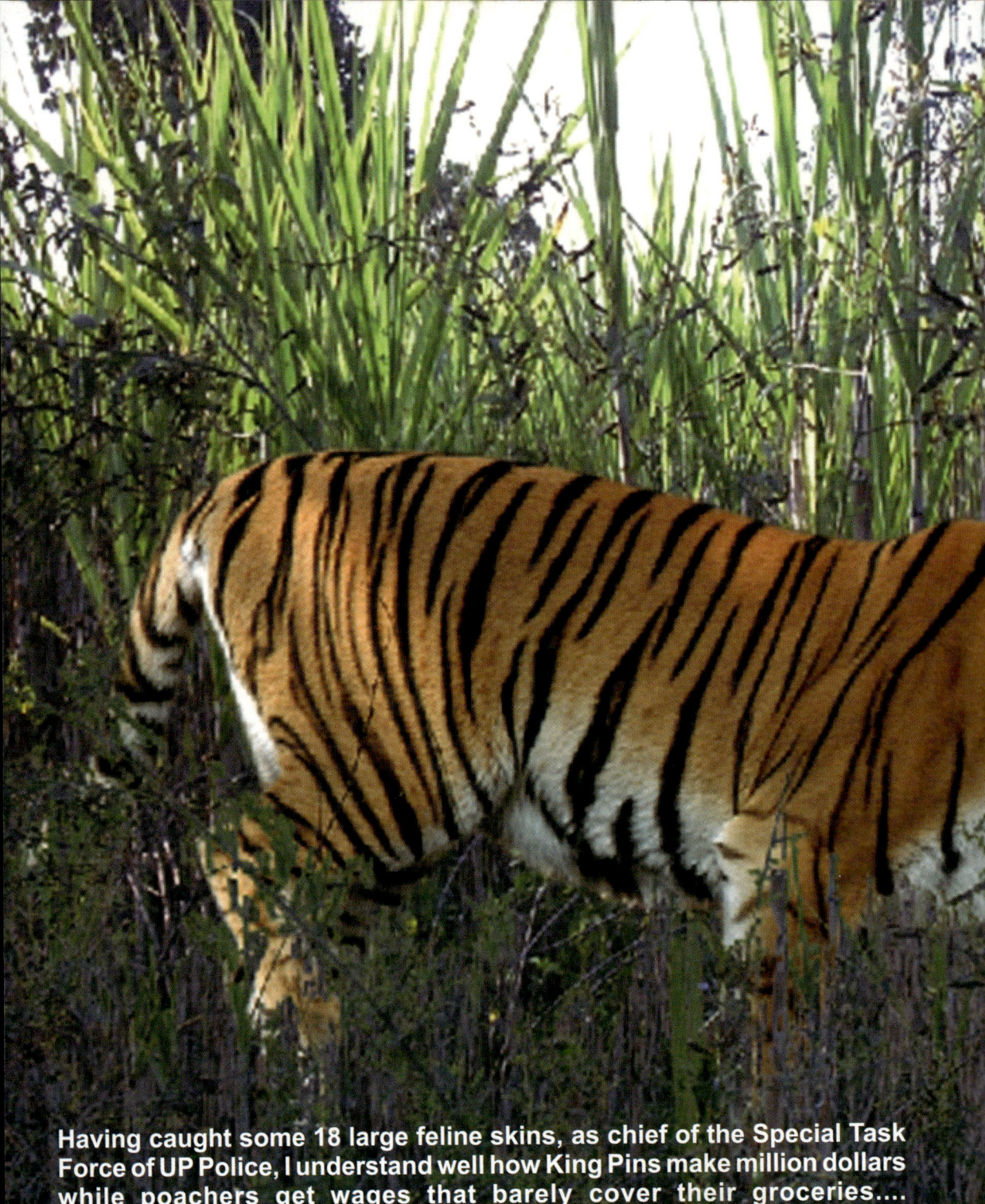

Having caught some 18 large feline skins, as chief of the Special Task Force of UP Police, I understand well how King Pins make million dollars while poachers get wages that barely cover their groceries.... 'Sugarcane Tiger' is a brilliant story of man and nature, its conflicts and reconciliations, as well as Dr Shukla's vulnerable daring to protect farmland wildlife.

- Amitabh Yash, I.P.S., Inspector General of Police, U.P.

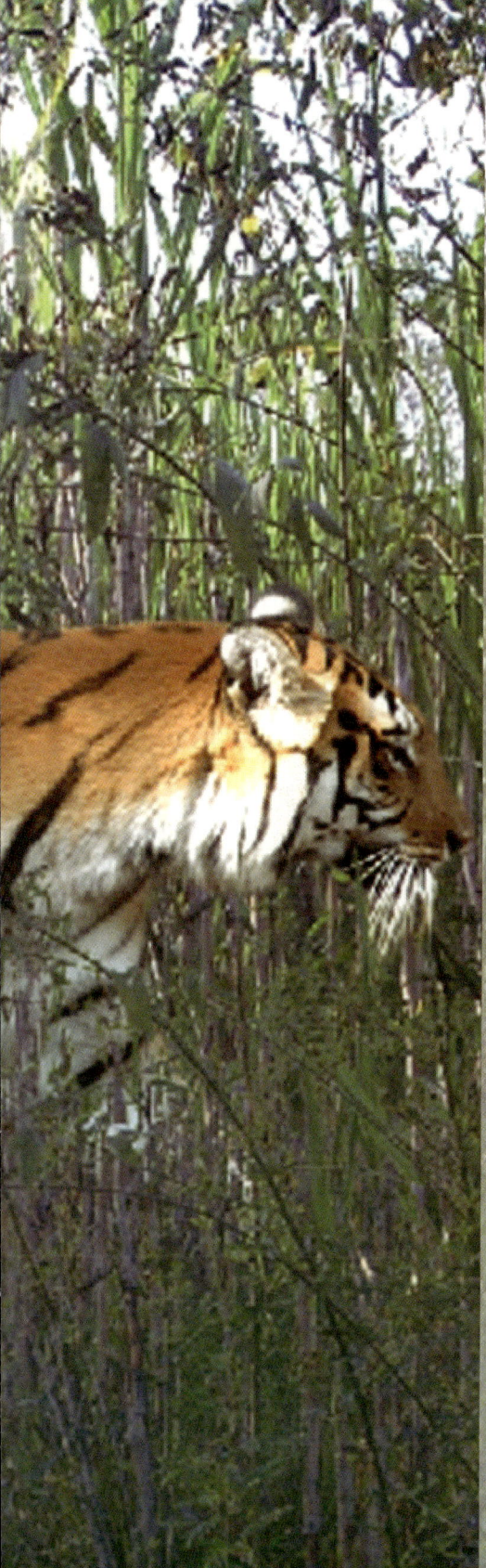

It is the need of the hour that some mindful biologists take pain to survey the great expanse of Tarai farmlands and consume this upbeat package of cane-tiger phenomenon which Shukla has brought to light.

— Raj Saran Verma, Indian Express

I have been associated with Dr Shukla in many of his promising ventures in Tarai farmlands. His findings about tigers in sugarcane augur well and proper with the awesome phenomenon. These set a new paradigm for tiger scientists.

— Wung Longwa, IFS, Chief Conservator of Forests, Uttarakhand

Lost in the far corners of India's Tarai farmlands, you are brought to a sudden appreciation of the universal nature of the tiger that infiltrate the sugarcane fields and live there. Without much verbosity, with precise, almost instinctive logic Dr Rahul Shukla strips the dogmatic knowledge about the predator with serious observations. India needs a political courage to sound out this knowledge and use it for the good of wildlife.

— Ranjit Bhargava, Padm Shri, Chairman WWF UP Chapter

An inducing portrayal of farmland wildlife; Shukla's attachment to Tarai is almost visionary and commitment to tigers is absolute.

— Ashok Kumar, Vice Chairman WTI

Rahul Shukla provides an entirely different research material from his contemporaries, both on scientific scales about tiger's comportment in farmlands and a new growing attitude towards their conservation by his pro-people instance that he calls saving men from tigers... the work has several clear flashes of important insights into day-to-day tiger actions.

— Sanjay Pathak, DIG Wildlife, National Tiger Conservation Authority (NTCA)

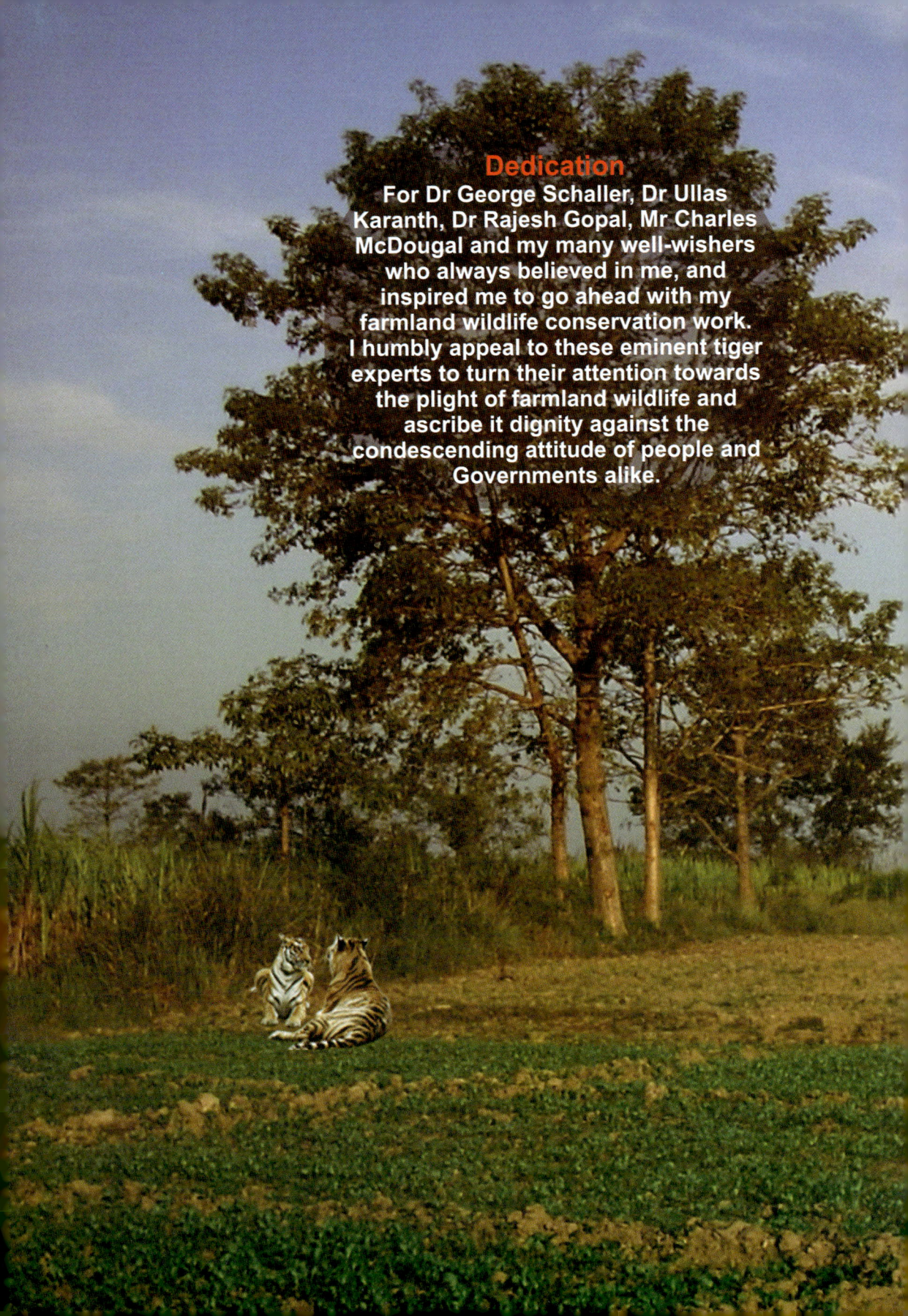

Dedication

For Dr George Schaller, Dr Ullas Karanth, Dr Rajesh Gopal, Mr Charles McDougal and my many well-wishers who always believed in me, and inspired me to go ahead with my farmland wildlife conservation work. I humbly appeal to these eminent tiger experts to turn their attention towards the plight of farmland wildlife and ascribe it dignity against the condescending attitude of people and Governments alike.

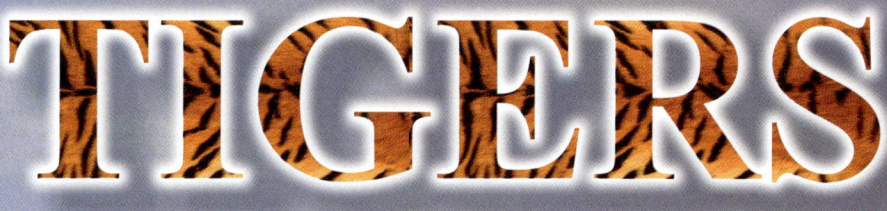

TIGERS
IN THE LONG GRASS

My Link with
Big Cats in Sugarcane

MAN EATERS and MITIGATING
MAN–TIGER CONFLICT IN TARAI

(A Sequel to Author's Sugarcane Tiger)

Rahul Shukla

Assisted by
Shrivridhi Shukla

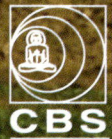

CBS Publishers & Distributors Pvt Ltd

New Delhi • Bengaluru • Chennai • Kochi • Kolkata • Mumbai
Hyderabad • Jharkhand • Nagpur • Patna • Pune • Uttarakhand

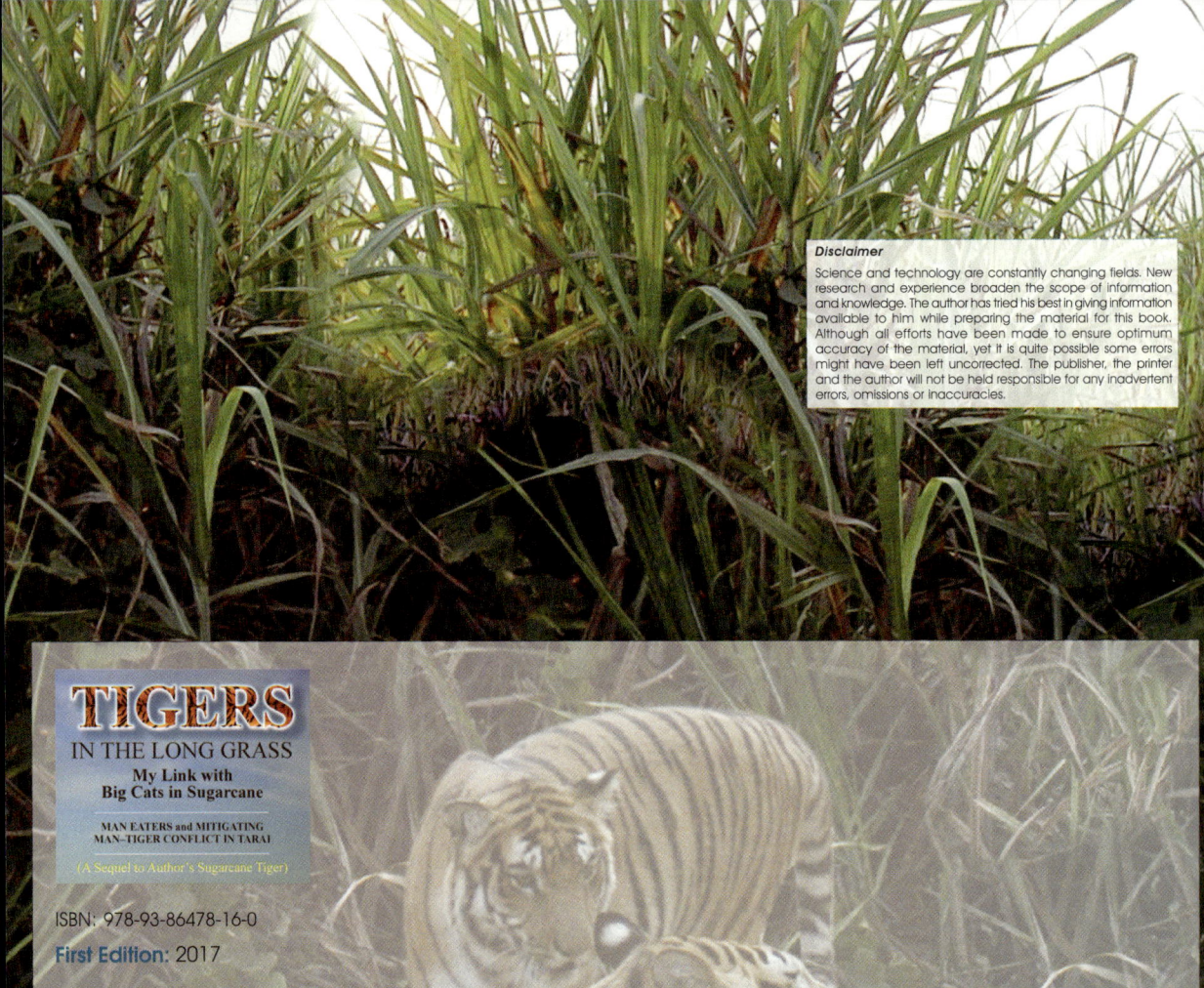

TIGERS
IN THE LONG GRASS
My Link with
Big Cats in Sugarcane

MAN EATERS and MITIGATING MAN–TIGER CONFLICT IN TARAI

(A Sequel to Author's Sugarcane Tiger)

ISBN: 978-93-86478-16-0

First Edition: 2017

Published by Satish Kumar Jain and produced by Varun Jain for

CBS Publishers & Distributors Pvt Ltd

4819/XI Prahlad Street, 24 Ansari Road, Daryaganj, New Delhi 110 002, India.
Ph: 23289259, 23266861, 23266867   Fax: 011-23243014   Website: www.cbspd.com
e-mail: delhi@cbspd.com; cbspubs@airtelmail.in.

Corporate Office: 204 FIE, Industrial Area, Patparganj, Delhi 110 092
Ph: 4934 4934   Fax: 4934 4935   e-mail: publishing@cbspd.com; publicity@cbspd.com

Branches

• **Bengaluru:** Seema House 2975, 17th Cross, K.R. Road, Banasankari 2nd Stage, Bengaluru 560 070, Karnataka
  Ph: +91-80-26771678/79   Fax: +91-80-26771680   e-mail: bangalore@cbspd.com
• **Chennai:** No. 7, Subbaraya Street, Shenoy Nagar, Chennai 600 030, Tamil Nadu
  Ph: +91-44-26680620, 26681266   Fax: +91-44-42032115   e-mail: chennai@cbspd.com
• **Kochi:** Ashana House, 39/1904, AM Thomas Road, Valanjambalam, Ernakulam 682 016, Kochi, Kerala
  Ph: +91-484-4059061-65,67   Fax: +91-484-4059065   e-mail: kochi@cbspd.com
• **Kolkata:** No. 6/B, Ground Floor, Rameswar Shaw Road, Kolkata-700014 (West Bengal), India
  Ph: +91-33-2289-1126, 2289-1127, 2289-1128   e-mail: kolkata@cbspd.com
• **Mumbai:** 83-C, Dr E Moses Road, Worli, Mumbai-400018, Maharashtra
  Ph: +91-22-24902340/41   Fax: +91-22-24902342   e-mail: mumbai@cbspd.com

Representatives

• **Hyderabad:** 0-9885175004   • **Jharkhand:** 0-9811541605   • **Patna:** 0-9334159340
• **Pune:** 0-9623451994   • **Uttrakhand:** 0-9716462459

Printed at Paras Offset Pvt Ltd., New Delhi (India)

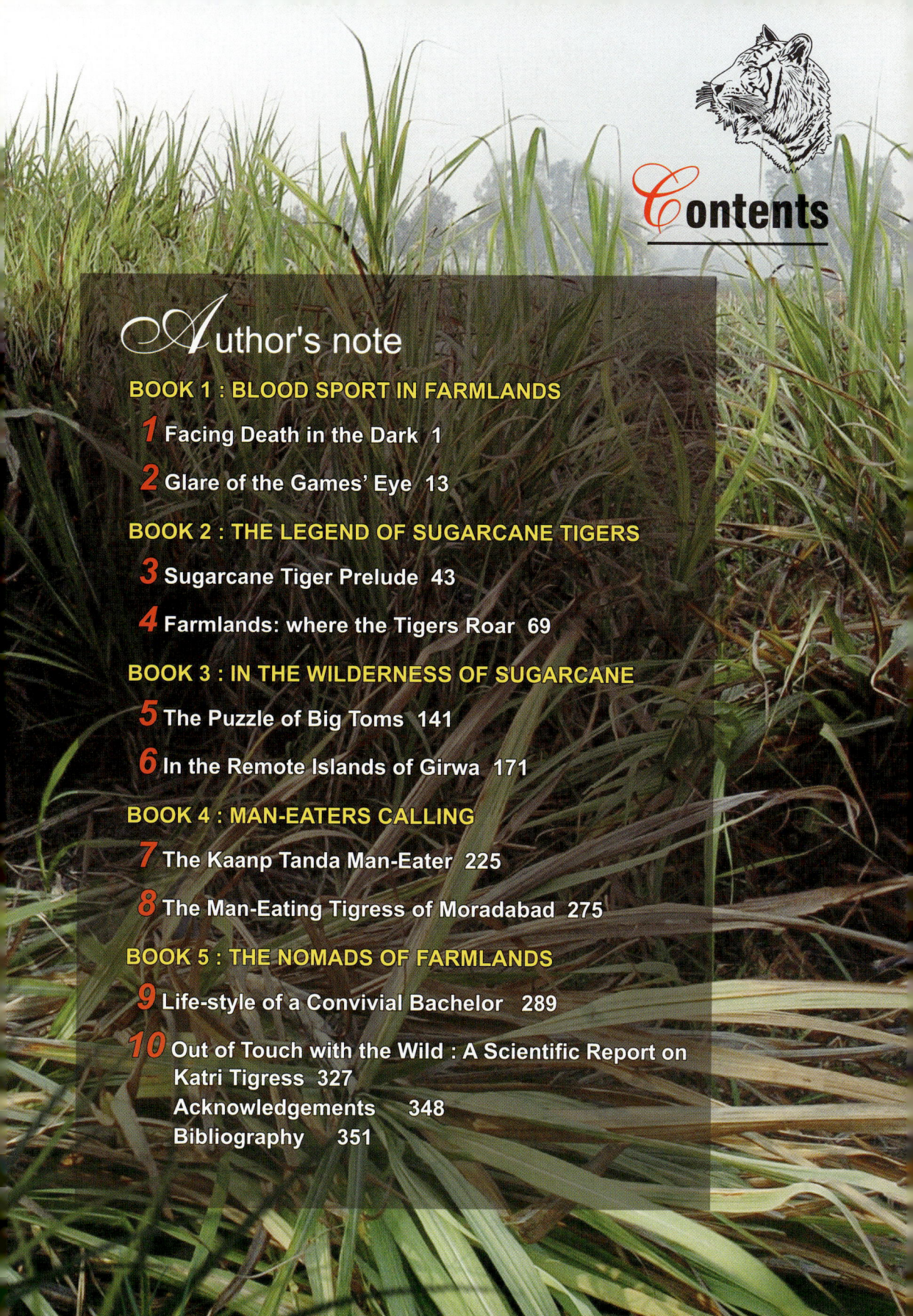

Contents

Author's note

BOOK 1 : BLOOD SPORT IN FARMLANDS

1 Facing Death in the Dark 1

2 Glare of the Games' Eye 13

BOOK 2 : THE LEGEND OF SUGARCANE TIGERS

3 Sugarcane Tiger Prelude 43

4 Farmlands: where the Tigers Roar 69

BOOK 3 : IN THE WILDERNESS OF SUGARCANE

5 The Puzzle of Big Toms 141

6 In the Remote Islands of Girwa 171

BOOK 4 : MAN-EATERS CALLING

7 The Kaanp Tanda Man-Eater 225

8 The Man-Eating Tigress of Moradabad 275

BOOK 5 : THE NOMADS OF FARMLANDS

9 Life-style of a Convivial Bachelor 289

10 Out of Touch with the Wild : A Scientific Report on Katri Tigress 327

Acknowledgements 348

Bibliography 351

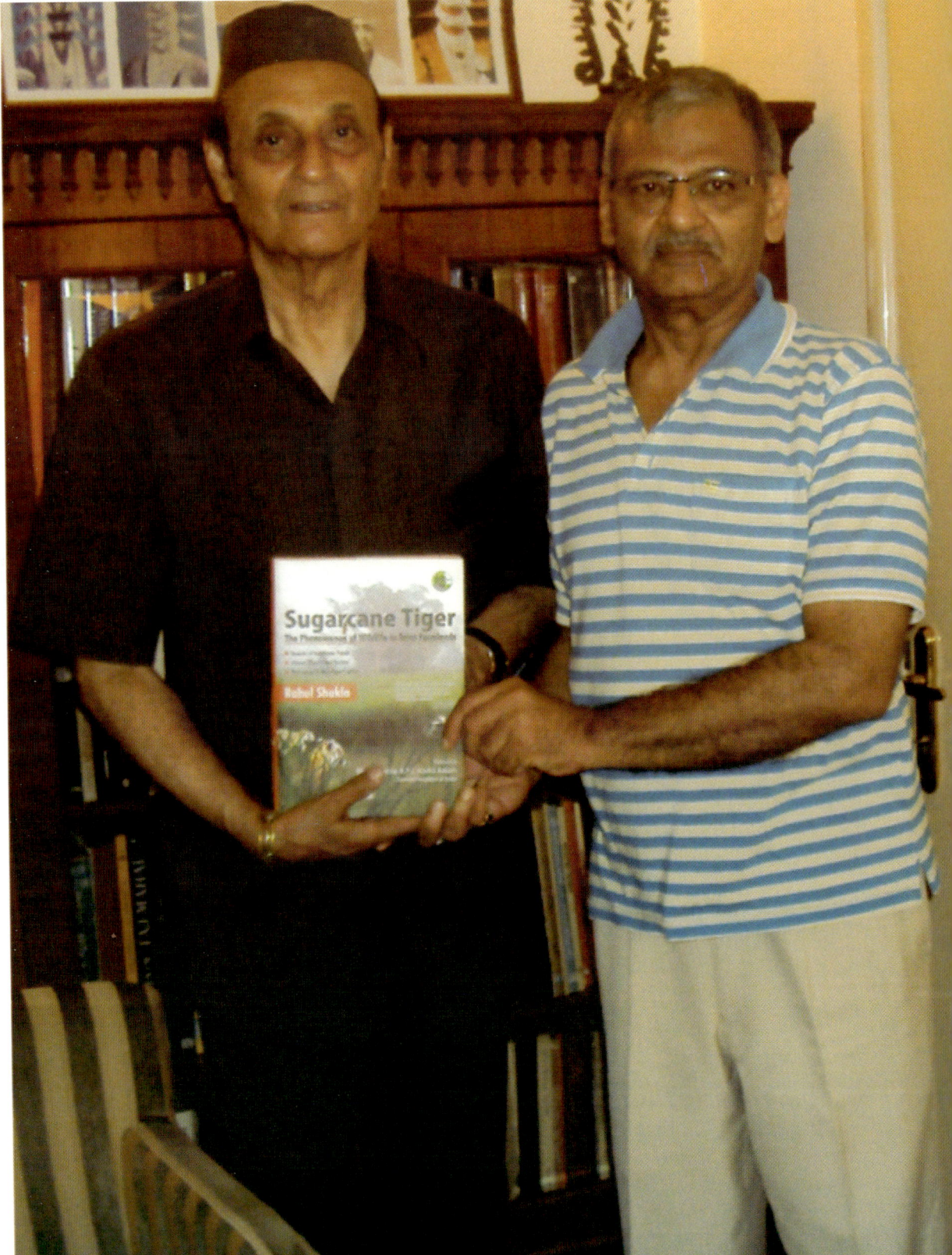

Dr. Karan Singh

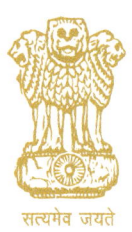

सत्यमेव जयते

3, NYAYA MARG
CHANAKYAPURI
NEW DELHI - 110 021

Foreword

A recent document of Environment Ministry reveals that there is plenty of farmland wildlife in several states of India. Yet, no state has ever hosted even a single research programme to understand the mechanism of their survival in such places. Tall crops such as maze and sugarcane offer dense cover to stalking predators, and perhaps this brings wild tigers into sugar fields and enables them to stay there.

Dr Rahul Shukla has researched the puzzle of sugarcane tiger phenomenon for years and through his writings has challenged the dogmatic conservation strategies, to present an authentic record of farmland tigers and other wildlife in the Tarai. He has found that any animal living in human dominated landscape, even an obligate carnivore like the tiger that cannot eat anything but meat, is there by the process of naturalization. It also implies that enough food exists there for both species – the prey and the predator – to subsist.

During his assignment as Honorary Wildlife Warden of Dudhwa Triangle, Shukla recorded tigers that move out to big sugar farms, travelling up to 20 kilometers away from their principal jungles and spend winter months in the cosy crops. He individually identified about half a dozen tigers that successfully travelled as far as 40 kilometers through human dominated landscape to reach other forest trails. His findings attracted wide disagreement initially, but 20 years later in 2015 it was proved by scientists that some tigers do take such long journeys. At present some 500 censor cameras are installed in Kheri and Pilibhit forests covering some 2000 square kilometers of forest for tiger census by National Tiger Conservation Authority (NTCA).

Till March 2016, these cameras had recorded the movement of no less than 4 grand male tigers, progressing through farmlands and forests of Bahraich, Kheri and Pilibhit districts including those of Shuklaphanta and Bardia in Nepal. Taking in all the intermediate areas of human population in this gargantuan undertaking, they not only pass through cane farm corridors but also stay there, living and hunting in them. This needs understanding that the sugarcane tiger phenomenon escalates in winters and dilutes during pinch-periods, yet continues all the year round.

Our knowledge base as how dangerous mammals agree to live in agricultural landscapes is very scanty because their life patterns don't show this living as a kind of passive adaptation of the terrain. It is rather the dynamic element of life that revels in the nature of life and needs to be studied by serious ethologists. It is only when we appreciate how carnivores live without creating problems, that we can understand the template that helps their survival and the possible causes of any abnormal behavior or aberrations from the otherwise normalized habitat.

There are convincing empirical findings which state that connecting tigers only with the jungle is unscientific. Large carnivores always do not necessarily need true wilderness for survival, and a viable population of mega-predators have always lived in the Tarai farmlands as an integral part of its ecosystem. For last 40 years, Shukla's studies in rural landscapes of Tarai, comprising some 400 villages, has covered observations of nearly 100 tigers, many of which were living so quietly that natives had no idea about their presence. Villagers were completely unaware of three tigers which he discovered between Suitanpur and Tulsipur sugar fields in Pilibhit district. This corroborates that big cats have the ability to go about their daily routine inconspicuously in human landscape for much longer periods than has hitherto been thought possible.

This well-illustrated book 'Tigers in the Long Grass", where long grass is a synonym for sugarcane plantations, is a sequel to the author's earlier introductory book on the subject: *Sugarcane Tiger: The phenomenon of Wildlife in Tarai Farmlands*. It is considered far ahead of its contemporaries in its ideas about farmland wildlife conservation. The author has performed a valuable task by initiating the discipline of farmland wildlife studies and brought the phenomenon of farmland tigers to the notice of the general public and specially wildlife lovers.

25 February, 2017

Dr Karan Singh, Maharaja of Jammu & Kashmir

Founder Chairman
Project Tiger

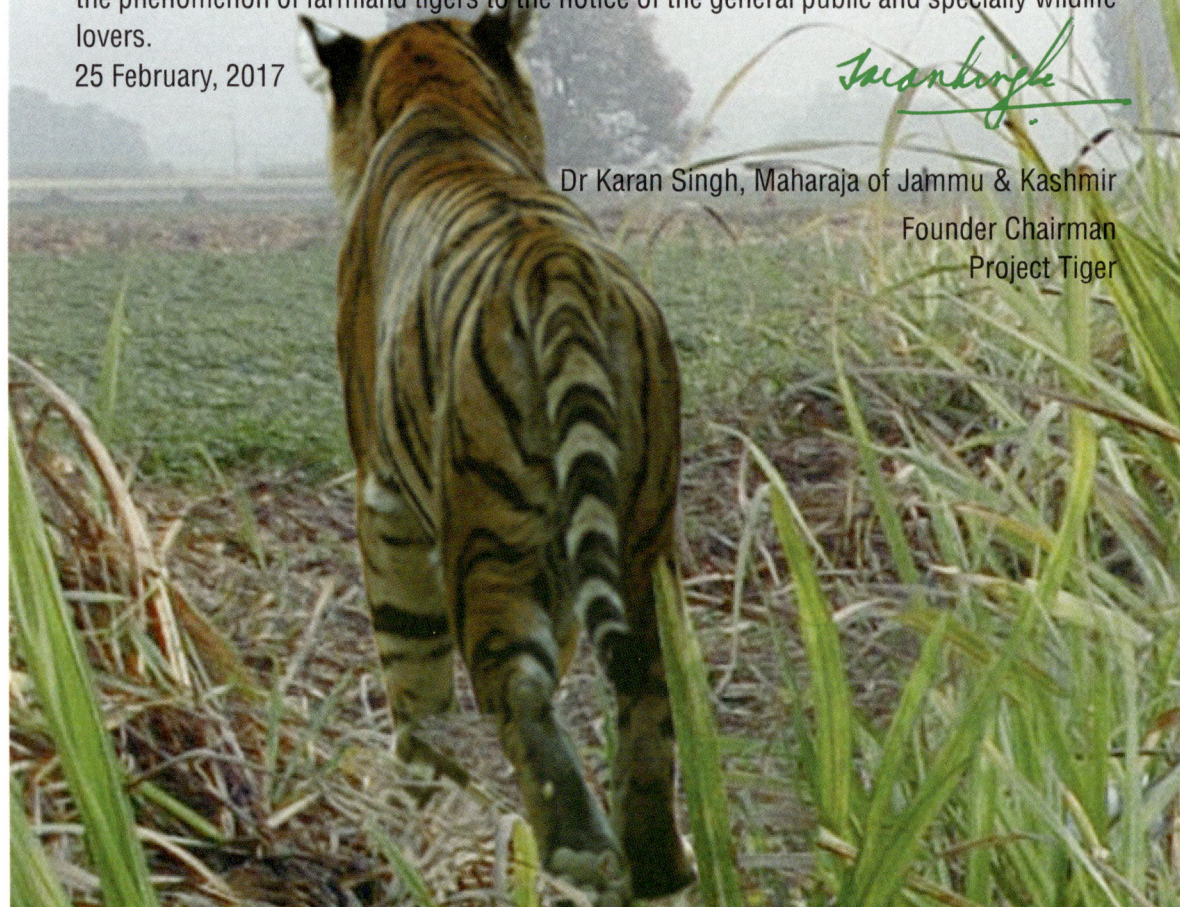

Dr. P.L. Punia

MP, Chairman
National Commission for Scheduled Castes
Govt. of India

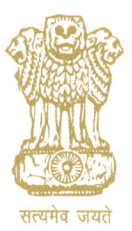

सत्यमेव जयते

5th Floor, Lok Nayak Bhawan,
Khan Market,
New Delhi-110003

Introduction

Wildlife in India is indeed seriously threatened. In the recent years their number has dwindled rapidly. The rising demographic pressure accelerated by poaching and deforestation has told heavily upon wildlife and its primary habitat. The Department of Environment, Government of India is fighting a very tough battle to curb this further unbalancing of eco-system and save its primordial wealth. At such time, Dr Rahul Shukla's pioneering work done for the preservation of farmland wildlife including tigers comes as a fresh ray of hope. The colossal data rather shocks us with information about the existence of tigers outside the protected jungles of Tarai.

There is no doubt that much wildlife lives in farmlands outside reserve forests. A sensitive and conscious environmentalist, Shukla watched this unremitting phenomenon through winters and monsoon, season after season for years and considering aspects of tiger

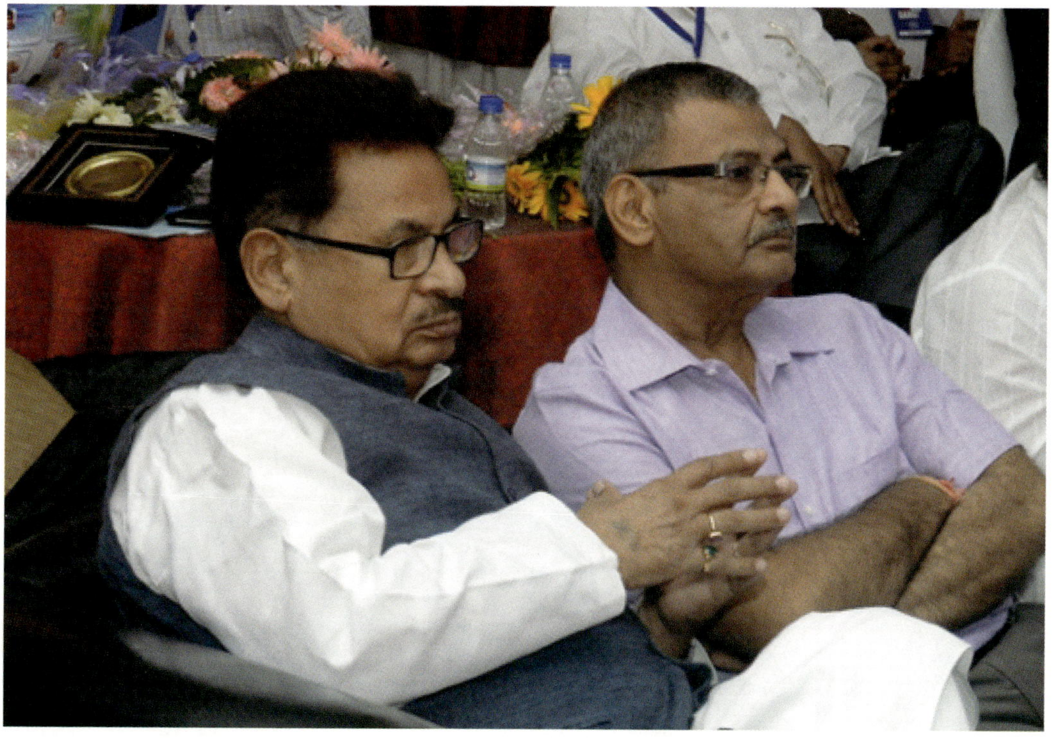

Dr. P.L. Punia with author

ecology finally came down to the conclusion that there are some tigers that prefer to live in sugar plantations by predilection. His approach towards the subject drew the attention of the Forest Department as he researched facts that supported the survival of tigers in sugar farms.

In the winters of 1998, unfortunately five tigers were poisoned in the Tarai sugar farms while nine mother tigresses were reported to be rearing their 17 cubs within these very fields. When the fact was brought to notice, Rahul, then a member of the State Wildlife Advisory Board, generated the idea of involving farmers whose cane crops these tigresses were occupying, into their protection. We declared some 18 farmers as Tiger Guardians, entrusting them with the responsibility to save tigers. The scheme worked well and the cub rearing mothers could be resuscitated.

During my double tenure as Principal Secretary to the Department of Forests & Environment in the state of UP, I took privilege of appointing Shukla as Honorary Wildlife Warden of Kishanpur Tiger Reserve with additional Honorary charge of Dudhwa National Park and facilitated him in many ways to conduct his studies and seek a systematic judgment on this problem.

Rahul's outstanding contribution is the discovery of Sugarcane Tiger. He has done immense work for their conservation. Though due to their vulnerability to poachers, their survival in farmlands has always been at high stake but the very discovery undoubtedly adds an important scientific dimension to the modern study of big predators' changing behavior.

For years Dr Rahul Shukla stood absolutely alone in his efforts but finally blazed the trail of agrarian wildlife research in India. The Forest Department of Uttar Pradesh is deeply thankful to him for venturing a selfless public service of 'Saving Men from Tigers' in nearly 400 villages to mitigate man-tiger conflict by thorough orientation of natives and also giving this 'one of its kind' study to understand as how tigers live in rural landscapes without causing harm to villagers.

'Tigers in the Long Grass' is the result of an enchanting obsession. Several thousand hours of tracking and observation are encapsulated in this single volume which portrays the natural history record of cane-dwelling tigers. This critical phenomenon investigated by a non-forester with scientific accuracy, offers a package of crucial knowledge for an overpopulated country like India, by exposing an unthought-of reality that tigers have always lived in Tarai farmlands and still do exist at remote points.

05 January, 2017

with deep regards

Dr P.L. Punia
IAS (Retired)
Former Principal Secretary, Department of Forest & Environment
Government of Uttar Pradesh

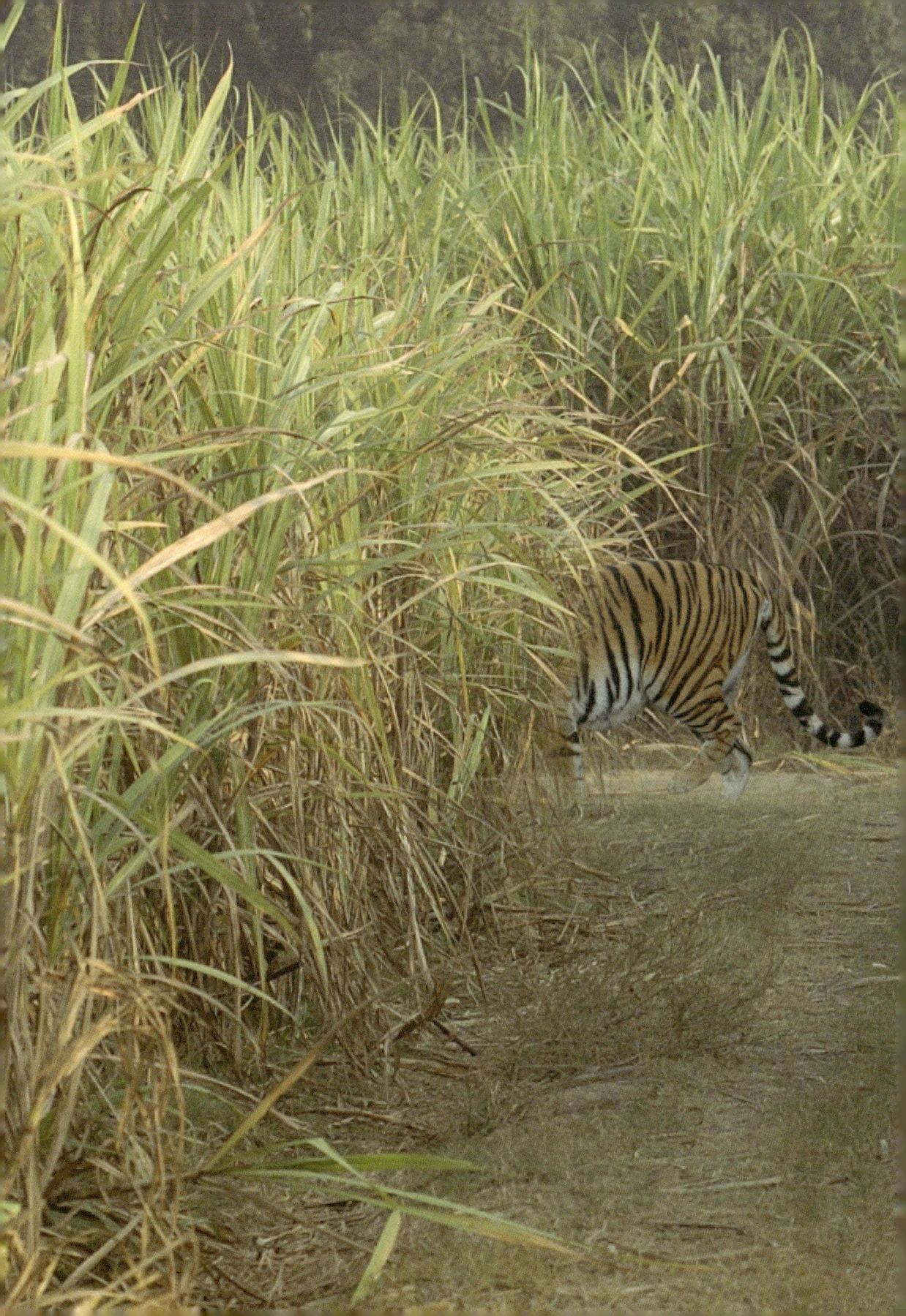

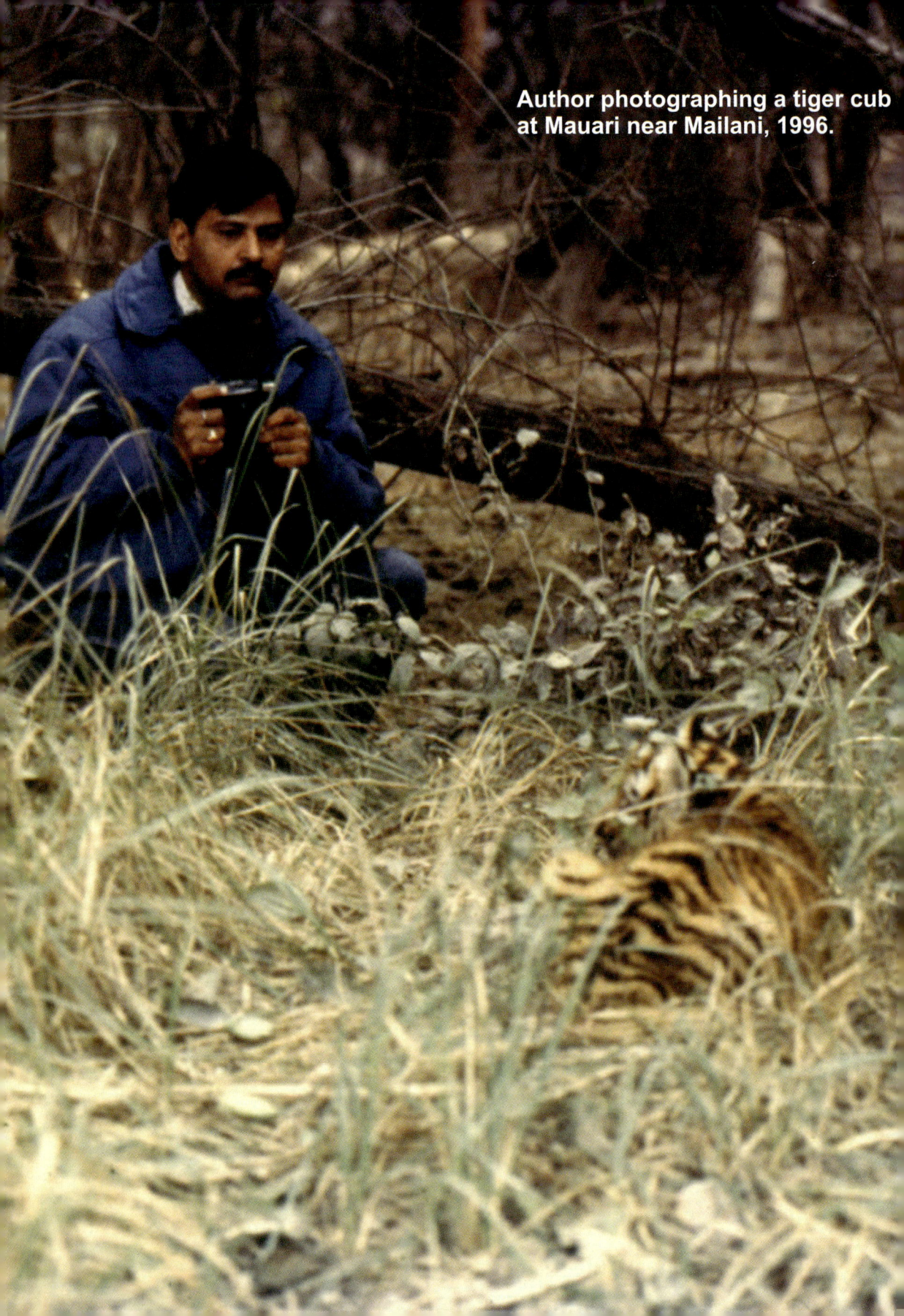

Author photographing a tiger cub at Mauari near Mailani, 1996.

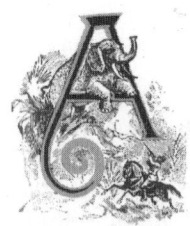

Author's Note

It may be strange for many readers to know that many a solitary striped wanderer of jungles have periodically walked down their long way to the city of Lucknow and lived cheek by jowl in its per-urban wilderness. Since my boyhood, I can recall no less than 30 leopards and 10 tigers camping near this bustling city. Such events – not incidents – have occurred in 1962, 65, 67, 69, 76, 79, 88, 2009, 2012, 2014, and lastly in October 2015, when the Katri tigress crossed the city border on her way to Ganga ghat in Kanpur.

All the tigers were essentially disoriented and strayers from Tarai's magnificent wilderness. They arrived during winter months and settled down cautiously in countryside forest patches. Caught between a strange concrete jungle and cultivated fields, they almost accepted the patchy wooded areas as their second home, when their closest home with resident tigers was over 100 miles away.

Nature, in its infinite wisdom of prey obtainability, carrion-eating and scavenging, had ensured their survival without much problem to humans but less-informed and inexperienced media persons maligned them as ravening monsters full of bloodlust that could easily turn into potential man-eaters. Hence they were intensely baited at their halting stations and then destroyed. The last tiger appearing in 2012 was the only lucky bloke that was immobilized and relocated in Dudhwa jungles.

The outskirts of Lucknow city harbor a number of patchy forests. The fragmented timberlands spreading on all sides of the city are known by the name of Kukrail Picnic spot, Malihabad mango trail, Moosabagh forest, Khurram Tola, Behna forest, Chak Ganjaria, Kajari jungle and many others. These forests are third-grade sub-optimal environments, some of which are properties of private owners, some fall under the territory of Gram Sabhas while the rest are a part of the state's protected area network. Tigers came into these jungles and lived peacefully with dignity and majesty making them home for months. Almost all of them operated economically on selective prey base, without interrupting their human neighbors. But a tiger's large kill, like buffalo or bull, is an important event. The sight of such a kill itself generates dread and a sense of danger from the predator; hence the killers were considered a menace and destroyed without a second thought.

I remember seeing the carcass of an ill-fated strayer, dubbed as *Bade Bhai* (Big Brother) by locals, that was shot at Kukrail Picnic spot hardly 5 km away from my home at Indiranagar colony. It was the forenoon of Christmas-eve in 1988. The mist was still clinging in the wisps to the sliver tips of elephant grass that abounds around Lucknow city. The body of the tiger, placed on freshly cut green grass, was being carried in a tractor trolley through a village path, when a passing group of Naga

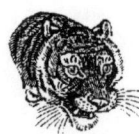

Sadhus stopped the procession in the way. They took out some flowers from their *Kamandals* (handy water vessels) and showered the tiger with petals. Their deeply revered gesture came from the belief that the tiger is the mount of Mother Goddess, while they sounded the holy conch shells. Then, in a touching gesture, they also touched the mighty paws of the animal godhead, placing their heads on them. The villagers instinctively raised the chant of *Jai Mata Di* in the praise of the departed soul. Amongst them was also a Muslim family whose milch buffalo had been killed by this predator.

Howsoever fearsome and terrible the super predator might have been, but at that moment its striped dead body and its visible spiritual force seemed no less potent to me than when it was alive. For a moment, a supernatural energy seemed to run through a continuum of time and the vehicle of the Mother Goddess, as though deeply in sleep seemed too enormous for the landscape. It remindeded me of Robert Ruark's comment, an American touch stone of African hunting, "A dead tiger is the biggest thing I have ever seen in my life though I have shot an elephant".

The scene hovered in my mind for many years. It made me wonder about the paradox that the bureaucrat in charge of the operation was given a 500 rupee reward by the Government for eliminating the persecuting menace even though the villagers had never reported any trouble from it. They had interacted almost peaceably with each other. This proved that the wildlife management ploy called lethal control often causes enormous harm to wildlife. He was a benign beast, revered by villagers as *Bade Bhai* and perhaps that is why the shooters' macho demonstration of triumphal flag march, like the prostitution of wild wealth by unscrupulous operators where any normal beast can to earmarked for destruction, had turned into a deeply mourned procession. The sound of resounding conch shells was indeed the persisting rattle of cordite salutes rendered to that awe-inspiring star.

❖

This kind of protracted sojourn of tigers near the growing city of Lucknow is not only mind-boggling but in fact it throws up a challenge to the ecologists' community as how intelligently the tigers survived here. This domain of tiger behavior, about which we know practically nothing, needs understanding and should be interpreted with caution. I am sure if the remarkable matrix of their survival without harming humans is properly grasped, it would call for a shift in the concept of conservation, which is focused solely on designated Protected Areas, as well as paradigmatic shift in tiger studies. The entire conservation philosophy then will have to be rewritten with a baseline fact that wild animals are eminently adaptable and if we leave them alone, wherever they are at home, they will survive well without disconcerting humans.

The conservationists were unable to understand as how these animals had created stable range occupations in this mixed semi-forested landscape, where trucks and cars noisily streaked past on the nearby road, and silhouettes of concrete structures lurked on the distant skyline as a mark of formidable power of human enterprise. To many it appeared fascinating to theorize that even a super predator

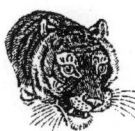

like tiger could sometimes conceivably change his role into that of a leopard that concentrates on peacocks, dogs and monkeys on the outskirts of large cities like Mumbai. But tigers don't live by theory: They live by challenging, testing actions creating their personal 'killing fields.' Hence it was something else that wildlifers had failed to catch on. Nevertheless it brought out a shocking fact that even rural landscapes have potential to entertain not only lesser lights of life but also have enough food for large predators. This includes highly-specialized diet comprising prodigiously of one type of prey – the ungulate.

The effect of environmental conditions on a predator's life is extremely important because exclusion from familiar hunting grounds contributes to high level of mortality in tigers whatever their age may be. The juveniles are most vulnerable to ouster but matured and old ones too are not immune. Displaced adult tigers, the earlier range holders, are dominant beasts. They especially turn dangerous when cornered because they are confident individuals. Such displaced animals often turn defiant and create problems.

However, none of these city-lurkers showed aggressive tendencies, never developed a sweet tooth for human meat, and never qualified to be shot or even meet their nemesis the nature's way such as dying from starvation. Indeed the presence of enough food served as a cushion against man-eating. It was no less than a wonder that puts one in awe, but to my amazement no records were generated on this mechanics as on what and how they lived here all the time and why none of them ever harbored the traits of man-eaters. However, their discoveries lead to an alarming panic in city. Scribes wrote about their innate savagery, providing recreational features with profuse poetic license, as futile chases by inexperienced foresters and boisterous city-dwellers troubled them without cause.

These hard-pressed animals were perhaps foolishly-happy that they had the precocity of living by the side of man, and were now exposed to the heinous side of this co-existence. On holidays hundreds of fun-seekers roamed about their fragmented habitats for their one glimpse as they were chased from cover to cover. Though the necessarily rare animals could have been captured and released in the forests but the result of the gibbering, populist mayhem was their tragic elimination at the hands of foresters.

No ethologist (the student of animal behavior from animal's point of view) used opportunities to record these animals' behavior, when they were constrained to live cheek by jowl with humans without their own relatives being around. No conservation scientist, ecologist or biologist, cared to bother as how the wanderers of extraordinary vast solitudes had agreed to live in a baleful co-existence with humans, where no expansion of space was possible. Fecal analysis is a recognized tool of studying a tiger's diet in the most comprehensive way. Sifting them under the microscope allows the scientist to pinpoint almost everything the tiger has eaten, including its occasional diet of lizards, frogs, grasshoppers and termites and other

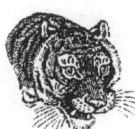

sorts of anomalous tidbits. But no one cared to collect even that, though it continued to fascinate them as revelation that the animal once destroyed by humans as competitor had lived so precariously in human dominated landscape, using almost any usable piece of land; with least resentment towards its persecuting pressures and with such a noteworthy aplomb.

Scientist Albert Einstein once said that each atom in the space is the centre of the universe. Keeping this in mind if we closely observe the animal world it was clear that these tigers were the centre of their own world; the world of farmland tigers. This signified the opposite that the so-called singular animal of dense jungles could also live in vast spaces of agrarian lands. Indeed it was a blind spot in our knowledge of tiger ecology and we needed to fill this gap in order to save this animal.

As my interesting annotations draw on, the highlights of half a century pass before my eyes. All this dispersal of tigers was taking place because an interesting, somewhat similar situation was prevailing in the Tarai. A substantial population of tigers had made home outside the protected area, inhabiting large farmlands of sugarcane that were sometimes 10 to 20 miles away from principal jungles. The making of modern Tarai with expansion of farms had abruptly shaped a new critical development paradigm for a soap opera of tigers. The great sugar farms cultivated by Sikh settlers that had arrived post-Partition from Pakistan had become like seclusion zones for tigers to flourish. In fact the deforestation of great grasslands and its replacement with sugar crops did not turn out to be habitat depletion of any kind, but it rather shaped up into somewhat categorical manipulation of habitat in favour of wildlife that finally commenced the phenomenon of cane tigers with great thrust. For a tiger the perennial sugar crop was a select, high-class auxiliary of grassland jungles.

During the sport days of big game, especially the first decade of 1950s after Independence, the state of Uttar Pradesh even allowed shooting 5 tigers on a single license. The fee was a paltry one hundred rupees, but despite this there were people who wanted to shoot tigers without license. They registered this 'outside jungle' phenomenon of tigers and shot them to their fill, hence their population could never increase. During the early 70's when a blanket ban on shooting was imposed, the tiger population increased. The trend escalated rapidly and covered a large extent of land. The tigers did not seem to be distributed in space only but also in time. They bred excessively and their numbers increased at a biologically unrealistic rate. This overflow led to a condition where more animals had shifted into farmlands to find slots as resident animals.

Whether we celebrate or lament this fact or deny it outright, but the tigers had again arrived to live in the sugar farms with no jurisprudence in their favour. The multiyear trend of their population revealed that their numbers could be as low as 10 and as high as 45, as declared in the booklet of Dudhwa Tiger reserve. The phenomenon was also occurring in the farmlands of my maternal family's Zamindari

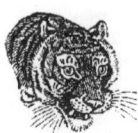

landholdings, abutting jungles of South Kheri. This interested me boundlessly, because I had been visiting these villages since childhood and had intimate knowledge of many odd un-tigrish slots outside forests where tigers had been shot during old days and were still being found living good naturedly, often with great secrecy. Furthermore, the scientific fact about tigers' territoriality in jungle or in farmlands is that they only settle down properly when the signs indicate the presence of few other tigers. Hence many of these represented a breeding population that were on an average above five years in age.

My passion for wildlife is grounded in the hunting and rifle-minded tradition of my family; I make no apologies for having been a student of hunting in my boyhood. It was a way of life for an elite little fraternity of people as well as a big source of revenue for the state Government. Hunting was called sport, wild animals were the game and their killers were sportsmen. Moreover, the rules governing the reserve forests did not apply on cultivation fields, gun licenses for crop protection were also issued to farmers thus the farmers practiced it freely and persistently. Anything going by the name of conservation, environment or ecology was completely unknown to people.

I grew up with this background, watching and assisting pursuit of big and semi big game. Since the age of eight I indulged in my love of hunting for next 12 years and then one day I witnessed a macabre killing of an antelope by villagers that offended my sensitivities repugnantly. No amount of argument could justifiably equate that perverse performance with that of a professional predator who kills only for food. The criminality of the act made me bid farewell to recreational hunting and put the rifle back on the racks. But the god of the jungle – the tiger – continued to fascinate me. Tigers gave me the cause to call on Tarai repeatedly and fulfill my heartfelt desire to see them up close and explore their world, know their ways as completely as possible so that I could discard many quaint misconceptions, woven around them as myths for ages – one of them was that these wild animals are pushed into marginal habitats by overloaded tiger populations inside jungles and their living in farmlands is accidental. How wrong I was – they seemed to be here by choice!

Tigers in sugarcane were no doubt wild tigers, flourishing in the agrarian terrain. Field biologists in consent with wildlife managers have long divided the term 'wild' and subjugated it by invoking two handy scientific phrases, in situ and ex situ to express explicitly the status of any given free-ranging animal. If the creature is wandering through the habitat from which either itself or its recent ancestors are born, it is said to be in situ (a Latin word for in position, meaning being in its original place); if it is anywhere else it is ex situ. These terms may appear alien to many, but these are in fact among the most informally employed jargon used by tiger conservationists everywhere. My argument was that if this factor of origin is applied on the tigresses that seek nursery to lay their cubs in sugarcane then what does the in situ status of cubs qualify for - a jungle or a farmland tiger? Tigers in farmlands

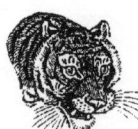

were constantly in situ for they were living here regardless of the fact whether the land is considered wild on scientific scales or not, but the animal in situ definitely remains wild as per the limits of the term.

This proved that sugarcane tiger was no intriguing exception, as these were not maladjusted in rural lands because despite man-initiated conflict with big cats, man-eating was extremely rare. This fundamental aspect of tiger biology and ethology, as why the tigers hadn't become really dangerous needed to be understood in this context. And if I was wrong in my interpretation then the scientific rationale presented in the terms in situ and ex situ is questionable. What for, then, the jargon is acknowledged in conservation circles?

With this view in mind I devoted a great deal of time to finding the answer about a segment of tigers having personal predilection to sugarcane farmlands. Like a devotee of big cat on pilgrimage, I spent hundreds of hours upon trees and knolls, watching them through binoculars in their natural state and in the end I concluded that I have found the explanation. This process was comprehensible on Malthus's analysis that had become integral to understanding of the phenomenon's evolutionary mechanism; in which the preponderance of prey animals in every terrain is cut down by nature's selective scythe by introducing some kind of predating agency with absolute aggression.

The baseline data I had steadily generated to make a few generalizations about the bio-ecological character of the entire cane tiger population that ranged large during the decades of 70's and 80's gradually turned into a hefty opus. It was both qualitative as well as quantitative material and by and large free of the subjective impressions documented in early natural history.

Of and on during all those years, spanning four decades, I came across over a hundred individual tigers, mostly females and juveniles in farmlands, watching and studying their habits in the human dominated landscape whenever an opportunity offered. A majority of them were cool normal beasts that never posed any danger to human life whereas there were a few who on account of their bad experiences with man including injuries caused by man had turned anomalous. These perforated carnivores had placed themselves on the wanted list and they contributed to some real gruesome threatening experiences in my ventures.

I admit that in the face of a long list of variety of ends that an adventurer can achieve in Tarai, I was more likely to fall victim to an overdose of normal tigers in thick cover than anything aberrant. I have come within waltzing distance of no less than half a dozen amok tigers and surprisingly I am still safe and secure because I have personally been incredibly cautious with these beasts. In two cases I have enjoyed a supernatural luck with notorious man-eaters in not having gotten the strike; otherwise I cannot say what I might have looked like with that extra advantage of my passion.

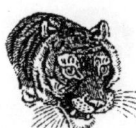

Man has reached everywhere on this globe, and when most of the wilderness of the world is already under the management - or mismanagement - of humans, as one may say, we have to acknowledge the importance of the human agency. In the context of Tarai tiger, the contribution of sugarcane fields in providing wild tigers with alternative grassland breeding ground and helping protect the endangered microcosm of this species may not be huge but is nevertheless unique. This truth was picked from the public domain with a data of tiger numbers and the prey densities and was still in the public domain yet the foresters had a problem with it. What was the bottom line of this matrix on the part of wildlife mandarins – total inattention?

My question was and even today is: If wildlife flourishes in farmlands then whose wildlife is this – people's or government's? Moreover, if presence of tigers and other similar predators and their normal prey (different-sized ungulate prey) are ex situ then the case is closed. For a moment I put aside my thesis of sugarcane tiger but if the answer is in situ then it must involve issues of wildlife management in farmlands and there is no escape from it. Ad hoc considerations for these are unlikely to yield proper methods of scientific management. Why can't we generate a wing for Agricultural Wildlife out of the main Forest Department like United States Department of Agriculture Wildlife Service and serve the cause?

The wildlife in all countries belongs to the government first, manned by their great set-up by law with commitment to the project. But here, in a paradox of destiny I was fighting a dirty battle with my own government's medieval policies to protect farm tigers, perhaps more intensely than with poachers, whose covert nature of activities – shooting, wiring, trapping and electrocuting animals – was continuing unabated all through the years, silently and clandestinely, making it difficult to evaluate the loss.

As I write this, everywhere in India much farmland wildlife is being constantly decimated. Sanctuary India mentions that in 2016 alone, over 250 *nilgais* were officially shot in Bihar, 5,000 animals killed by tribals, including 1000 iguana lizards in West Bengal during hunting festival, over 200 wild boars shot in Odisha, 300 boars and *nilgais* shot in Chandrapur in Maharastra. Human in intraspecific competitions operate without legal limits and there is not much supporting justice for the animal that eventually leads to their genocide. It is like an unfathomable juggernaut where the administration doesn't know which way to go and what is best to do but we must deliberate that India is an over-populated nation and we cannot afford to take such chances with wildlife, at least near tiger range jungles, where it works as cushion for humans against big predators. For after all, farmland animals prevent tigers from nurturing any motiveless malignancy against humans. I won't be surprised if a spurt of man-eating starts in these lands sooner or later.

I may be pardoned for using shorthand terms like 'graziers' for cowherd boys, 'wildlifers' for wildlife aficionados, 'tigarine area' for sound tiger habitat and 'strayers' for the lost ones. In addition also for the opening chapter of this book that deals with past episodes of shooting in croplands, which was considered an established form of

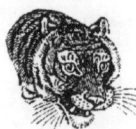

semi controlled culling. Shooting and research don't go together in modern writings but my recapitulations of those long past days, its log fires and daring stories of family icons that were told and retold wrapped in species of distant glamour contributes towards fulfilling the purpose of this book, because in present shrunken wildlife scenario, it is hard to realize such descriptions as cold facts. From my judgment, this record also authenticates the unmistakable historical existence of tigers in farmlands. Now sadly, when the state government appears to be abdicating its responsibility as an effective protector of farmland wildlife, this writing reasons why it should be protected against various onslaught of pro human dispensation and medieval polices that administrate this specialist subject.

Dr. Rahul Shukla
E-mail: tigersoftarai@gmail.com
Mob -09450544546

Book 1
BLOOD SPORT IN FARMLANDS

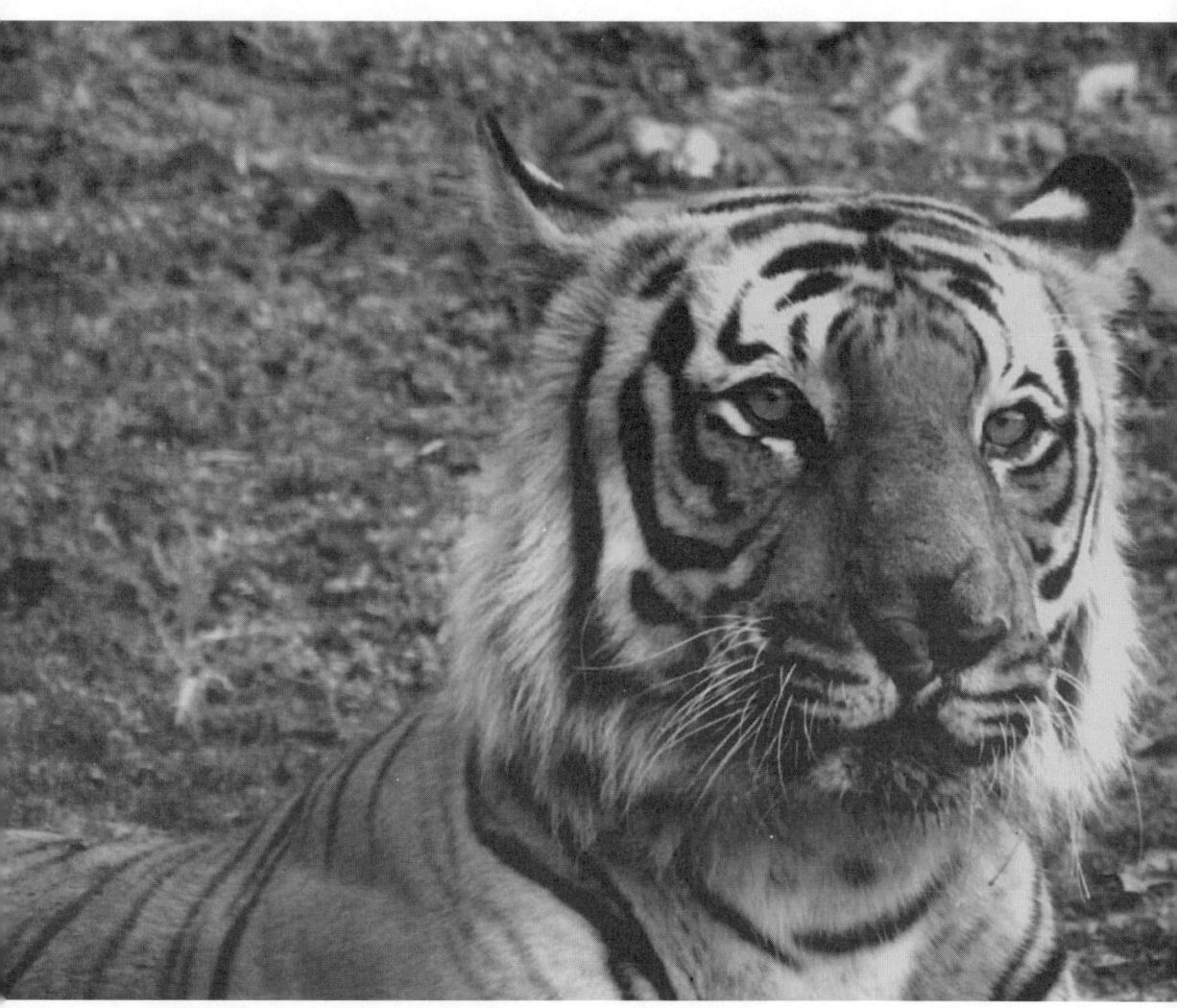

CHAPTER 1
FACING DEATH IN THE DARK

Chapter 1

Facing Death in the Dark

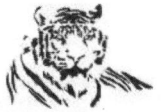

"Man has tasted tiger's blood for centuries without having been tasted much in return. Now it is the time for them."

- Billy Arjan Singh

THE AFTERGLOW OF THE SUN LINGERED OVER THE FARMLANDS OF GHOLA and the air was cold. The two men settled in the front seat of the Gypsy were Billy Arjan Singh with his brother Balram on the driving seat, while I alongwith Aftab Wali, the Assistant Wildlife Warden of Dudhwa National Park, and my old native tracker Phagunia were seated in the rear boxbody of the vehicle. I had a .416 magazine John Rigby rifle loaded with heavy caliber bullet of 410 grain, metal covered, with 70 grain smokeless powder that generates a striking power of 17 tons; an immensely potent wallop for any large sized, dangerous animal including elephants.

Phagunia had a .32 Indian Ordnance pistol holstered at his waist, while Billy had lent Aftab his Holland & Holland .375 Magnum rifle. The fatal weapon had a very tough safety lock but an exceptionally weightless trigger that fired at the hair touch of the finger and even our protagonist Billy was unsure as how to operate its tricky mechanism. The gun's reliability had so deteriorated that it often fired upon at the sheer unlocking of safety catch.

The ungodly weapon was as unusable as a cricket bat against a tiger and juxtaposed to Billy, this act was also uncharacteristic of him for as a rule he had always kept his firearms in excellent condition.

We were on our way back to Tiger Haven (Billy's residence) from Sathiyana forest range. No one spoke much. The radiation fog that usually settles in the night had begun to take over the tract. The sound of the Gypsy's engine as it moved off seemed to drill into the peace of the evening. We had driven about a couple of miles, when we passed close to the hutments of a small village Gajraora. Daylight was on the point of withdrawal and the brightly pinpointing stars had begun to lurk here and there, when we saw a figure silhouetted gently against the fragile light, sitting in a squatting form with its back towards us. Distinguishable as large animal, it was looking towards the lonely hamlet. The headlights and extra lights of the vehicle were instantly put on.

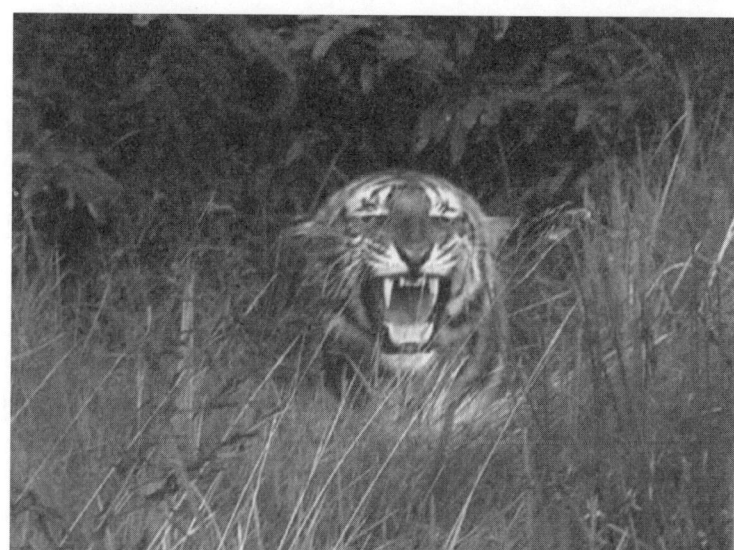

An injued tiger, hit by a truck that the author rescued near Gola Khutar Road, Lakhimpur Kheri.

Disturbed by the cutting beams the animal turned his face towards us, his eyes reflecting the glare with the ambiance of burning fire. This was the man-eater of Ghola that had terrorized the villagers and squatters of the farmland for over a month.

Aftab had often seen this tiger earlier; he immediately recognized it, confirming its identity and the hunter's problems were enormously simplified. Our unanimous thought was to deal with it immediately; a right moment to give the quietus to this terrible menace. Not bothering as who shall shoot the tiger – Billy, Aftab or I – I rested the gun on the open iron bar and aligning on the tiger that was some fifty yards away slowly slipped the safety catch off to fire. The gun was dunked with hyper lethal bullets, proven tiger killers that mushroom inside the body as they carom around slashing everything in their path. I was about to fire when Billy reached his hand, grabbed the barrel crosswise and pushed it vehemently down with force. It shocked me awfully, stopping me from pulling the trigger.

"Nooooo, this is not the man-eater," he said emphatically, turning his neck and looking into my eyes. Though Aftab ruled out the possibility of this being the wrong tiger and even Balram questioned if it was not the man-eater then what the hell the fella was doing so close to a human habitation. But Billy by some peculiar process of deduction, declared it to be a tigress and as resolute as ever, appropriated the Rigby from my hands. He even unwittingly evoked his sarcasm upon me: "This is your sugarcane tiger boy, and you want to shoot it!" Billy was thoroughly critical of my sugarcane tiger theory, because I had branded his pet tigress Tara reintroduced in wild, not as wild but as feral tigress, just as pet cats readily go feral, and this nomenclature was a pain in his neck. However, this was no good moment to scoff a sniper shot at me when the tiger was there.

Save for the old man everybody was dead sure of the animal being the actual man-eater, earmarked for annihilation. For a moment I thought that the old fuddy-duddy will slip down the car noiselessly, track with heroic skill and shoot from my gun as his gun was quite useless for any emergency. I sat quiet but no shot rang in the vista, moments later the tiger slipped into the thicket of sugarcane and silently dissolved his stripes into it.

All five of us got down from the vehicle, Billy holding my rifle like a broom, which he didn't put back in my hands despite my asking. Aftab led the way breaking trail with that ungodly gun, while I followed him literally disarmed, feeling the absence of the reassuring weight of a .416 in my hands. Phagunia was behind me with a ready pistol in his hands, which in any case was virtually useless against a dangerous mega fauna. The tiger had indeed vanished like ectoplasm though the ammonia of his 'very musky' urine, much stronger than normal squirted on a tree slapped us in the face. A farmyard could be attar of roses in comparison with the vile stench that saturated the ground and atmosphere because the marking fluid with its base in uric acid is loaded with many chemicals like cadaverine, phenylethy-lamine and putrescine including pheromones that stimulate sexual activities in opposite sex but reek pungently. We examined the tracks, which showed to be definitely of a male and by all possibilities the right tiger. Darkness had set in. Beyond the radius of thirty yards, the inky blur of nightfall hid everything in its fold and at such a time rooting the man-eater out of thick sugarcane was not our idea of good fun.

The Gypsy's headlights shown brilliantly on the undisturbed vista while the only shadows cast by Billy and his brother were falling upon us long and wavering. There was no indication of the killer being around but under the circumstances he could have easily taken any one of us at a point blank range in a single stride.

"Professor Saheb, I don't think we need to follow blindly along the trail with this dum-dum gun," said Aftab, "in case the tiger has not moved away and makes up his mind to launch an attack at this moment, we will be in trouble." I also felt the same. Perhaps the tiger was still around and fully aware of our presence, perhaps watching us clearly or might even have taken a position of advantage by now. Evaluating the danger involved in this performance, when I had no weapon for self-protection, and our tracking could influence its behavior made my skin crawl. We immediately left the tracks and came back to the vehicle.

Our return journey to Tiger Heaven was a bit frustrating; Balram was absolutely unable to rationalize his brother's incorrigible stand which was perhaps an impossible opinion. Though he and his brother were well attuned to each other in jungle matters but now the identity of the man-eater was no longer in jeopardy, he grumbled all the way and was thoroughly critical of Billy.

Despite an impressive know-how about all tiger hunting expertise available in the Tarai represented by our confirmed killer team, the end goal, however did not harmonize at all. In fact it turned out to be a fatal mistake on our part to let the stamped killer past the worst.

The tiger hadn't gone anywhere. He was actually very much close at hand, veiled in the deep darkness of sugar, avoiding us, thinking on its legs and watching us intently. About an hour after our departure, he didn't waste much time in sorting out a human victim. The petty farmer, named Budhai was leveling his field, in the semi full moon, just behind his hutment with buffalos yoked to a plank when the tiger suddenly materialized from behind the thick trunk of a *Neem* tree, seized the man, and without pausing to kill, dragged him into a sugarcane retreat. Hearing his shrieks, the rescuers ran protesting and the killer jogged away leaving the man but in that short time, the scissor shaped incisors had created large holes in his neck and chest and sheared away a huge chunk of meat from the back. The man was rushed to a dispensary five miles away but he died in the way from the rupture of major blood vessels bleeding excessively.

Next day when the news of human kill arrived, the place and the timing of the kill directly corresponded with our presence on the spot and we all including Balram and Aftab felt shocked as if reduced to impotence. We felt the answerability of Budhai's death rested squarely on our shoulders for had we availed the fine opportunity last evening, the man would not have met this gruesome end. There was nothing we could do about it but to wince and admit the setback, as the sight of wretched man's remains haunted me for many days.

The end message of the story is that tiger matters require subtle judgments and a hunter often has to fall back on his own resources of instincts, based on subconscious accumulations of past experience. Under the influence of the old man we were rather guided by his predispositions and hadn't done what our real instincts told us.

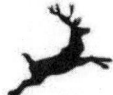

Thunder Claps and Tiger Roars

"If a man proves too clearly and convincingly to himself... that a tiger is an optical illusion- well, he will find out he is wrong. The tiger will himself intervene in the discussion, in a manner which will be in every sense conclusive."

- G. K. Chesterton

The day after this tragic incident a heifer was tied towards the afternoon close to the spot where Budhai had been condemned. I with Phagunia and Aftab –designated to lead the shooting team – perched ourselves on the *machan*. Our armoury on that day comprised a .12 bore shot gun, a 30 Springfield rifle and as usual my .416 Rigby; the gun that was once the emblem of Nairobi based Norfolk Hotel, where the most colourful bunch of professional hunters ever draw together for sundowners.

The gun was needed to qualify for an unrestricted professional hunter's license in Kenya besides years of hard big game hunting experience that constituted a most serious business.

Extended before me was the immense sugar biome of Ghola, 3000 acres of old buffer area, the land configuration of which is in a shape of a cup; with a lake in the center that stretches immediately outside the park opposite Sathiyana range. It was once a favoured haunt of swamp deer, and now had been cleared of *ratwa* and *narkul* grass and turned into prosperous cultivation fields. Every year during winter months, tigers came to live here without break in the sugarcane crops, which are planted right up to the boundary of the forest. But this time the tiger that had came to live here had developed a sweet-tooth for villagers, taking to serial human killings.

This tiger later branded as the Ghola man-eater, operated in an exclusive farmland area falling between Puranpurwa, Gadaniya, Mehangapur, Gajraora and Padua. It was this phase that while visiting Dudhwa, I became involved in this man-eater's hunt for a week's time. My accidental short stint provided me with a class-apart spectacle of conspecific tension between adult tigers. The squabble of great cats -no mock fight but a lethal encounter- that occurred beneath the glimmering umbrella of the thunder god was an experience of a life time.

It is generally accepted that once a tiger has adapted to a particular area as his home range, he strenuously resists any attempt on the part of any other tiger to infringe upon his preserve. This does not happen often but when it does, there usually is a fight to decide which animal shall remain in the disputed territory and which shall leave for good. These are, I believe, the only occasions when fights occur, except during the breeding season. However, the experience left me believing that even resolute man-eating tigers that deliberately seek human prey and don't land in territorial competition for prey with normal tigers, do *not* prefer crowding in their range and, for many other reasons, guard their territory equally well. Even though man-eating is not a natural phenomenon, the tiger, in essence, remains a tiger insofar as its natural instincts are concerned.

That day we had been on the *machan* for over four sunny hours. As dusk fell, the February evening started getting chilly and soon a storm begun to build up over Sathiyana range. Enormous piles of clouds appeared in the east, obstructing the golden rays of the declining sun. The clouds grew like a brown rose that flickered splendidly from within. The sky blazed with most vivid lightning and a drizzle started slowly cooling the earth.

Not long before, the winds escalated and a ferocious thunderstorm rolled in. The torrents of rains waved over the boundless expanse of cane and a heavy sheet of water drenched us to the innermost. There was no use sitting for the man-eater so we decided to abandon the vigil. Phagunia packed my rifle in a plastic

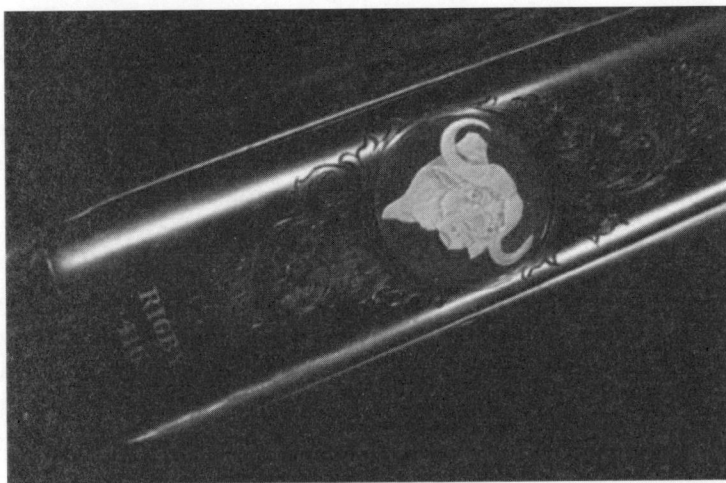

Rigby .416, Author's family souvenir and a classic heritage rifle.

cover and we started the walk back to our camp in Ghola. The village was some two miles away as the crow flies. We took the cart track that wound past the sugarcane fields. It was an unusual evening with strange lights and thick brown clouds, and the village was half an-hour's walk away. After walking for just about five minutes, I was like a drowned rat as streams trickled inside my jacket, giving an uneasy sensation to my body. It was too dark to distinguish objects on the ground that had become fairly watery and there were splashing sounds as we put one squelching foot behind the other. Walking in the incessant flashes of lightning and thunderbolts was quite a toilsome experience. Intermittently the farmland glistened green, as the vault of heaven rent asunder and then it would be dark again, as dark as the inside of a black sack.

During our trek with lashing winds adding to our woes, we sensed quite a few dark inky masses of wild animals crossing our path. They appeared uneasy and apprehensive, moving like specters in some fearful disturbance and there was no misunderstanding about it. More animals followed. We heard the characteristic trampling of their hooves on the drenched ground. None of us were actually able to identify the passing animals when a flash danced in the sky, and the light did not seem to illuminate so much as to penetrate the wild animals, which was in fact a sounder of wild boars.

As we toiled forward we came upon lots of swamp deer in a green wheat field. They had come out on their nightly feeding rounds, standing like phantoms with their backs to the driving winds and rains. One swamp deer fawn never moved at our sight though we passed it within 5 yards. He was shivering with cold and standing with its head down between its forelegs. It gave the impression of a dim ghost that was praying for stillness and peace to return.

The expanse of Ghola farmlands falls in a low-lying band where the water cascades down from higher surroundings creating a temporary deluge. The water level had suddenly risen and its unbroken sheets appeared to threaten us with inundation. My men, though used to severe thunderstorms, were apprehensive and wanted to hurry back home and I am also not exactly among those who might be called afraid of the dark, but I do not deny that a certain percentage of my boldness disappears with the passage of daylight. It was this moment when the nature's deadly drama began.

There was silence for half a minute when the interjection of a tiger floated in the air. I heard a clear a call *h-oo-w-m- aauangh-aauangh* that was much different from the gurgling rumbling of clouds. It sounded so loud that it was difficult to guess the direction it was coming from. But I felt sure that it came from very close to my left. The call had an instantaneous effect on an unseen herd of blue bulls. There was consternation in the cane fields, followed by stamping of several hooves as several antelopes crossed the cart track before us. Their shadowy silhouettes, parallel to huge phantoms, bounded forth in a mad flight. My heart leapt to my throat. No hiding of the fact that they crossed so close and at such a pace, that I was afraid. The blue bulls are toughened animals which might make even a Jeep overturn should they hit it on the road. A man on their stampeding route would stand no chance.

All of us halted in our tracks and letting the blue bulls pass, moved our torchlights over the fields. Nothing was visible clearly in the pelting rain as a sheet of blurring haze covered the objects around. But soon to our left, the outline of a head became clear as a pair of burning eyes reflected the glare and we all recognized them to be that of a tiger.

The environment was not conducive for any meeting with a tiger, when my rifle was in its cover. Very slowly I uncased the gun but I had to load it since per habit I had not left a cartridge in the chamber while covering it. The surroundings seemed to be charged with a nervous tension as I loaded the gun swiftly and mechanically. Unfortunately the cunning beast understood my gesture and before I could line the beads he retreated slowly. His dark shadow shifted up to a *neem* tree and then vanished.

After a few minutes' silence, the short loud calls of *auaangh, auaangh* again emanated from the diametrically opposite direction of North. The solo singer, perhaps a different tiger growled quite a few times then his calls ended in a long drawn staccato *huh-uh-uh*. Shortly after, this rumbling call was responded from the South; deadlier and angrier than the first and roughly from the same distance as that of first.

Quivering with adrenalin we listened to ferocious growling's. There were apparently two tigers, located some hundred yards away from each other. A straight line drawn between them would have crossed my stomach. But all this was only a prologue to a drama that was about to begin. The darkness was thick again and it was hard to realize that we had inadvertently reached in the midst of two great cats that were not finding themselves fitting to co-exist with each other. The rain lashed strongly, a blinding flash ran zigzag in the sky and a terrific crash of thunder boomed. With that, their real dialogue started. The two giants steadily increased measuring the colossal strength of their lungs. They roared their questions and replies so aggressively that the confab soon turned into a deafening serenade, awesomely terrifying.

Our every nerve was drawn tight. It seemed that the balance of power was being tested by vocal means rather than force. There was another exploding *aaom* that temporarily seemed to hold the forked sheet of lightning suspended in the sky. This was no long distance communication. The tigers were keen to meet and were approaching dangerously closer to each other. Roars, growls and coughs are specific signs in tigerine language, and since I don't speak it, I could not understand whether it was meant to convey rage, hunger or love. It could also be just their capricious temper, which can change from good to bad like sunshine to thunder; or perhaps by co-incident their royal route had just collided tonight.

There is a vast difference between tiger roars emanating two miles away and twenty yards away. In my forty years of proximal jungle time, I have heard enough of their roars, having experienced some half a dozen similar dark hours in the past. But I had never witnessed anything frighteningly adventurous like this. In April 1977, when treed by a cub rearing tigress at Bela village that moved around my tree showing displeasure, I had faced tiger roars from closest quarters. I could stand them because I was on a safe perch and when the story was revealed to the press, I had daringly stated that no music is more beautiful than a wild tiger's roar in his home. But 8 years after that incident, this instant experience when the predators were hounding around us unseen, gave me a feeling of being in a theater where the play had started but the curtain had still not lifted. My opinion about tiger roars was fully altered.

Defiant tiger roars are stupendous, that might dreadfully equal the vibrations of a supersonic plane taking off. These spatial warnings, preserving the sanctity of a tiger's freedom, have an uncanny power to full-fill encompassing space, sometimes so wholesomely that they make you feel fearfully small. Unsure of their accurate location, you sense 'a premonition of death' and the loud growls begun to reverberate in your stomach.

The hair on the back of my neck tingled. Phagunia wiped the rain water from his face and was the first to fire his gun, followed by Aftab, who boomed quite a few rifle shots in the direction of the roars. Under such wild conditions of weather and place, I would really have preferred any other kind of sound imaginable than this 'chilling to the bone' music of power struggle, in league with the gut-wrenching powers of darkness which then seemed as if it would never end.

Interestingly, the big cats were not concerned with our presence; even gun firing had achieved no effect on their aggressive postures. Aftab was sure that this offending tiger was *the* man-eater. He said the attention of rogue was so engrossed in chasing his rival that "the risk of we being attacked by him was reduced to zero."

The tigers were now thoroughly involved and baying for each other's blood. Tiger fights are rather like a squabble between domestic cats, in which far more time is spent in bounding, snarling and threatening each other by growling rather than engaging in actual physical confrontation. Blows are exchanged only briefly and are divided by long periods of posturing and maneuvering where the real purpose is to chase the rival away and not to kill it. After enough of a verbal duel, the stronger one started chasing the weaker which ran away, apparently not wanting any kind of physical confrontation.

Next we heard the characteristic thumping of their paws on the swampy ground, as the curtain partly lifted on the play and the actors passed from close quarters. Then suddenly there was more crashing of canes, shrill screaming and snarling as the tigers passed through dense canes. By far sugarcane is the worst country to face dangerous predators and a hopeless vegetation to be enveloped in when matters are serious. It is especially so when one is dealing with irate tigers, which have been known to cover hundred yards in just over four seconds when charging. But such chase is intermittent, and the speedy bouts last for a few seconds. They tire easily and after a few moments, sprint again.

However, no human being can withstand these powerful animals and if the devastating killers collided with us headlong, the enormous projectile energy of their terrible claws, with hundreds of pounds of their weight, would instantly inflict fatal wounds.

The situation was not to our liking but Lord Hanuman's grace kept our courage high over fear. Phagunia again boomed the .12 bore shot gun, the lead ricocheted in the clouds that appeared normal with the raging hurricane but the tigerine chase remained unaffected. Perhaps the weaker one, being pursued with insatiable furry and having perceived human presence, was trying to seek protection through our intervention. He was not ready to leave our neighbourhood.

The climax of the drama had begun and it seemed wise to put ourselves further out of reach. With mingled astonishment and unease we slowly squelched our way, through the stubborn clay, furtive and bedraggled in the pelting rain when the hectic runaround completed a few more circles and the sparring continued for good ten minutes around us. Like madly sputtering rockets, they circled twenty to thirty yards in canes and then crossed the cart track. At every one to two minutes, I would hear the distinctive thudding of their paws as their ghostly forms crossed the road. Sometimes from our back, sometimes from the front, sometimes sliding through the mottled murk and sometimes literally air-borne – but they were never more than 20 yards far from us.

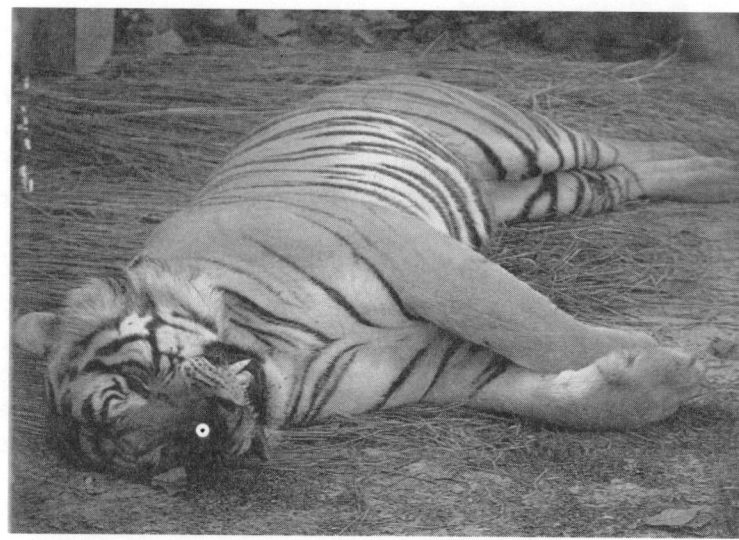

Ghola man-eater shot dead by Raja Somu. (Photo Credit : Aftab Wali)

The sugarcane was as thick as the human wrist and often so tangled that it was impenetrable at any pace, yet it broke like matchsticks against this ferocious struggle. I could clearly hear the splashing paws, the panting sound of air being sucked in through their mouths, admonishing each other in a piercing falsetto. The electrifying experience held us mesmerized in the awe of super predators.

I dared not put my rifle down for it was my only life insurance. The unique conversation of super cats was more of a tolerable zephyr as compared to this high voltage chase which now seemingly foretold an earthquake. It was remarkable that the strong paws with tough springy cushions that allow tigers to stalk their prey with deadly silence produce so much of sound when running.

I did not want to experience as to what it feels like having a tiger's large body across my neck, yet the sounds of those thumping paws were a trifle more communicative than the brain-paralyzing impact of their ultrasonic dialogue. Those who know tigers closely would understand what I mean to say.

A streak of flame, in the meanwhile zoomed in the clouds and like gigantic white splinters of broken glasses, wrecked from a cosmic window, it dispersed here and there in the sky so that everything visible was bathed in pure white light and the shadows were pure black – no less.

We were sure that the chasing tiger was the man-eater of Ghola, while the other one, driven out of the jungle by the raging savannah fires, had just arrived in the cane fields. Phagunia was mumbling gibberish, "Goli Maro Phouran", (Bust him without delay). He wanted us to attempt just plain bum shooting at the chaser. He had been a lifelong hunter. In his view if we three stood ready together and fired a fusillade as soon as the tigers broke cover, the bullets might strike the man-eater's heart and lung from the broadside. But I was partly hesitant because my earlier jungle training had tutored me to not to take running shots at unwounded animals. Moreover, there are many uncertainties in tiger hunting; outstanding sporting qualities were demanded of the man who should bring down the chaser neatly in the dimming lights without plugging the wrong one, which at least I did not possess. And above all in such weather conditions, there was a fair chance of being maimed or killed by tigers than succeeding in busting them. Finally when Aftab also declined to handle the man-eater, I gave up the thought.

The play was drawing to an end. After hanging overhead for an hour, the rain suddenly stopped as unexpectedly as it had begun and with that the sparring and growling also attenuated. The storm passed and the period between the flashes and crashes denoted its movement towards west, where the tigers also followed and went away into the depths of larger sugar farms. The temperate growls of the benefactor, perhaps still in chase grew fainter as the duo faded out in the vast sea of sugar grasses.

The relief from enormous tension was palpable. We restarted our journey back for the camp-house watching the pall of clouds that was suddenly divided into two as the silver sickle of the moon and a few stars began to peep drowsily from the floor of the heaven. The combined light of heavenly bodies dispelled the darkness and shed a faint glow over the vista of sugar fields that seemed all silent as if nothing had happened there.

A week after this incident, I was in Lucknow when the Ghola man-eater was shot dead in a joint operation of Forest Department, managed by Aftab Wali with Raja Somendra Shah and Billy Arajn Singh. Billy claimed in his books to have shot the man-eater himself that was later perforated by unrestrained feu de joie firing; however foresters and locals maintain that the tiger was done away by Somendra Shah, fondly dubbed as Raja Somu.

BLOOD SPORT IN FARMLANDS

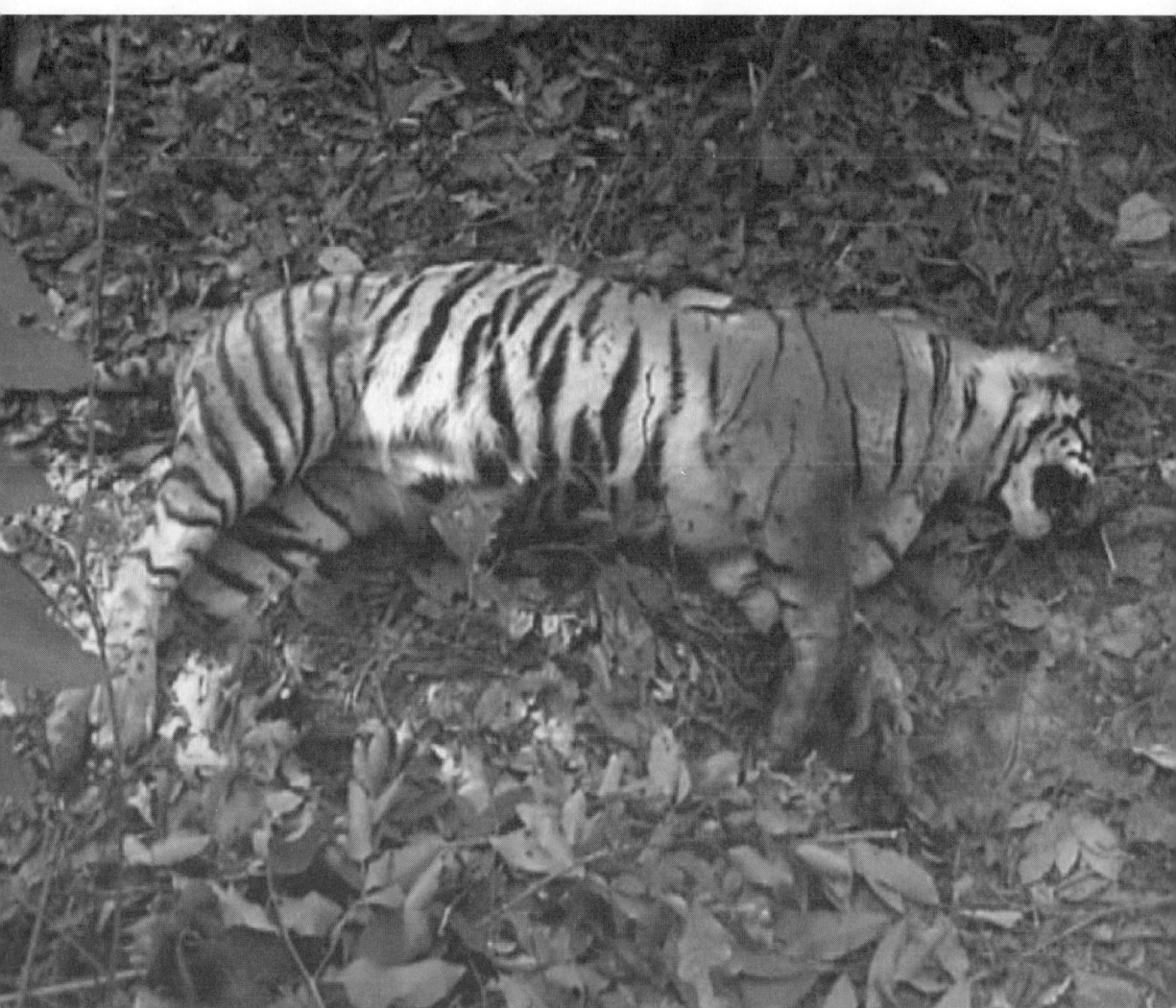

CHAPTER 2
GLARE OF THE GAMES' EYE

Chapter 2

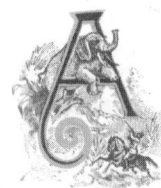 **uthor's Note**

(Wildlife conservation is basically a post-1972 phenomenon, before that there was no government law to control shooting outside the protected zones. Crop protection was taken as the fundamental right of the farmer. Permit-holders caught monkeys for export and gun licensing was liberalized in many states. Wild animals were chivvied from field to field; and were invariably killed by troubled farmers. Hunting of species comptetive to man was an unwarranted exploitation of animal wealth that resulted in a virtual carnage of agricultural wildlife. The Killer Ape Theory -a post Second World War hunting hypothesis suggests that through sophistry and legerdemain man has evolved as a ferocious hunter killer. Though his carnassials have become grinding teeth yet this recreational murder for deatery demands has immense hold on the psyche of the human race. This calim was justifiably accepted in the academic consciousness of policy-makers.

We hunt because generations upon human generations have evolved this way through an evolutionary selectivity that compels us to follow that course of action, making us an instinctive killer. It is sometimes with the same compulsions as the descendants of saber tooth and the nimravines that roam this earth in forms of lethal cats and other predators, having attained their present day specialist excellence as killing machines, perying upon herbivores. All that man has done is to modify murderous instinct with ethics and rules under the title of sportsman, where the death of a prey even in most inhuman manner is the most logical conclusion. The theory had deeply influenced the incipient government of India that had more justification in favour of crop protection hunting than the poachers themselves had.

This story may smack of a teenager's self-eulogizing adventures, too decidedly a swagger for a modest man to describe in the first person singular, but in fact this is a first-hand account of my introduction to the plethora of Tarai's agricultural wildlife and its absolute richness.)

Glare of the Games' Eyes

"Wherever men gather and talk of brave deeds, so tales of the hunt of the ways of the animals, of hair breath escapes, of stirring adventures and perils hold the fascination of young and old in all lands."

- Arthur Musselwhite

MY FATHER HAD PASSED AWAY WHEN I WAS ONLY THREE MONTHS OLD. My mother was twenty then. In the mid-fifties, life was difficult for a widow in a conservative Hindu family. She decided to return to her parent's home in Lucknow and there she settled down for good. I was brought up in my maternal uncle's home. It was a paradisiacal family where I could never feel the absence of love and understanding. My childhood was that of a happy carefree boy who had everything – a lovely house, affectionate uncles and grandparents and more than thirty first cousins. Ours was a towering Brahman family of Lucknow. Its members occupied various important positions in administration and universities. But its roots lay in the villages of Tarai where feudalism was still practiced and power flowed through the barrel of the gun. In all of these villages shooting was a recognized form of recreation and for many an objective well worth contemplating. There, the roars of cordoned-off felines still dominated the trumpeting of the frightened elephants and ponderous guns still boomed on big cats with great precision. I had witnessed the glory of big game hunting, its sportsmanship and bravery since early years of my life and felt bamboozled by all its powerful veneer.

It is said that a child without tradition is a child crippled before the world. But my pride was the family title. I had 'possessed and absorbed' the incendiary passion of my maternal family so much so, that I was proud of it as a child.

My maternal great grandfather Pandit Chhotey Lal Dixit, fondly called Kunwar Sahib, was a Zamindar of high status. He owned thousands of acres of land comprising agricultural fields and forest ranges. He had bought and established many villages of which three major settlements were Selhua, Larti and Phatteypur. The old veteran was an undisputed leader of early settlers in this area. He was an excellent shot. His accuracy with his favorite gun .303 was proverbial and his fondness for hunting was innate. He hunted tigers purely for personal challenge and would rather hunt than eat or sleep.

He had bought Gadhiyar, a *charagah* (grazing grounds) village having shot a rogue elephant there, bought Larti having accounted for a man-eating tigress inside the village and bought Phatteypur in 1889, after confronting a powerful group of Rohela bandits in which their 19 horse riders were mowed down within half an hour and their horses captured. In recognition of exceptional honour and bravery of his forces the great veteran had allowed his commander Ram Singh and his men to keep the looted weapons and horses with them. The defeated Rohelas were members of a former feudal clan and the story of this vendetta, no less exciting, is a pride record of my maternal side of family.

In 1960s, the segment of Phatteypur landholding was manned by an uncle named Bahadur Lal Dixit, who farmed on nearly 1000 acres of land. He was a pleasant hardworking man, a folk hero and a literal virtuoso with light rifles. His reputation of fearlessness and his calculated bravado had helped enhance his charismatic appeal. He always used his gun with deadly effect and having banged eight leopards in a single night was widely regarded as a leopard specialist. During friendly sessions of gun handling, he often pricked flying migratory ducks with his .256 Mannlicher-Schoenauer with such ease as if they were sitting targets and never missed them even once. The very spectacle made his peers dumbfounded in stunned disbelief.

Hunting Ventures at Phatteypur

"Hunt, like love making, takes place in a timeless zone where all outer actions cease to apply".

- A Taiga Proverb

It was in December of 1968 that I reached Phatteypur with my grandmother. Those were hard winters and the sprawling farms were subjected to the raids of wild ungulates, which was a rudimentary yet perennial problem of Tarai. Night was the ideal feeding time for wild herds. Until the crop was near fully ripe the villagers could seldom spare the time to guard their fields during the hours of darkness. But as it neared maturity, they spent most of their time in protecting their crops and passed several sleepless nights, shouting clamorously and beating metallic cans to drive away the marauders.

Taxonomically the animals involved in plundering pillage were varied. *Nilgai* (blue bull), *chital* and black bucks eat wheat, millets and rice, porcupines eat vegetables, jackals and sloth bear attack sugarcane, maze and fruits, wild boars eat all the crops including peanuts and dig for tubers, while *Hanuman langoor* and rhesus monkeys digest all vegetables and fruits. Sometimes stray elephants also passed through the area, feeding on grain crops and sugarcane. The damage resulted not only from the animals feeding on the crop but also from trampling by large ungulates like *nilgai*, uprooting all vegetation and leaving other forms of waste was the work of wild boars. During nightly walks, the sound of brittle cracks of each personally reared cane-stick being uprooted by wild boars – that ate less and

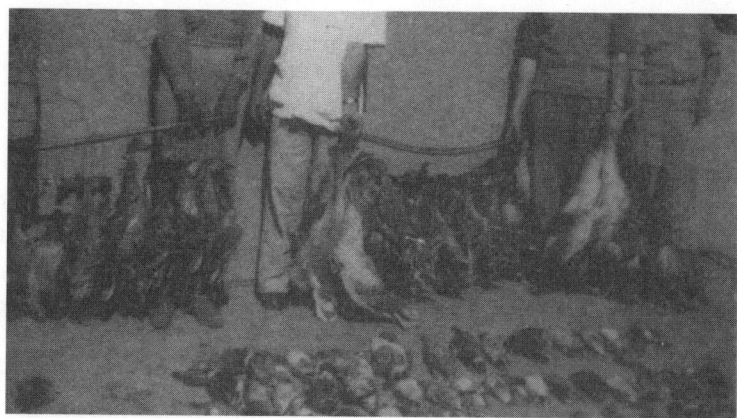

Phatteypur water ponds were famous for providing large feather game to hunters.

destroyed more – was akin to breaking of their own bones for the encumbered farmers.

Such damage adversely affected the production of staple food grains and as no farmer could stand such losses, the pragmatic solution of problem lay in lethal control of the marauding animals. It was simply an expedient approach to satisfy farmers for a brief period at best – perhaps an attempt to set the balance straight under a forced admission that the animals took an appreciable portion of crops.

Shortly after the closer of my school during winter vacations, my arrival at Phatteypur was a welcome event, where the family was always happy to entrust me the responsibility of guarding the fields from the nightly visitors. It was indeed the right thing for me to do, just as a signal honour had been conferred upon me and far from lacking in enthusiasm, any such assignment for which I was physically fit was a comfortable business. I admit I had never been an air rifle boy who relentlessly pursues avian population but I had started handling Purdy shotgun from the age of eight. During my early teens I gradually shifted to light, medium and even heavy caliber rifles, dedicating a good time in learning the art of gunmanship. I had lived through this kind of pastime at Larti which was the hub of Kunwar Sahib's domain. In that village, I had associated native hunters in their poaching escapades, learning the native language to be able to understand them and be understood; of course while enjoying my jungle apprenticeship and absorbing a great deal about the ways of wild animals. Hence I was not a newcomer to the game.

Night shooting was a time-honoured practice in farmlands. The prime time for the sport started with the onset of winters by November and ended with spring – by mid-February. As was the case in Larti where ace hunters like Chhotey and Phagunia were deputed to guard crops by Uncle Blaster (a cousin of my mother about whom I have written in my previous books), the scene was much the same in Phatteypur. Here, Dularay and his crew of watchmen comprising Gopi, Gokul and Hemraaj were entrusted with the job.

Dularay by his own account was a good hunter and Hemraaj hailed from the criminal hunting tribe called Musahar. He was an inveterate dacoit who had been imprisoned several times. Last time when he was being taken to a magistrate for the purpose of interrogation, he escaped from police custody and landed in Phatteypur where uncle immediately ensconced him and employed him for strong-arm jobs, mandatory for feudal style of management. This carnivorous hominid group from the 'Killer Ape Background' had built themselves a few smallish wooden platforms, about ten feet high, in every direction of the village. These creaked and swayed noisily with night-wind when they sat with their guns waiting for animals to show up.

My first hunting venture at Phatteypur was exciting. The sun had gone down and the preparations for the *shikaar* had begun in right earnest. Gaiety and a sense of excitement grew in the atmosphere as fires were ignited in courtyard and, back from their day tie-ups, a goodly company of farmers had gathered around it. They sat narrating their tales and swapping village gossips. With the elation of a blatantly tempting hunt rising in my veins, I waited for real darkness to descend, when Uncle Bahadur Lal entered the scene. Sporting his enormous waxed moustache that was his trade mark, he put his hand on my shoulder and said laconically, "Listen kid, ours was a tough bringing-up. We were not made accustomed to the comparative safety of a home by night. This is our wildlife management job. We did this when we were even younger, now it is your turn, take a gun and go with my hunters."

Uncle's taste in rifles was conservative to the extreme. As a deer hunter, his favourites were old fashioned light bores, .250 Savage and .275 Rigby. These delightful little weapons with their 140-grain bullets killed like lightning all the smaller varieties of thick-skinned game. Uncle called this weaponry his 'crop protection darlings' and when I was asked which one I would like to use, I chose to carry both guns. Their weight not over 8lb was comfortable to carry on long nights triumphs.

To feel familiar with guns, I was advised to first test-fire them. A mango orchard lay outside the village where half a dozen tin boxes had been hung on a tree for the rifles to be zeroed. The boxes were swung and in my sporting enthusiasm I emptied the entire magazine shooting as many targets in as many shots. Both weapons suited me admirably as I turned from one to other oscillating box with a "take that" with every trigger pull, scoring neat. Such swinging target drills sharpened my reflexes and gave me a very good idea of lead and deflection and also perfected the synchronization of the hunter's trinity – the eye, the trigger and the brain. However for skillful hunting, I was preached caution, stalk the animal as close as possible and fire from some dead rest whenever available. Well it was my hope that I should not disgrace myself by poor performance when in company of adept native poachers.

Two hours after the dark had set in, Dularay and Gokul picked the pigskin bags filled separately with rifle and buckshot cartridges, a gun bearer would carry a .12 gauge shotgun and a spare rifle .275 Rigby or .333 BSA while I armed myself with .250 Savage and went out. I even stuck a nine inch long hunter's knife in the belt of my leather jacket and with all this paraphernalia hung about my person I felt confident to meet any eventuality. We carried half a dozen fixed-focus torches that were painted black. We walked out of the village and entered the crop fields. I strode in front with the gun ready in my hands while my team moved behind me in a single file, sweeping the torches in the either direction. Light rubber-soled shoes helped all of us to move lightly and almost soundlessly. Several tracks winded into the cultivation fields and we turned in through any one of them to enter the by-lanes of standing crop. The dark always brought out hares, porcupines, foxes, jackals and even occasional hyenas. We encountered scavengers every now and then but leaving them alone, we looked for the primary despoilers of the crops like wild boars and *nilgais*.

The most fascinating feature of this landscape was the colossal numbers of wild boars. Sugarcane was their perennial delight. They arrived as soon as it was planted. They would dig up the sets which are planted and covered with earth. After the sets had germinated they took shelter in the crop itself and as the cane matured, they made shelters against rain and inclement weather by piling cane leaves in extensive heaps; getting under the pile of trash, they elevated it to form a kind of igloo. They even dug up the fresh earth to form breeding shelters, and bred outrageously large families, as is the wont amongst their kind. They lived in their larder and ate at all hours with their tribe growing in geometrical progression, increasingly competing with human beings for livelihood.

Moving noiselessly through the crops we walked for a short distance and then stopped in order to listen in case the sounds of the night had something to tell us. When the boars chew the ripe paddy grain with their big teeth it sounded like the chatter of innumerable chestnuts. We did not keep the torches lighted all the time. We walked for some distances in the darkness and then switched on the lights, swept beams at the edge of the scrub, over ripened crops and the grass borders in a wide arch, not forgetting the occasional sweep behind and then shut them again. We did this at an interval of every two to three minutes.

At times our spotlight picked out a whole constellation of gleaming animal eyes. These would be usually Chital or porkers. Startled by the unusual light, they generally stopped feeding and gazed steadily into its source. A few of them may temporarily look away but when Dularay dipped and swept the light from one point to another or just moved over the herd in circles, they were hypnotized. They turned towards the light and stood rooted to the spot. While two trackers held torches, I and my entourage would open fire.

In case of porkers, the tenacious animals presented a tough proposition. Though their eyes shown at incredible distances but their shooting only took place at ranges varying between 15 and 40 yards. There was no excuse for not killing clean with every shot, because if the first shot was badly placed one could fill them with lead and still lose them. Wrongly placed shots often also provoked charges and if by chance the hunter happened to be on the ground then there was nothing petty and half-hearted about it. Wild boar pursuit was indeed, a skillful job bound to transform anyone into a qualified sport killer.

These rounds were a regular affair and no evening was bereft of adventure. My cousins Sudheer, Lakheemo and Mahesh, all rifle-minded boys, often accompanied me and our selectivity in shooting was only scrutinized when there was the question of the relative dimensions of the trophy, otherwise we were free to shoot any pot game as we had to kill and it was no matter how many critters escaped wounded. One moonlit night we were returning to village on a bullock cart locally known as *lehru,* when a sounder of wild boars materialized on the dirt track road, some sixty yards away. The safety catch of .333 BSA was already on and the oversized bead of elephant ivory as night sight was flipped up when I selected an oversized item and shot it. The terrified sounder scattered in the field, jostling and shrieking while the big boar went down instantly, but only to gather strength and spring up. It meant that he was only stunned by my shot. It then whirled in the air and faced us. With a speed that belied his bulbous bulk, he came all out at us. All the six gunners fired simultaneously and we heard the wallop of bullets taking his entire body as he fell as if pole- axed and covered some distance, sliding in momentum.

We thought it was over. We jumped down the cart to collect the trophy but the boar was made of tougher stuff. He got up like a prize-fighter, his face and chest covered with blood, and gathering his force for a rush came at us like an express train. Its eyes fairly blazed and every hair on its body stood on its end. The anger and fury of a wounded boar presents the most aggressive sight and sound that man can face save for tiger and elephant charges. My cousins and I lined up abreast again and fired as the bounding animal drew close running parallel through a gram field grunting like a brass banshee. The track was deeply rutted and ankle deep in dust yet the heavy beast weighing close to 300 pounds took a volley of bullets, and rose in the air as if practicing wind sprints when a shot took it on the foreleg and it fell down, going over a series of somersaults.

A cloud of dense dust rose at his fall and we were unable to see where he had exactly fallen, so six of us walked into the choking dust, and the commotion brought him to feet again. Wiggling himself to a facing position, he got to his three feet like a punch drunk boxer, swinging from side to side with foam blowing over his boiler-tank chest; he again attempted a charge when a volley of shots, more in vain of *coup de grace* settled his accounts for final. Later we walked up to the boar and found that his chest cavity had been fully devastated, his heart, lungs and even

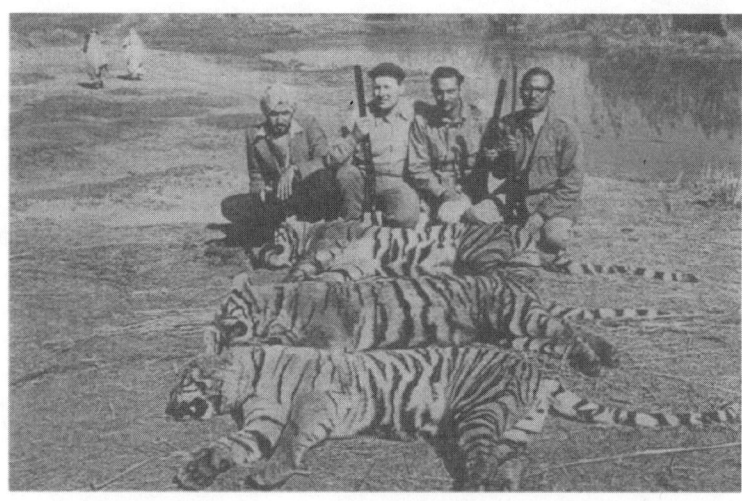

A camp shoot near Phatteypur, 1967, Family Archives

his entrails had burst out but the gallant warrior had enough oxygen stored in his brain to continue until a slug in spine eventually scuttled him.

A full adult wild boar is a classic game animal and if one does not drop him stone dead or mortally wound him with first shot, he gets the idea that he is invulnerable to bullets and keeps coming despite wounds that would disable any strong animal.

In totality, this hardy beast had taken 17 shots to finally surrender to his destruction and it was no mean feat of the rifles too for each shot had found its target.

Wrath of a Leopard

"Wounded leopards have been reliably reported as having mauled as many as seven armed men in a single rush and then melted back into the grass before anybody could do anything but bleed."

- Peter Hathaway Capstick

A watchman who had been guarding his crops from a *machan* had a grandstand view of the whole drama from his post. After the shooting was over, he came running to us and said that he had heard the guttural sawing of a leopard near his post who was feeding at the kill when in the chaos of the slaughter the escaping wild boars had passed only 20 yards away from him. They were squeaking and grunting in nervousness. The leopard took his lead from approaching boars and also ran away for his life. This is common occurrence in a shooting country. Animals see other animals in flight and evidently decide that there must be a reason for running so they also join in.

The man's watchpost stood some two hundred meters to the north. While the behemoth carcass was being tied to poles, I decided to check the watchman's information but Gopi said we must complete this job first, the leopard will not be affected by this, saying "indeed he would come back and wait for us." I could not withstand a little disagreement over the improbability of any animal staying put during so much of disturbance when several rifle shots fired at such a close range followed by struggling commotion of wild boars. To this Dularay's answer was "Bhaiya, leopards are different material."

We moved back with the watchman, intending to follow the wild boar trail which would lead us past the spot where the leopard had been chewing his meal. We left the cart and walked the road in a single file, dully lit by the slinking silver of moon. Our rifles were pointed at the fringe of sugar plantation some 10 yards to our left. There were no blood marks on the trail, which meant no critters had escaped injured. Once more I wondered aloud whether in this turmoil, the leopard might have cleared out but Dularay was emphatic: "No Bhaiya, just wait, he must be somewhere very close."

We moved slowly on the cart track, one cautious step at a time, peering into tall sugar patches when we came upon a dead *langoor*. Leopards seem to place monkeys high on their prey list. A critter from the same group, partly eaten lay on the bare ground over a parapet of ploughed field. Dularay walked carefully around the carcass and asked us to be organized to catch sight of the animal. He declared roving the torch, "Even if *gulha* (colloquial for leopard) has full stomach he is more likely to return to collect it. We will just ensure seeing it and that's all", and then he mumbled caution to not to fire for he didn't want to take any chance with the animal.

If it were true that the leopard was the kind of animal that would not condescend to back away from the fusillade of bullets then we certainly were toying with trouble as we were disrupting his dinner by standing on the very spot; an interruption to which they do not take lightly. Gokul picked up a few pieces of semi-solid mud and threw them into surrounding crops trying to flush the leopard out. We edged slowly away from the carcass, each man hurling an occasional mud ball into the wheat crop and sugarcane that lined the either side of the cart track. The idea was just to spot the animal and not to challenge or nail it. Many men have made fools of themselves while trying to frustrate leopards. However, the comforting thought was that we were armed with five rifles and a shot gun, and if any charge took place, we had enough guns to get dead on flying target.

But we had forgotten that semi-dark and dark nights are a critical factor in increasing the danger from felines and a leopard by the day and same leopard by night are not the same. They are two different animals.

Five minutes passed but nothing happened. Because of the earlier barrage of firing on the boar all the natural noise of nature was still hushed. We could feel that silence but for the whisper of the tall crops in the night wind when right in front of us the sugarcane shook and parted and a blur of black and golden lightning streaked low across the open ground uttering a deep continuous guttural growl. In three lightning leaps it covered two-thirds of intervening ground and went after the watchman. The man ran like a hare with the leopard after him and was about to pull him down when I with the stupidity and foolhardiness of a young novice, slipped onto the safety and snapped two hasty shots from my .333 BSA double rifle that apparently missed the target. It appeared dammed strange to me for in that phase my gunmanship was at its peak form and my bullets were always precisely placed, never more than three inches away from where I intended.

However, having knocked the watchman flat on the ground by the impact of his bump, the leopard abruptly turned back and rushed towards the kill. In the way it encountered Hemraaj who pushed his stave in front of him for a mouthful of wood's initial bite, but the beast ignored the pole. He didn't halt to grab it; rather in the vein of a polo pony player who hits the ball with well-aimed stick, it reached the kill and hit its paws, sweeping, good and hearty at the dead *langoor* that went flying inside the sugarcane and the leopard followed, plunging into it. In a second the night swallowed him up, spooky in its awful silence.

Everything had happened in a flash. The entire incident had concluded in less than ten seconds and everything was now deathly quiet. Though all my associates were particularly adapted to shooting at random, killing some and wounding other animals in process, but here none got a chance to line up his gun except me. The jungle ninja had not only maneuvered a tricky tactical situation into his favour but spared our lives, when our team's killer instincts –pull the gun and fire automatically – had gone cold but for Hemraaj's alertness that had pushed his stave in front of him. Dularay's face was red and eyes as wide as poached eggs. He was bearing a mad grin. He said he had never done this before and he will never be guilty of repeating such folly. For a fourteen year old boy like me it was an adventure of toying with the real possibility of death rather than to actually die. It was all our doing for entertainment and spectacle; the leopard had never asked for it.

There can be no better instructor than on-the-job experience. We had just been lucky to escape the penalties exacted from our unwise behavior, yet unable to grasp the actuality of our providential escape from being severely injured. Moreover, a lacing from the cat's claws, particularly dewclaws where layers of rotting meat are embedded, generates a deadly risk of septicemia that can mean almost sure death within a few hours of infection.

I refilled the gun with soft points as we beat a hasty retreat, discussing the feline's flashing temper and especially about five things in a leopard's charge: the suddenness of things, lack of warning, the high speed rush, the deep tone of the sawing growl and his ultra-fast reflex in tossing the kill inside the sugarcane to get away with it. Close range charges of spotted cats are so unbelievably fast and unexpected that even potential rifles are often reduced to uselessness.

Our conduct shirked aloud for disaster. Perhaps the saving grace was that the hunger-crazed leopard had not been harboring some old perforated wound otherwise that pure charge of nitroglycerine would have taken a good care of his tormentors; and some of us might have got some radical redecoration of their faces or may be worse, our lives forfeited.

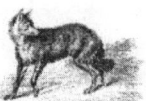

Jackal Commotions

"The shrieking orgasm of sounds has left the ear outraged, numbed; and the silence falls doubly sweet, as the night reasserts her gentle sway; swinging back to her quiet course."
- Col. A.I.R Glasfurd

Towards midnight, jackals put up a great commotion. Their weird cackling yowls started from all around. The howling was taken as a signal and repeated by the other pack. The unusually noisy chorus of rising and falling echoes was eerie and agonizing. Yet I felt enthralled by the magical pull of yowls and chortles floating in the chill of winter. *Woooo... ooh... Where-o-where? O- Where?.. O- Where? O- Where? Yes, where? Where –where -where? Here! Here! Here! Here! Heeeeeeyah!*

Over the length of time I have spent in Tarai, I have come to believe that the sound of landscape is not the blood-chilling rumble of a tiger or the thundering trumpet of a bull elephant, in actuality it is the voice of the jackal that gropes through the coy virgin darkness like the charm of the land, seemingly coming from nowhere yet everywhere. Like the croaking of frogs in South American Pantanal, the world's largest continental wetland nearly ten times the size of the Florida Everglades, the laughter of prowling hyena in Africa, the yowl of coyotes in Prairie and howl wolf in Taiga, the jackal's caterwaul is indeed the apex spirit of the Tarai.

When the sun sets, jackals lose no time in announcing their presence by the side of villages where pariah dogs give them a hot reception. This nuisance, like a regular ritual of rural India continues for long hours until both parties are completely tired. Then comes the grand finale with a strange sing-song howling, a unique ululating from both sides as they thank each other for the entertainment. Then the cacophony abruptly stops and a deep silence comes to prevail over the vista and quite accustomed to this feature, we moved alert and imaginative, taking in and exhaling the Tarai air as quietly as a baby in a crib.

These ventures were tough and wearisome affairs that demanded a thorough going-over in the field. We needed committed trackers, who should not abandon the troop in the middle. The men who had spent the previous night in rounds and felt worn out for want of sleep could not continue to join. So each day a couple of new recruits were taken without fail. Dularay was indeed the only companion, never

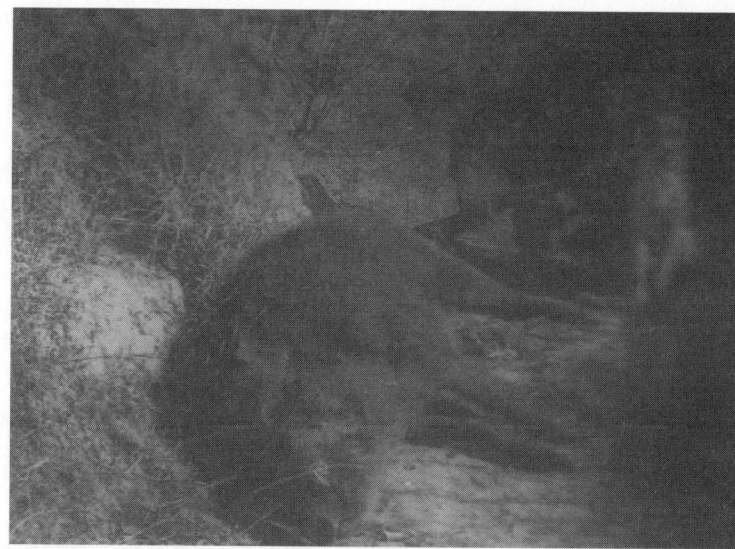

Hunting rounds never drew blank; one or two wild boars were always on hand.

tired, who joined us assuredly. An hour before sunset, he would enlist the names of men who were to accompany us on that day. The names of those interested were picked up from the circle sitting around the bonfire and respective roles were assigned to them. One of them was to show the torch, the other was to carry the rifles, and a small team was to cart the trophies to the village.

Unlike wild boars where we could at once start shooting at them, deer and antelope herds demanded a differentiation between males and females. At the indication of black buck or *chital*, I left the torch bearers on the spot and crept closer from the other side, organized for action and careful to keep away from being silhouetted in the paralyzing beam. The poor animals failed to sense my presence as they were approached safely and unhurriedly. Four of my best *chitals* with antlers exceeding over thirty inches were taken almost at a point blank range.

Once it was a pitch-black night without moon, and earlier in the evening several light showers had fallen, when giving a thorough going-over to immediate surroundings with my torchlight, I saw a long-bearded black blue bull standing near a dense thorn break. The beast presented me with a fairly good target. I pumped in two shots of .330 BSA in his shoulder. The shots struck true with a heavy thud as he slumped flat on his belly in full stride. My little experience said that such determined effect of shots quickly brings animals on the point of death, but this was an exception. Gokul ran and grabbed his horns and the animal began to struggle hard and almost threw him off his feet. Gokul didn't let go of his horns, for the fear that he might probably get up and stab into his stomach, so he hung on with both hands and tried to tilt it nearest to the ground but the animal's neck won't twist. Then suddenly with a jerk the bull got up and threw Gokul some five feet away. I wondered how the bull having been hit hard through the lungs and shoulders had so much of power left in him. Had he happened to have been only very slightly wounded, Gokul would have become his dessert on the moment.

It was not the end of the story for then the bull got up and dived in the matted undergrowth. Clearly the animal had just gotten the notion that he had recovered and there was nothing that could stop him. I hastily sent two more shots after him but he quickly disappeared. I must say that the growth was tangled enough to stop anything on its four legs and despite that, he had gone strong some hundred yards off before it collapsed. It took a full half day's operation for Muslim villagers to retrieve its carcass. I was completely mystified by the night's events, learning that wild animals have great tenacity in body and power in their necks. The god's honest fellas, such strong beasts as blue bulls, should be treated with respect.

This case is a practical example of the psychological impact of adrenalin on a wounded animal.

Needless to say, crop protection in itself was a valid point and a subterfuge to shoot animals. It was no poaching for poaching was done in jungles so crop protection was a positive word. There were privileged natives who had done no other work for years than this high-volume productive job. The animal shot down in the crops was considered the property of the farmer. The substantial protein it provided in form of fresh meat was a much bigger compensation to the farmer against the meager loss of his crops. The price paid by the poor creature was ultimate as this hunting supplemented the consumption of meat from domestic animals and was also traded locally.

Uncle Bahadur Lal, like his younger cousin Uncle Blaster of Larti, had given me several orientations on the escapade. "There is nothing as painful as seeing an animal limping about in crippled condition. The great thing is to pick the spot at the animal and put the bullet there -- not just anywhere at all into the brown of the beast. The bullet at the right spot is the basic need of the night hunting. Shoot with moderation and don't grudge an extra cartridge in putting animal out of pain. Do not open fire until you see the object. It ensures that you at least know at what you are firing. Moreover bullets with their high velocity are easily deflected so care should be taken to shoot between twigs and strong grass like sugarcane if it falls in the line of fire." For a student of hunting, these nuances were gospels.

One night while negotiating through a paddy field for a wild boar sounder we passed in close proximity of a lone hyena. Without a threatening, warning yowl, the animal abruptly rushed over Gopi, who turned and ran away. The hyena chased the man, lowering his neck several times and trying to snap his jaws at the running man's legs and calf. His efforts were so determined that we could clearly hear the jaws closing with vicious sound, when Dularay blasted the animal with his shot gun. The bone crusher's terrible bite might have resulted in a smashed foot for the man. We examined the body and discovered festering wounds with oozing pus. The scavenger, perhaps mistaken for a buck at night, had been perforated with low velocity, weak load of muzzle-loader.

Identifying Games' Eyes

"Who can believe that there is no soul behind those luminous eyes!"
- Theophile Gautier

In my early phase of night shooting, I did not know how to differentiate between the eyes of different animals. Almost all the eyes shining in the torchlight looked similar to me. But as my experience of nocturnal expeditions grew I gradually developed the ability to recognize wildlife by the shine of their eyes. Now today, I can name most of the animals at a single glance in the torchlight. I know how certain other factors are to be taken into consideration when the identification of the animal is to be ascertained. The first is the general background whether the animal is positioned in a dense or sparse cover, whether he is masquerading from a depression or is standing on an elevated ground or he is just on the usual level of earth, the normal conditions of camouflage light and shade in which he is standing. Also important are the season, the weather, the land terrain, dry, wet or swampy, the movement and the colour of eyes and above all, the height they are positioned, for it tells the height of their owner animal. Although the difference between the spaces of eyes also serves the purpose but it is not easy to determine it at fluctuating distances. Nevertheless those who have the ability to judge it minutely, rarely commit the mistake of firing at the wrong animal.

Animal behaviour against the light also helps understand its identity. Big eyes belong to ungulates whereas a carnivore's eye is slightly smaller with more brilliant reflections. The eyes which abruptly slide upwards and downwards, through a wide circumference belong to deer and antelopes, whereas the eyes that stare unblinkingly back at us and move quickly from side to side like that of a leopard, never jerking and suddenly seem to dip while focusing intently on the source of light are always the eyes of tiger.

The tiger has a highly evolved system of defense within the eye. Its pupils contract in bright light and protect the eyes from the glare whereas in small carnivores the pupil contracts to a narrow perpendicular slit. The tiger's eyes appear like a small circular opening in the torch light. In the dark of the night the pupils dilate and permit a great amount of light to enter into the eye. The tiger has in depth vision that is particularly tuned to detecting the movements of his vesper prey. His eyes are accustomed to work in dark hours.

Amongst nocturnal hunters, a tiger is probably the only mammal which possesses a highly developed optical system that is capable of reflecting the faintest streak of light. His eyes show flames in the setting sun, lambent in rising moon, and are translucent against the feeble flicker of earthen lamps. Occasionally a reflection lights his eyes even under the faltering mellow sheen of stars. When light falls on his eyes, they hold the languid beam suspended and it seems that the tiger's eyes have their own light.

The ungulates feel obfuscated by the light and do not move at all. The leopards take to cover sinking to the ground but continue to stare back at the light giving themselves away, whereas the tigers show a tendency to approach them. This may appear determined or even dangerous but I think that their only motivation is curiosity and not the intention to harm as is generally supposed. The world of shining eyes provided a great thrill and unusual entertainment that makes me remember the Tarai nights so filled with mystery and romance of uncertainty.

First Date with Farmland Tiger

"You have to give the tiger a room. If you don't give it, it will bite you."
- A Tarai Proverb

These nightly hunting rounds taken at odd hours from 8 p.m. to 12 midnight and then again from 4 a.m. to 6 a.m. were exhausting affairs but a high success rate in kills always made them come up to my expectations beyond doubt. I was surprised to find myself in unusually good form as on an average I shot two animals a week. I shot one *chital* to three wild boars and one hog deer to three *chitals*. The occasional addition to the score was sometimes a blackbuck or a blue bull that was mostly for the Muslim population of Kolhu-Gara village that fell nearby. They were our subjects during Zamindari period. The goddess of sport was generous and this ratio always kept the meat situation at ease. As soon as the kill was done it was tied on a bamboo pole and dispatched to the village whilst we went ahead in search of more animals.

Needless to say the rural landscape then was scantily populated with humans, and the game animals of commoner-kind were plentiful. Though the closest jungle trail was no less than ten kilometers away but there were some patches of reedy swamps around, called Banukiya and Dhanega Nala that harbored a variety of wildlife and a good presence of game attracted carnivores. There was a resident leopard and visiting tigers were also reported.

One day we received the news of a tiger's sighting in our fields. This interested Uncle Bahadur Lal and he decided to go looking for it. He had a long experience in hunting big game but since the death of his two brothers by a tiger in the neighboring jungles of Mala range in 1966, he had given up shooting for good. His brothers, a magistrate and an Indian Police Service officer, were immensely powerful and fine

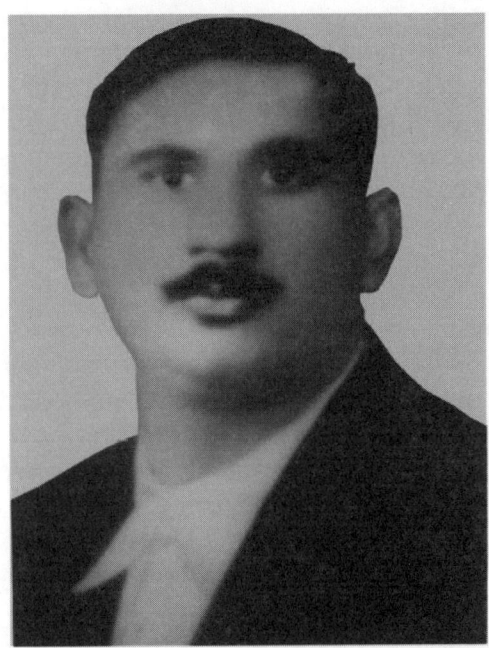

Folk Hero, uncle Bahadur Lal;
A born shot, he could prick flying partridges with .256 Mannlicher-Schoenauer as if they were sitting targets.

shots, it was unbelievable for him that they should lose their life this way, henceforth he was only interested in spotting the tigress – that's all. Beautifully dressed in tweed sports coat with riding breeches and long boots that had seen better days, he came along. His hunting outfit had a peculiar effect on him. Looking younger and energetic he fitted the mold of Gregory Peck or Robert Preston, the macho gun slinging stars of African Safari movies that were produced by Hollywood's MGM studio and were largely shot in Africa's Masai Mara triangle. Uncle handled his heavy gun .475 No-2 Jeffery's double-barreled express rifle with ease. The classy gun had settled some half a dozen tigers and elephants in the past and was potentially an undisputed killer.

We walked through wheat fields expecting to catch the cat in our torch lights. The abreast formation was assumed with Dularay on the right wing, Gopi on the left, while Uncle and me were in the middle with two armed guards covering us from behind. The barley crop was high for me, some of it level with my neck, while it was up to uncle's chest. We could see up to 30 feet clearly in torch lights; the length of just two nice springs for a tiger.

The events of that particular evening are indelibly stamped on my mind as though it happened yesterday, for it was my first live date with a farmland tiger. My shot gun was loaded with LG Alphamax cartridges that I held chest high and there was considerable optimism in our team. We moved slowly, I remember my susceptibilities and their impulse mechanism had never been tuned to such a pitch earlier, learning that danger not only adds zest to all forms of sport but also tends to sharpen the faculties. The excitement and fear hovered over my young mind. During swimming lessons at school I was led to believe that the brain of a drowning man develops greater activity at the moment when he hovers between this and the next. Thus danger is understood as something that you are prepared to face. I discovered that this moment was much similar to that situation. Twenty yards of our advance brought nothing. Another forty yards produced nothing. The barley crops seemed as innocent as sugarcane, when Dularay and Hemraaj simultaneously happened to apprehend the tigress in the flairs of shooting lamps.

Framed in two powerful beams, she stood amongst the wheat stems, which were white with the frost. Soon she began to move from south to north diagonally, approaching closer to us. It was fascinating to watch her this way as she covered some eighty yards in a smooth stroll. Time and again her eyes disappeared and when they reappeared they seemed to have come closer. Both the men kept the torch focused on her as she took to scanty cover and slowly settled crouching on her belly, stone still, looking smack at us – as though wondering what a pair of moons was doing on earth. Her eyes were like electric bulbs, showing green at angles.

This gave us some real thrilling moments. She had approached within twenty yards of our crew, Hemraaj kept the torch on her. I took an unusually careful aim under the circumstances, consuming extra seconds, for it was not the time to do a haphazard job of trigger pulling. Her head was slightly raised and extended, when Dularay turned the torch beam from the tigress on his own face so that she could spot him properly. She stood still and stared at him with a quizzical expression on her face. Dularay then steadily waved the light on whole of the crew and several times up and down on Uncle's profile. This came as a shock to her. She had probably not expected to see so many humans standing in the darkness. Looking at us with a questioning gesture she bounded back in the sugarcane that lined the cart track and was engulfed by it.

Like Uncle Bahadur Lal, we all had stood still before the tiger. I was holding the trigger of my shot gun, wondering why no fire had come from the seasoned uncle. A heavy bullet precisely placed from the magnificent double-barreled express rifle would have done the job well and properly. But everybody held his fire. When the tigress was gone I asked uncle why didn't he shoot when we all were ready with a repeater? Uncle first removed the cigar-size 500 grain cartridges from the chambers and handing the gun to Dularay, answered, "Kiddy, during winters tigers invariably live on our farmlands. Then my sugar farms temporarily belong to them and we become fellow citizens sharing a common turf, so we must try to live on friendly terms and respect each other."

A more gentlemanly thinking would not come up from an old man, whose outstanding ability with guns and lifelong experience in shooting big game was immense. Like a gospel of truth it registered on the clean slate of my mind and became the abiding principle for life.

One morning a week later, false dawn had begun to turn the trees into contorted monstrosities and I was passing along the edge of a dry Nala when I came across the tigress again. She was lying in a hollow where there was some grass about four feet high. I passed the hollow about thirty paces ahead of my men and kept out of the grass, where I am sure the tigress had watched me track past. Then my crew came after me, speaking loudly and walked through the grass and put up the tigress, which bounded on the track and passed the open channels between the

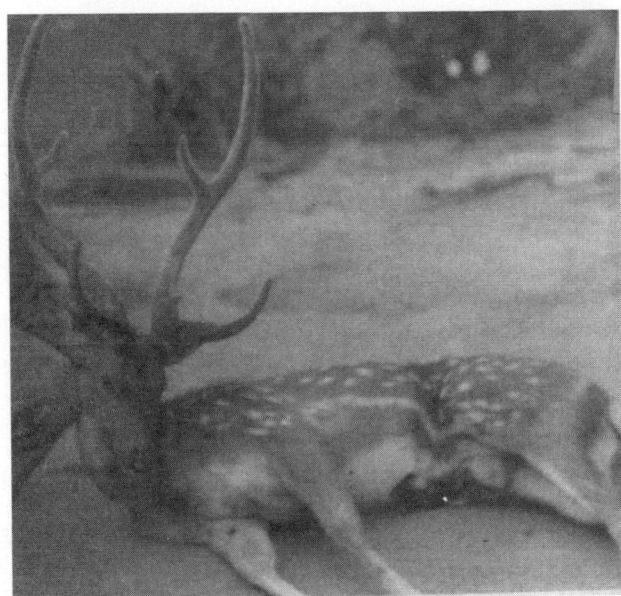

Chital were a fair game in sugarfarms.

heavier plantations of sugarcane. Hearing the thumping sounds of heavy feet and people shouting warning, I swung my big six-cell torch and probed the opening. In the flash of the beam I could just catch the rear of her tawny back moving like a blur off into the sugar field. She was hardly 5 meters away from me.

The best thing about this incident was that I had no gun in my hands but only the torch. A few minutes before, having carried the rifle for over five hours, I had already handed it over to Dularay. Else, being an adolescent teenager I might have stacked a bullet into it with undetermined effect. At any rate be it a boy or a senior, reckless-foolhardiness and jangled nerves do make people commit howlers and they often pull trigger in excitement to which I was no exception.

When uncle learnt of it he felt happy. "It was good that you didn't have the gun. You saw that the tigress did not disturb you because you stood cool. All predators are wise cowards. Appearance of timidity and weakness offers a strong temptation to their ferocious instincts. They also know what a man can do to them, so assume a bold bearing in their presence and you will find them tolerably safe neighbors. Anyway, any pot game is welcomed but don't look for extra excitement with tigers. That's insanely dangerous."

As an old timer, uncle represented the finest traditions of hunting ethics. Like a teacher who keeps his pupil away from misguided notions and corrects his tiny teensy errors, he had given me an important lesson – build-up of personal experiences on common everyday occurrences. What could be a better lesson than this for a teenager, ensuring his apprenticeship in field-sport with such veterans? These words I will remember for all my life – avoid extra excitement with tigers.

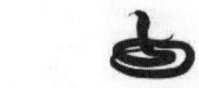

The Serpentine Ordeal

"I'd like to make it very clear that getting bitten by a venomous snake is dumb, clumsy and nothing to be proud of."

- Romulus Whitaker, renowned herpetologist

Snakes seemed to swarm everywhere in Phatteypur. Their preference to live in the village fields is generally attributed to the crops grown there. Millions of rats frequent the field, living in ground holes to eat the grain. They formed natural food for snakes that occupied their holes and accompanied them all the year round.

One day, dusk was about to settle when the calls of peacocks prompted my 'meat hunter' (not sport hunting) instincts to shoulder the gun and go in the wheat fields. Drawn by the calls I reached near a huge *pipal* tree and found the bird there. Its heavily feathered tail was partially projected out but the body was covered in thick foliage. Trying my best, I looked from many directions but could not manipulate a killing shot. I circumvented the trunk to get a better view of the bird when it sighted me and took to rapid flight. But as darkness was deepening it alighted on a banyan tree, some 100 yards away.

The colours had intensified in the west and hardly a minute of twilight was left, when I again located the bird on a branch. Its bare chest was prominently exposed. I steadied myself against the tree trunk slowly aligning the gun when a sharp hissing sound emanated around me and slowly transformed into a sonorous whistling. I knew that such sound is released by an angry snake, preparatory to striking. I hastily glanced over the tree trunk but there was hardly anything. A few seconds later the low hiss slithered again like a cold, thin blade. This time it seemed to rise from the very spot where I had been standing. I looked below and an icy chill ran down my spine. There, between the space of my legs was a half-coiled cobra, the ultra fast and deadliest snake in India which can strike thrice on a single point just in one second.

I stood rooted to the spot. By sheer luck I had avoided trampling upon it. My foot had crossed over it and the reptile had sensed my vibrations. The snake was thoroughly disturbed. Its swelled hood stood erect up to my knees, its two-forked tongue darted in and out of its open jaw that was recurrently whipping past my legs. The light was poor but I could perceive its movements unmistakably. Profuse rills of sweat burst out of my body. Like they say in the wild west - it was a real McCoy.

I do not know for how long I stood there transfixed with fear, my heart pounding hard against my ribs, gazing helplessly at the snake as it moved its hood in search of danger. It looked around for some time then feeling satisfied that there was no immediate cause to worry, it closed his hood and slumped down on his half coiled body. Perhaps it had mistaken my legs as stems of some plant or shrub, and I had thus escaped its attention. I slowly brought the muzzle of the gun down from the peacock and turned it into the direction of the snake, taking a time which seemed vast like eternity. Finally as the gun bead came in line-up, I pulled the trigger, blasting the reptile into pieces. The peacock fluttered away, squeaking in the darkness as I heaved a sigh of immeasurable relief.

Cobras are prolific breeders and generally give birth to thirty to fifty babies. From the moment of birth the mother usually leaves her offspring to fend for themselves, as the little unpleasant devils are born with a near lethal dose of poison in their fangs. Two hours after being born they can kill a fowl and at the ripe old age of one day their venom is so fantastic in virulence that they can inflict a fatal bite on a human being. A solid bite, even with anti-venom at hand, usually means a rapid singularly horrible death. According to some herpetologists, a cobra can strike up to a distance that is forty percent of its length.

The terrible ordeal was over; I had not only had my share of high adrenalin but it seemed that I had monopolized all the hair raisers.

One of Phatteypur's great fascinations for me was to hobnob with its wildlife through my favourite field glasses. As dawn broke and the rim of the sun showed fiery red, seemingly coming out of the ground in the flat country, my cousins and I would sit on the roof of the two-storied mud fortress and watch the extensive stretch of yellow and green, like a wide open veldt. This was the grazing ground of wildlife, crop-eaters and cud-chewers, as well as their hiding ground. While enjoying breakfast we would view the wildlife; a jackal running away with a brown partridge in its mouth or make out a colony of *Hanuman langoor*, sixty to seventy in number, making a chattering commotion on a *gular* tree and their strange acquaintance with spotted deer herds.

We would descry a pair of hog deer and further away on the gold flooded horizon a sounder of wild boar, snatching their last morsels on the paddy or gram before retiring for the day. On the other side of horizon would be blue bulls standing under the clouds enveloped in pink vapors. The slate coloured males, much darker and larger than their beige females, with their distinctive white stockings would first make for the shade of timber, while the females followed them a little later.

For half an hour we would spot the game and study the behavior of practically all the animals visible to us, drinking our fill with the field glasses. As the sunlight grew stronger and heat shimmered, the wildlife disappeared, as if it were never there. During the heat of the day they lay up in the bush and crops and came into open about four o' clock in the afternoon. Soon the human activities and their livestock took over the landscape and the black bucks that and were still upholding their night grounds, would also shift in cover. On far away Assam road, occasional passing trucks disturbed concentrations of more black bucks that hadn't yet taken cognizance of blazing sun. As if startled they instantly took to a steeping and floating action; with the sun glancing off their rich black hides and horns; tails up, legs flying and hooves hitting the ground with pattering rapidity. Their racy bounds, raising a lot of dust seemed to reflect the symmetry of movement one sees in larger birds as they cut the air.

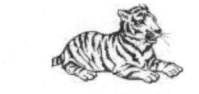

Glimpses of Tiger Cubs

"Tigers, except when wounded or when man-eaters, are on the whole very good-tempered... Occasionally a tiger will object to too close an approach to its cubs or to a kill that it is guarding. The objection invariably takes the form of growling, and if this does not prove effective it is followed by short rushes accompanied by terrifying roars. If these warnings are disregarded, the blame for any injury inflicted rests entirely with the intruder."

- Jim Corbett

Some vegetable farmers, like small ranchers, had made enclosures around their fields to protect the farm produce, raise livestock and keep out the unpleasant nocturnal visitors. But the flimsy fences made of dry thorns, thumb-thick rope and wooden dowels didn't offer much protection. A predator could easily jump over them and big grazers like blue bulls easily knocked them down. And in case a straying elephant wanted to see just for a change of his taste what the farmer is growing, he had no problems. Its great stride is designed to break paths for other animals, its trunk to uproot trees and its huge feet leaves pits deep enough to serve as water holes for small fish and fowl. In case the enclosure was found broken we were advised to check inside it.

Once we entered the broken fence of an enclosure, hardly a five hundred square meter plot in which cauliflower, beans and spinach were growing. A medley of squeaking sounds attracted our attention; advancing in the direction we found the newly-laid litter of a sow, comprising over 20 piglets hardly a week old. The mother had gone to look for tubers and the piglets with their just-opened eyes, had come out of their corner to explore their world. Dularay wanted to stuff his bag with the piglets, but seeing my reluctance he gave up. Sow mothers are troublesome and the dark nights tend to make them more dangerous for they move about more confidently and pose threat to interceptors. This was the climax of the hunt and we left the place without losing time. Later we worked harder for hours, hoping to catch eyes in our flares but nothing showed up and we returned empty-handed.

The first half of the round was finished by midnight. There were several wooden watchposts in the fields, we would retire on one of them, the watcher there would provide us with blankets and quilts, we would have a short sleep then again, as the cocks voiced their morning calls, we would start our second innings. This was an

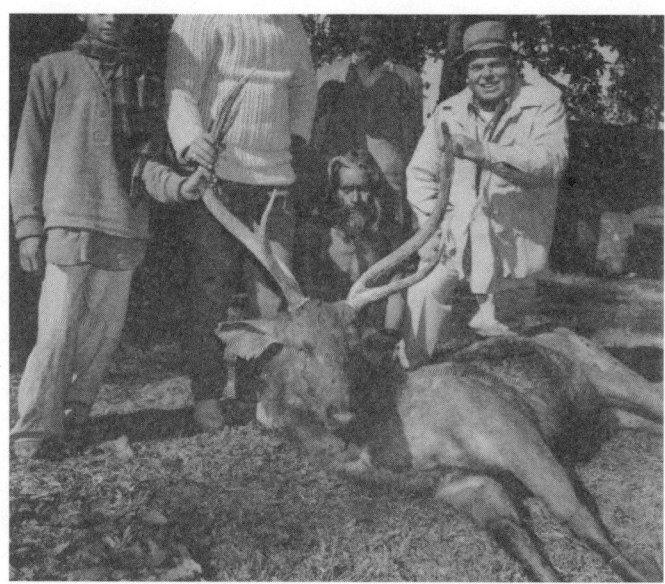
A sambhar shot in Phattaypur farmlands

ideal time for swamp deer, which also strayed to Phatteypur farm during rains for breeding and often stayed there in surrounding swamps and lakes where their fallen horns were found by villagers. I encountered quite a few of these deer in the fields but they all being does, I could never shoot one.

A *gauhari* (cow herder) named Banwari, had kept his fifty-odd cattle heads in an enclosure, which was raided in the night by the guest tigress I had encountered with Uncle. She was the resident of a swamp called Banukiya. The tigress had killed a small calf and consumed it then and there. The panicked cattle stampeded in the enclosure and broke out, scattering in all directions. The bellowing calls were clearly audible to us from a mile away in the night. Banwari had even better audition, for his hut was only a few yards from the enclosure, while the sound of the tigress's chewing the meat was like soundtrack aired from hell. Possessed of no better weapon than a stick and no appropriate light equipment to aid him in the circumstances, Banwari decided to stay indoors and leave the predator alone.

The moment I neared the place, scores of cattle eyes reflected in the beams of my torch and it was impossible to distinguish these from that of the tigress, if she was indeed there amid them.

The panicked cattle had thundered far from their enclosure. Next day a few oxen returned by themselves but the others had joined a mixed herd of blue bulls and black bucks. It took me three days and a good walk of over 40 kilometers, to separate his cattle from the antelopes. Every time the wild animals sighted or scented us, they made off at high speed and the dumb cattle followed on their trail.

My last meeting with the tigress was in February 1969. At the first suspicion of daylight we had started retreating for home. The stars were paling in the east and light over the vista was so faint that we could barely see beyond two hundred yards. We were moving quietly as we always did when the pungent smell of a dead cow that had died a natural death and had been thrown in a large depression, assailed our nostrils. From the high ground I could just see a spot of white profile.

We converged some ten yards before the spot and threw the lights on the cow. There was nothing near the carcass, not even a jackal. Then we roved the torch around and found the tigress lurking at the edge of the depression with some four cubs trilling around it. They had apparently sensed us coming while approaching the carnivores' food and stopped in their tracks.

They were the first tiger cubs I had ever seen outside a zoo or a circus. Their glimpse electrified me, coming with the suddenness of an apparition as they stood there, with the smoky haze of the night still behind them. It was too early for the birds or most of the sounds that come with the light.

The tigress did not go down in the depression. She rather immediately reversed, not in a panicked retreat but in a dignified trot as her cubs followed her without slightest hesitation. The ground was almost bare for almost a hundred feet in the direction the family was heading. After a few seconds, she stopped and looked back at us and also her cubs that had now broken into a run. We swept the lights over them. Obfuscated, they again stopped and looked at us. They did this quite a few times, though kept gaining distance from us with every little jog. I watched them retreating towards the swampy slot of Dhanega Nala, those four yellowish tawny beasts, the bouncing balls of fur who would soon rule this vista and whose speed will mean capture and whose fangs would mean death.

Sometime after the daylight broke and began to spread over the vista. A jackal howled a tapering wail, and a crazy mocking yammer of a fox rose; as the scavengers retired to their hideout for the day.

After the sunrise, a whirlpool of great lammergeyer vultures circled over the depression. The rising air currents had transferred the pungent smell of dead cow to the soaring birds and they were coming down to investigate the dish. They soon gathered in a milling crowd, hopped on and off the body flapping their wings, and gorging on the carcass in their insatiable hunger, finished it in a day. That night when we passed through that depression only the skeleton of cattle had remained on which a family of hyenas was feasting. The leading male showed a stretched bloated stomach, which seemingly had crushed bones inside. We took our hats off to the hyenas' digestion and went ahead.

This way the rounds, never a wasted effort lasted for the entire night crammed with little thrills. Finally when the moon paled and the long winter night came to an end, we called off the hunt and retraced our steps. A buck or a boar swinging by his feet from a branch borne by two sturdy trackers was a common sight when I returned. By this time an orange glow would have lit the sky and the morning risers would be out in the field, and seeing my bag their compliments would come my way. "What a large animal, what symmetrical horns, what a good kill?" They would grin in admiration. "Bhaiyya is a determined pursuer; he will not come back empty handed." It flattered my ego and I felt something like the great white hunters of African veldts, Bill Judd, Allan Black or J.A. Hunter returning Hollywood- style.

Farmland hunting had two clear benefits: one could safeguard the yields and also keep the villagers supplied with solid fresh protein. By the time I reached the village the rim of the sun would be showing and people who wished to share the hunt would have arrived in uncle's compound. A hot water bath at home rejuvenated the energies. A quick breakfast and I returned to the compound where by then the trophy was set for the dissection under the *pipal* tree. I supervised its skinning and distribution, keeping the choicest parts for the larder that would furnish us with the delicious roast for lunches. I would then return to bed and fall into a deep sleep.

There came phases of a week or a fortnight when literally ten to twelve hours of the day were dedicated to this atavistic passion. I think that shooting in the field at night and superintending the dissecting of the carcass in the morning, and following the trail of herds during the day, then again preparing meat for the smoking ramps was a job of considerable magnitude. Yet, it was a top assignment from the perspective of a teenager that he did with surprising ease and in fact enjoyed it. It was living adventure to the fullest. I have some times read about the momentous years of a person's life, and I think that as far as I am concerned, my early years in the Tarai qualify for that appellation.

In the feel of a teenager, I liked Tarai as my home and when I came to my residence at Lucknow I felt like a guest. Least I knew that it was the beginning of a kind of obsession for outdoor ventures that would admittedly be carried too far all my life.

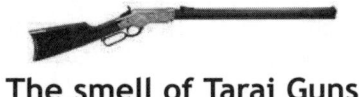

The smell of Tarai Guns

"If you take guns away from legal owners then the only people who would have guns would be the bad guys".
- A Tagline from the American Wild West

Around Phatteypur area, there were some half a dozen native hunters which were operating with antiquated old model muzzle loaders including Enfield rifles that were used in the Indian armed forces' Mutiny during 1857. It was not known as how this weaponry had found its way into this area but by educated guesstimates their users, who made living exclusively by hunting, killed two hundred to three hundred animals each year and wounded more than twice that number. During my nightly hunting rounds, I came across scores of wild animals which were wounded by the insensate natives and left to die a lingering death. Some of these held so much of decomposed, smelly abscesses on their perforated bodies that even after being killed these were inedible for natives. They were literally rotting yet living animals, sometimes infested with maggots and iridescent green flies swarming over them. I once shot a hog deer and extracted a large jagged piece of six-inch long iron bar, embedded in its stomach. The unpleasant souvenir was obviously fired with the weak-load of a native gun and this had set up a ghastly festering eruption.

Dogma demands that every effort should be made to eliminate a wounded animal, not because if it is a dangerous animal its behavior would become unpredictable and pose threat to mankind and others, but more particularly for humanitarian reasons. Even game department laws made it mandatory that wounded animals be dispatched. Under this hunters' intrinsic code, that must be honored, I took the job seriously and tried to track wounded ones on priority. I often went to infinite lengths to make certain that the animal is not bequeathed to die a drawn-out death from gangrene, starvation or weakness. Though tracking and hunting cannot be done at the same time but this acme of sport, exercised during day light hours made the combination of both possible to some degree.

Though it was all for non-dangerous pot game but the same ethic of hunting is also responsible for many tragedies within hunters fraternity. Many were mauled and got new looks in retaliation by potentially lethal predators, while some met their catastrophic end in the implementation of what they considered to be the commitment of sport hunting. Human ego is a strangely complicated singularity when it comes down to single minded qualifications in sport killing. One may justify it as a compassionate process but to many it is an aggressive ploy of embracing one more bloodthirsty adventure as final confrontation with a dangerous animal and relishing its entire array of emotions.

I have no recollection of ever finding any particle of pleasure in it, only discomforts in unfriendly environments, heavy sugarcane and swampy terrains where wounded ungulates, retreated with stoicism in the acceptance of death. Now with the present day maturity, considering the ruthlessness and insensitivity in which I indulged like an evil little boy, I think it was my clan of compulsive killers known by the honored name of over-burdened crop protector was basically driven by fraudulent dictum of miming and killing for pleasure. We as representative of the resentment of local inhabitants in direct competition with wildlife were indeed the real cause of wild animals suffering. I have had deep compunctions ever since and as I write this with more than a little bit of embarrassment and chagrin, I sometimes tell myself: "Well, the Killer Ape, all this male recreation was occupation of your ancestor's primal drama; a result of interminable macho stories of family icons, where licensed killing increasingly justified the illegalities, so you were impatient to walk on their footsteps."

But again this was perhaps the reason, that as a growing adolescent, ignorant of such debased overtones, I had no hatred for hunting but only a great interest and a great curiosity. All my suppressed sense of adventure, my instincts and my desire to discover my extent of physical courage, had been aroused by the great amount of sport in Tarai farmlands. I imagine that when myriad wild animals competed with human beings for agricultural crops my role was the holder of a thin red line and my feeling was very much that of the average boy who enlists; perhaps as a killer with conscience.

❖

At Phatteypur, I got the spot-on opportunity to make acquaintance with the veritable arsenal of Kunwar Sahib, a part of which was possessed by Uncle Bahadur Lal. The great veteran had more than 150 guns and most of the sophisticated weaponry of this lot was hoarded at Larti, which was indeed the depository of arms and ammunition for family members. The household shooting guns kept at Phatteypur, numbering over twenty, were from the same line of heirloom. This arsenal may sound incredible to a modern reader, but such collections were conventional amongst Zamindari estates. There were many large and medium bores in Uncle's armory that were considered more of status symbol for the family than of any practical use. Many of these were rarely fired since the old veteran's demise. Even their brass shells, stocked in cartridge boxes, had lost their shine. But in altered modus operandi the guns were worth their display, supposedly as the source of feudal power.

I used uncle's collection of guns freely. Every week I took out a different rifle from its case, of course with permission and set it right by blazing a couple of shots. There was an old catalogue on rifle ballistics, *African Rifles & Cartridges* by John Taylor, lying casually in the dining room almirah. No one there knew English hence no one read it. I spent a good time in studying the details of muzzle velocity and foot pounds. I still remember that the velocity declines with the decreasing weight of the bullet as the muzzle energy persuasion and foot pounds increase.

During this period I discussed with uncle the use of different guns, their velocity and wallop and handled a variety of heavy, medium to light bore rifles. For some days, I used .318, .256 and .275 Westley Richards and .275, N02 Rigby extensively and swore by the weapon. These accurate hitting firearms, with animal engravings, had a positively terrific reputation in the hunting fraternity, for a clean one-shot kill by these was a practical certainty.

I did not know this fact then, but now I understand that light caliber rifles always worked better than any canon. Even that super tough little Scott WDM "Karamojo" Bell, the veteran of African savannahs, used light caliber rifles on tuskers. In all his writings, he does not mention a single close call. He wrote that he could not ever remember using more than one shot on any elephant, buffalo or lion. He knew as how to shoot by anatomy with small bores like .256 and .275. These are even lighter rifles than many that are used for deer hunting in America.

Learning to shoot by anatomy from any angle with solid bullets was the deadliest and evidently the most merciful way of hunting and as I learnt the subtleties of hunting the quality of weapons assumed greater importance. I added a medium bore .330 BSA and an all-rounder .375 Holland & Holland to complete my battery that covered long range, with high velocity and consequent flat trajectory and extreme accuracy up to 250 yards with bare eyes and more than 500 yards with telescope. It was hard to get 300 grain soft point ammo in old loadings. Uncle solved the problem. He carefully prided off the alloy tips of slugs, exposing the bright soft lead beneath so that the bullet does not cross the body but stays in. The rifle was then loaded with three rounds in the magazine and one in the breech. One cartridge less in the magazine was to avoid the jam, which might occur should the bolt of the gun is worked very fast in reloading.

The .416 Rigby is a family souvenir for dangerous game, weighing 12 pounds to even the recoil; barrels of this rifle are deeply indented by tiger's teeth, the story of which is already recounted elsewhere in this book. There is also a Belgian made Rahillon .416 magazine rifle Once I rapidly emptied its entire magazine on tin cans at the mango-orchard, only to find that large rifles have substantially slamming recoil and firing more than a couple of shots is not only unpleasant but also unsafe.

However, if I were to go man-eater shooting tomorrow it would be taken in preference to any other gun. It takes five drams of powder with 440 grain hardened bullet having a thick cannelured base and hollow in the point to contain a copper tube stopped at the outer end. The bullet has now become a rarity and is not obtainable at a reasonable price. Interestingly there is also a .404 Jeffery magazine rifle and a triple barrel by Ferlach of Austria. It is a combination of a rifle and a shot gun; there are engravings of hunting scenes on the side lock plates, with a pistol grip and a cheek plate on the selected walnut stock. The gun is certainly a unique example of exceptional craft skills.

The quality armoury continues to grace the gun-racks of old mud fortress. Odd heavy caliber streamlined guns without ammunition are just reduced to showpieces but those tin packs of Kynoch nonexpanding solid bulleted cartridges with empty brass shells inside them, fired from these guns are sincerely maintained, much because legacy symbols are of enormous gravity for renowned families; these shells weighing in tens of kilograms and some of them still softly smelling with Nitro-cellulose powder, cordite and nitroglycerine explosives are an abounding reminder of a rifle-minded past. This, however, recalls me of Nancy Mitford's punch comment, thriving with poignant humour that an aristocracy in a republic is like a chicken, whose head has been cut off; it may run about in a lively way, but in fact it is dead.

❖

The most romantic feature of these nightly rounds was a deep hiatus of silence that ruled over the fields. It always started towards midnight and continued up to the false dawn. It used to be strange and a uniquely comforting time of hush, which often intensified to the level of being unearthly. The predators' fear borne out of the inherited distrust of the darkness prevailed in its full sway over the human settlements as the people slept in their huts, doors fastened and windows shut and their bonfires burning dimly.

Above the pulse of the sugar grasslands, the occasional bell of a startled *sambhar* rose from far across the Sharda canal, only to be responded by pariah dogs from a village. The distant whistles of railway engines, as the up and down trains clanked their way slowly from Kurraiya station to pick up speed for their journey to Bareilly or Lucknow or the short, rapid and prolonged hooting of coal engines, as the trains rumbled to a grinding halt at the outer signal, infrequently shattered the silence of the night. However, even the sounds of such a magnitude were soon swallowed up by the immensity of surrounding silence and utter stillness set in again, brooding in its concealed enigma.

These nightly circumnavigates were not a sort of experience that fade with the passage of years. I discovered a great deal about nature and gunnery in these rounds. During hard winters fog settled soon after sunset and thickened in layers. It hung low and heavy, reducing visibility and remained so till it was burnt off by the sun at the daybreak. There were times when the cloudy weather persisted and the fog did not clear off for many days and the fields lay covered under the hazy effluvium. Even the beams of the most powerful torches then shone like mere glimmers from five yards. At such times the crop protection expeditions came to an abrasive halt.

But I refused to acknowledge fog as a deterrent and roamed freely in the field for I had realized that the fog was beneficial in many ways. It dulled the senses of animals and our reactions on coming face to face with them were invariably quicker. Even migratory birds were forced to settle on the ground. They flew low and were slow to amend their mistakes of direction. This made me procure a good bag on foggy days.

However, such cool times drifted uneventfully and Uncle Bahdur Lal enjoyed them immensely. He sat in the midst of the throng on his deck chair and spent his time smoking his inevitable hookah, tightly loaded with several ounces of jaggery-sweetened tobacco. As the water gurgled in the pipe, he acquired some small measure of comfort from this apparent purgation with the clouds of coarse acrid smoke floating round him.

These excursions were a never-ending affair. As the next evening would set in, uncle would hand over a rifle to me and say casually: "Boy! Wildlife is thick on the ground and we are short of meat. If you see anything good, shoot it."

And that would be the initiation of yet another round for crop protection and meat supply to uncle's sulky and listless labourers. For them, a full flesh-pot and a good brew of sugarcane-wine was an infallible barometer of their working mood.

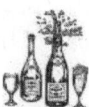

The Champagne's Fizz

"Looking on the happy autumn fields, and thinking of the days that are no more"
- Tennyson, Princess

Farmlands of Tarai, mysterious, uncertain and contradictory, provided a fascinating setting for adventuresome events and though the years have passed, fields of Phatteypur still serve as a great holding ground of wildlife. Perhaps the nature sees to it precariously that the feed of the predator might be reduced, individuals might suffer and die but species and their cycles must live on this special turf. Hence the land is much like champagne that hasn't lost its fizz. Tigers still crouch in tall sugarcanes with archaic regularity. Small family groups of *langoors* dot the landscape and *chital*, black buck and hog deer frequent the terrain in small bunches; and to underline even wolves appear periodically. Poaching over recent years has hit the colossal sounders of wild boar harder than any other species but their small assemblies, mixed with blue bulls, can be seen huddled together in gram fields, and migratory birds fly in the moon's reflection.

It is argued in conservation forums that out of 150 million years, it is only in past 150 years that mankind has seriously challenged the wildlife's claim to its land. All the natural treasures of their turf have been usurped by man; but the wild animals, adaptable as they are, have not evolved to acclimatize this change in their environment. This lack of tractability, when combined with high quality firearms and man generated animal-husbandry, is an incorrigible recipe for disaster. However, it seems strange that despite ever-increasing demographic pressure, Tarai farmlands can contain much of wildlife including tigers susceptible to modesty and the antithetical leopards – that can take any pressure from human civilization (until molested), and remain wild to the last breath.

This story may well be taken as my first introduction to a rich man-made ecosystem that shielded wildlife, with concealing care and then gave it up to potentially meet the subsistence resource needs of the people and also to gratify their hunter's dream. There was so much of vegetation offering nourishment to herds of grazing animals. Not to bemoan the passing of an era – it was this phase when the spell of tigerine farmlands took hold over me and I happened to taste the wine of excitement that the real countryside provides.

Book 2
THE LEGEND OF SUGARCANE TIGERS

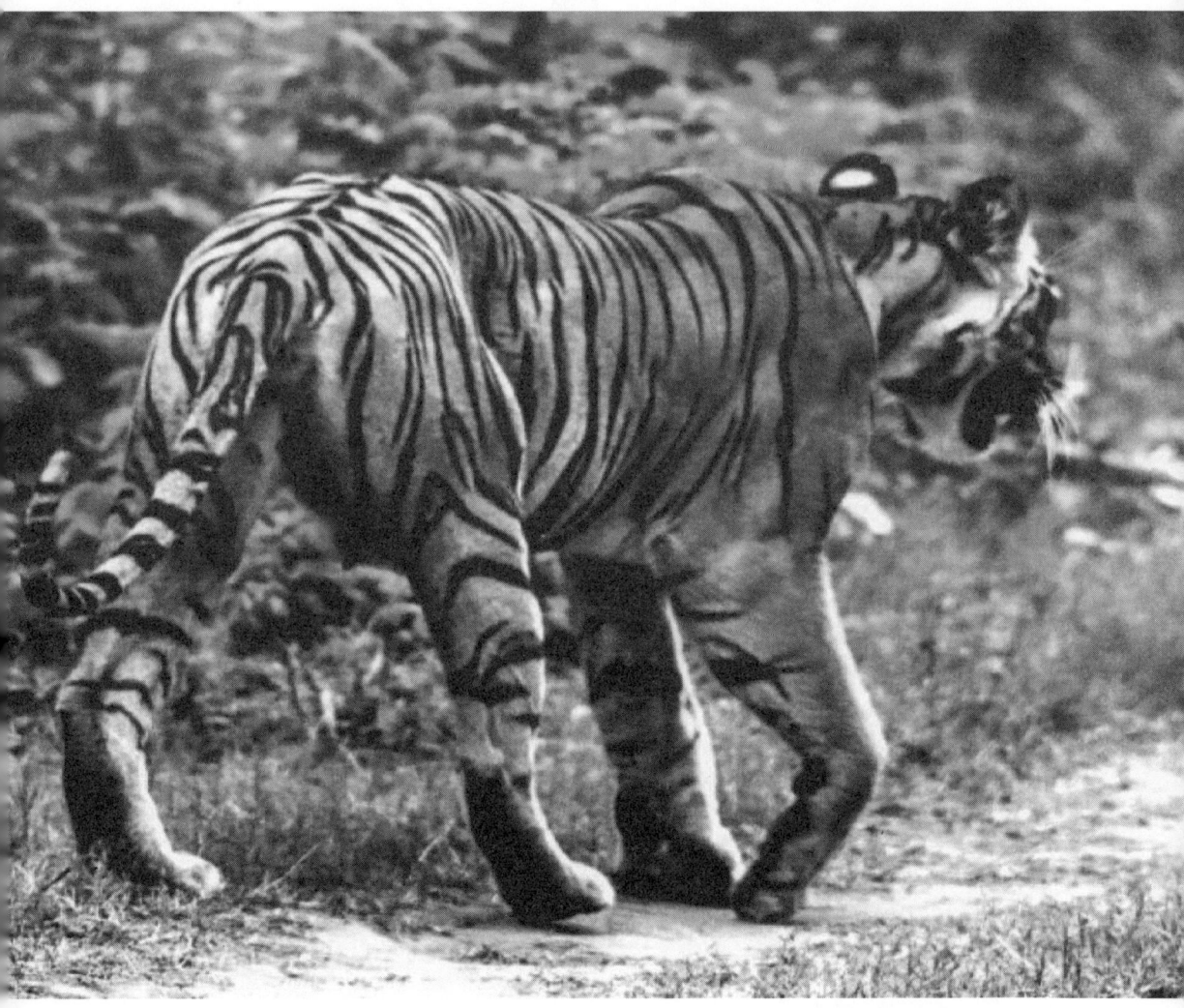

CHAPTER 3
SUGARCANE TIGER PRELUDE

Chapter 3

Sugarcane Tiger Prelude

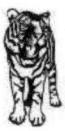

I CREDIT MY EXTRAORDINARY FASCINATION FOR BIG CATS TO THE LEGACY of my family that regarded big gameshooting as part of normal life. The love for wilds, handed down from generation to generation, has now become a part of my personality and indeed, my thought process. Years ago and later year after years, I had witnessed abundant destruction of big game. When such trophies were brought home in Larti or Phatteypurwhich I alternatively visited during winter and summer holidays, I also pulled their tails, bounced and played over them as a child without fear, while elderly members of family measured and admired them.

As a lad of 12, my Larti and Phatteypur forays had given me enough opportunities to participate in the hunts of native poachers in different forests in Mailani and Khutar. The tiger was the most potent being of the wild world, and the most conspicuous quality of the poachers was their ability as tiger-trackers. This naturally included the trail of its prey. These people were a special breed and there was a professional touch to everything they did. From childhood onwards their eyes were accustomed to notice the smallest signs in the wild and to draw instant conclusions from these observations. Where a normal man's eyes would see nothing but everyday trifles, the natives read their surroundings as an open book of dramatic actions and tragic events. A bent blade of grass, a fallen leaf and a mark on a tree helped them swiftly construct the chain of events with unfailing certainty which no detective in the world can possibly imitate. During these sojourn I also acquired the knowledge of the ways of *shikaar* and expertise required to bring down marauders.

I believe that boyhood impressions live on within us to guide our adult behavior. In later years when shooting was banned and I gave up the gun – or the perverse thrill of sadistic entertainment – the same principle guided me to take up farmland tiger research. Like a seed buried deep in the soil finds the strength to germinate, shoving its way up towards light and life, my entire wildlife experience of the past

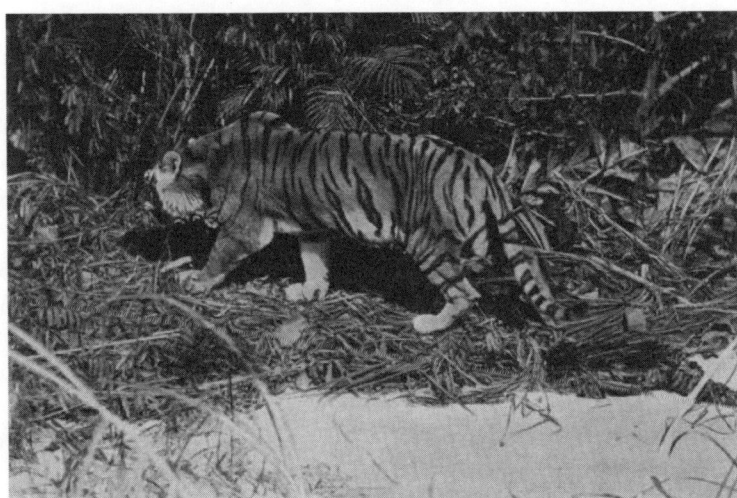

A tiger near a water pond
from family archives.

encouraged me to go in for this new enterprise. It finally centered on the rural areas of Tarai, where outside the boundaries of protected forests, it helped me crack the matrix of farmland wildlife. I stalked many tigers through the savannah of sugarcane plantations. I met many of them face to face at close quarters while on some occasions I was also stalked by a few of them.

Once a fugitive pair of juveniles followed me for a good twenty minutes and that was the longest mile I had ever covered. Ordinarily tigers seldom wander around during the day and certainly do not stalk human beings. But as they came up to our camps behind us proved that these were no ordinary tigers. I believe they had overcome their natural instinctive fear of man and had every intention of becoming man-eaters.

In those years I had no motor transport of my own and I had to walk lengthy distances except when I was ferrying from one place to another in the waters of Gomti, Sharda, Suheli, Mahona and Girwa rivers. Sometimes I had the luxury of using a friend's vehicle. This allowed me to see the real Tarai up close, including its people, farmlands, water ponds and a plethora of wildlife in isolated grass patches and swamps outside principal jungles. Falling in remote, hitherto inaccessible areas, many of these self-maintaining biological units were known to shelter specific fauna. These included monitor lizards, mouse deer and four-horned antelopes including black and brown partridges, red fowl, peafowl and porcupines.

Tarai farmlands had never been taken seriously in wildlife studies. However, one could always appreciate the presence of the surfeit of wild animals in the space of sprawling fields. The phenomenon of their co-existence with humans becamea pertinent question for me to solve. I sought to accomplish a long-lasting study that could open a new window to other wildlife activists as well as foresters, so that they might learn to understand its strength outside protected areas and respect it.

Tigers were the icons that challenged my courage, as their charisma again and again pulled me to dabble with them. Cane tiger research gradually changed the dimensions of my life. As I roamed the Tarai farmlands on foot with my old poacher' screw, now transformed into reformed protectors of wildlife, I stumbled upon an amazing fact about tiger's prevalence in sugarcane. Their population never seemed to expand, although at the same time every favourite niche of the habitat remained invariably full of tigers. It was almost magical on the parameters of tiger study.

As a prelude to the story it is interesting to note that in pre-independence times, the continuing living of tigers in farmlands is widely accepted in wildlife forums. Many unattached accounts of their hunting and undisturbed living are recorded in diaries of feudal Estates. The farmland wildlife under discussion was relegated to an ancillary position since the circumstances under which the animals lived in many of the surrounding human tracts were so small as to be negligible. But the havoc wrought by them upon standing crops often did find mention. The objective of diary writing was to supply information to a sportsman to meet the problem rather to invite a field naturalist to understand the prevailing conditions.

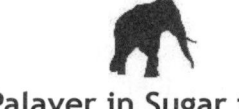

Palaver in Sugar fields
Kunwar Sahib's Hunt

"The old shikaartales do not only selfishly describe about a hunter's resolute valor and heroism but side by side also speak of the notability and renown of the Tarai wildlife."
- Author in his autobiography *Through Tiger's Den*

Having left Phatteypur, my maternal great grandfather Pandit Chhotey Lal Dixit settled down near Mailani jungles, and established a village named Larti exclusively for the purpose of hunting. Nestled amidst abundant *sal* trees, the village was the capital of his domain where he lived for 40 years and hunted tigers and leopards to the fulfillment of his heart. Needless to say he miraculously survived many a last ditch encounter in active big game pursuits.

The old veteran had domesticated four elephants for the purpose of shooting. These pachyderms were trained in tiger hunting. They were supposed to overcome their natural fear of the tiger and stand boldly against a tiger's charge, and not to flinch when heavy cordite rifles were discharged from those seated atop their backs. I say 'supposed to' because I feel that no elephant can be entirely devoid of fear where the tiger is concerned. Elephants give warning of the proximity of a tiger by throwing up their trunks and trumpeting, or often kick the ground with their forefoot, followed by the short impatient trumps that invariably tell that the tiger scent is fresh. Some, who feel real tension of the super predator's presence, bang their

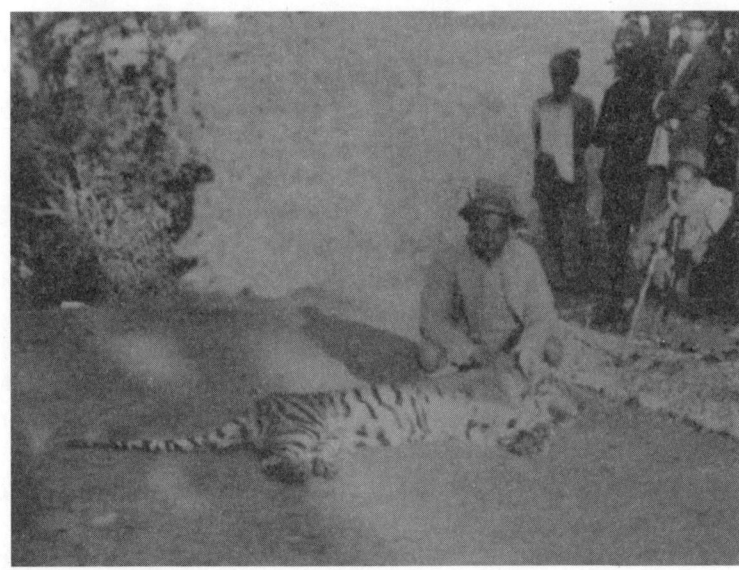

Kunwar Saheb with man-eater of Khutar, shot in March, 1925

trunks on the earth or trees as their bodies quiver in excitement.

Elephants were useful not merely for actual hunting, but for carrying home the shot game. Family stories mention the scores of animals that were brought home when grasses were being cleared for agriculture and how hunters hunted for the entire day. At dusk the elephants walked down the village in a stately fashion with plentiful carcasses of small and large game loaded on their backs. The great veteran also patrolled his domain on elephants as these beasts, essentially good swimmers are very useful in passing tangled marshes or wide and deep rivers.

In 1964 I was eight years of age when I reached Larti for the first time with my maternal grandmother. By that time only one cow elephant Ramkali had survived from that formidable assemblage. She had the reputation of fighting with a thoroughly enraged tiger that had plucked out her left eye. I remember seeing this octogenarian specimen in her stable. She was grazing placidly on the crushed lengths of sugarcane; and the nasty signatures of tiger's claw made some forty years back were still prominent on her forehead and much of his handwriting was even now visible on her trunk. I was struck by the friendliness of the cow elephant. I was seemingly no stranger for her as she rubbed my head with the tip of her trunk, staring at me unwinkingly from her single eye as if she fully understood that I was the direct blood line of Kunwar Sahib, her great past master. I fed her with fresh spinach and established a silent friendship with her. Alas, at my next visit her shed was empty for she had breathed her last after attaining a great age.

During my stay at Lartire counting of several hair-raising, gut-pulling accounts of Kunwar Sahib's prodigalities was part of daily conversation. The most fabulous account among these was not about the old man but about the valour of Ramkali's hair-raising duel with a man-eating tiger. The account was obtained from an octogenarian Kalicharan who had witnessed the scene as an errand boy. It is so fervid and heart-stirring that it is difficult for me to overlook its flutter and piquancy. This is how the old man recalled the entire episode:

Towards the end of November 1920,Kunwar Sahib camped at a village called Roushan Kothi, where MacDowell's liquor factory is now established. It was purely an agricultural zone then, near the city of Shajahanpur, with no tiger range jungles around. There was persistent information about a pair of cattle-killing/man-eating tigers operating in the neighborhood. The game in the area was abundant but the female had developed a personal predilection for human flesh. The male was a pure cattle-killer, though not known to feed on human body. Still both were happily going together. Although many efforts had been made to destroy these hardened offenders but all had failed in achieving the purpose and as is normal with the simple-minded folk with strong belief in supernatural, the men had begun to regard these tigers immune to punishment by any human agency.

Notwithstanding, Kunwar Sahib felt keen to test his luck in contriving the destruction of this scourge. The veteran put together a team of 15 members, in which I was also included. We reached the village and on that night camped at the edge of a mango orchard. I built a bonfire outside Sahib's tent and all men observed the precaution of remaining within the orchard in the immediate vicinity of the bonfire. The cozy warmth of the fire lulled the trackers to sleep.Kunwar Sahib and his deputy collector friend, Hanson McDonald, a British official, decided to commence their operation the next morning. I was asked to keep awake the entire night and be vigilant about the mighty marauder.

Towards midnight the deputy collector awoke and looking through the open tent door was shocked to see a pair of very bright sparkling eyes peering at the scene from across the fire. As he looked intently he marked out a pair of tigers standing at the edge of the circle of light made by the bonfire, where it merged into darkness. The servants were lying all around fast asleep,blissfully oblivious to the proximity of the potential danger. Very stealthily and conscious not to attract the attention of tigers, the deputy collector got up, collected his rifle and taking a careful aim fired at the nearest tiger. The spasmodic jerk with which the tiger lurched forward made it obvious that he had registered a hit. He let out a terrible growl and before the deputy collector could fire the second shot the slinking form of cats vanished into the darkness. At the gun report Kunwar Sahib had already awakened and so were the servants. They were now lustilyexercising their vocal chords.

In the bad light conditions and having no adequate lamps that may be used in hunting it was not possible to chase tigers in the night. The duo had successfully evaded the hunters by creeping along a sugarcane field for its full length which quickly carried them away from the danger zone.

Next morning KunwarSahib mounted his recently-acquired male elephant

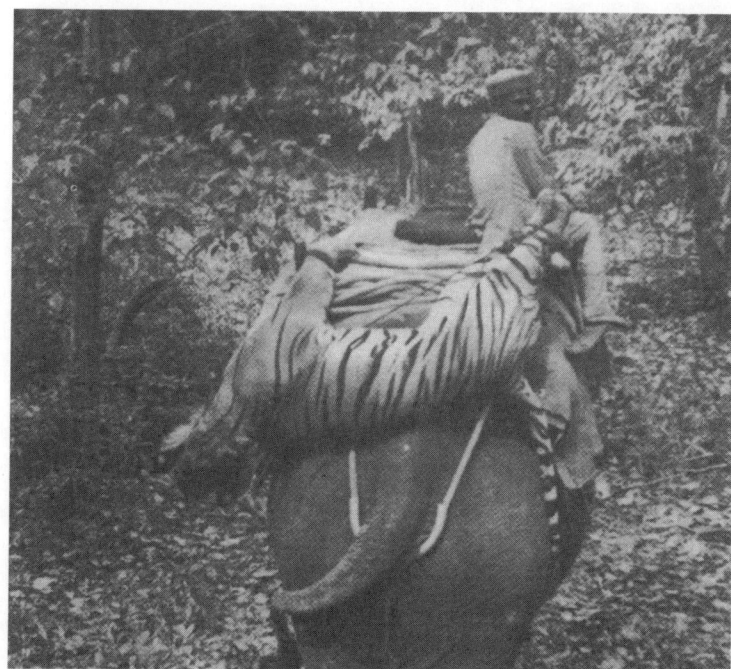

A large tiger being carried
back home.

pompously named McDonald Bahadur after the British dignitary of the same name who had gifted him. It was the pachyderm's first-ever tiger shoot, while the deputy collector took his seat on Ramkali. The head tracker Paeemen Pasi, the father of Chhotey Pasi who later taught me jungle craft, followed the blood trail on the ground with a spear in his hands.

The deputy collector had taken fancy for old veteran's. 416 Rigby, which he duly kept for the day while Kunwar Sahib armed himself with Jeffrey .400 HV double, made by Thomas Bland & Sons. Soon they reached inside an immense plantation of sugarcane, stretching like grass forest in all directions interspersed with wheat and paddy crops. As the beaters disturbed the grass the pair of tigers emerged in the opening of approximately 100 yards in a wheat field. Kunwar Sahib fired his heavy cordite rifle and killed the female instantly. It was an exceptionally lucky shot but this infuriated the male and he made a savage attack to devastate the offender.

He turned upon the elephant like a madly sputtering giant rocket with strong coughing vibrations. The gun had been reloaded and when he came within a sprinting distance two shots were fired simultaneously upon him but the shooter got the gleam of sun in his eyes and none of the shots succeeded in finding the target. Seeing the tiger's bare fangs Kunwar Sahib's elephant McDonald Bahadur gave a loud snort of fear, swung around and bolted back for the camp. He was running off at such a speed that it was better to jump down than to risk banging his head against the bough of a tree that might fall the way of elephant's escape. Though Kunwar Sahib again managed to reload and fire upon the chasing tiger but the speed of the galloping elephant hampered the accuracy of aim and the bullets again missed the target. The mahaut vigorously applied his steal goad to stop McDonald Bahadur but by then Kunwar Sahib, finding a patch of boggy soil, had already jumped out of the *howdah*.

Meanwhile at the other end,Ramkali went berserk. She emitted a shrill scream of hate and vengeance and charged all out at the coming tiger. The actions of both the elephants were unanticipated and all this had happened so quickly that the deputy collector sitting in his *howdah* was shocked and benumbed into inactivity.

The tiger hurled its heavy body through the air and landed on the forehead of Ramkali, embedding his fangs on the joint of her trunk. He hung down there with all his weight, clawing with the talons of all four feet.

The 65-year old Mahaut Kippha Khan had lead many tiger shoots. He first tried to pierce the tiger with his steel rod but when it didn't work he turned and neatly pulled the .416 Rigby from the dazed deputy collector's hand and tried to shoot. But the tiger caught the gun barrel in his mouth from the side and almost munched it, breaking one canine tooth in the process, and jerked it out of Kippha's hands. With both rod and gun gone from Kippha's hand, the tiger struck his claws in the thighs of Mahaut and pulled out a part of flesh. But the brave man only took a back leap and shifted into the Howdah. He retained his senses and, bleeding and sitting over the deputy collector, continued to drive the elephant and keep the pet's moral high.

It was a nightmarish spectacle being enacted in all its fearsome and nerve shattering acuteness. The mahaut vigorously shouted but the tiger continued violently to jerk his mouth tearing the flesh of pachyderm along with his thunderous gurgling sound as undaunted Paeemen, the tracker, moved here and there on the ground, giving his war-cry and desperately attempted to goad the spear in the cat.

Despite being badly mauled Ramkali remained undaunted and met the tiger's onslaught without flinching. Spreading her ears in a threat display like a windjammer in a line squall and screaming like a railway engine she tried to throw him off by coiling her trunk but it was not possible as her trunk wouldn't coil upon tiger for its long body literally covered the entire length of her trunk. Thereupon she rushed towards a tree to dash her head against its stout trunk.

Kunwar Sahib had already jumped down with his gun which had suffered no harm and its mechanism was in perfect order. He rapidly covered the distance and running behind Ramkali tried to maneuver near it for a mortal shot at the tiger, but both the combatants were so fiercely locked in fight that it was utterly impossible to drop the tiger without causing a serious harm to the elephant or worse to the deputy collector and Kippha still mounting on it. He observed the drama as a mute spectator feeling absolutely powerless to intervene. By that time Ramkali closed

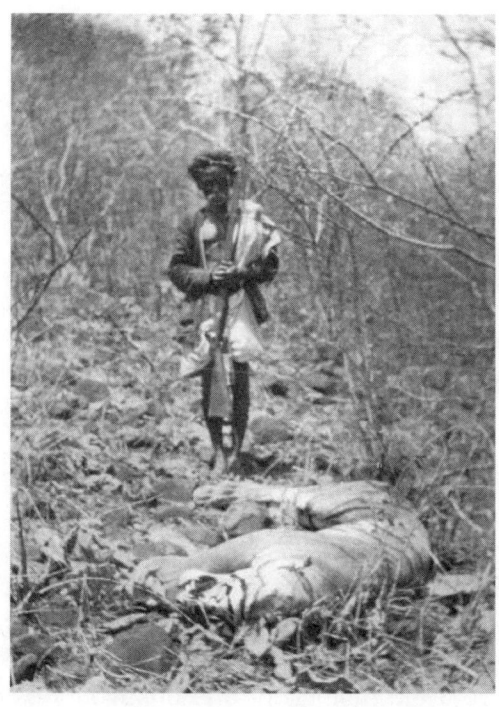

Paeemen Pasi (Chhotey's father) standing with a tiger shot at Maharajnagar Dhamar in 1934.

upon a neem tree where she dashed the tiger mercilessly at the trunk of the hard wood.

A painful *whoof* came out of the tiger's mouth and in just two mighty bumps, like that of a stone crushing bull-dozer, the super predator dropped down on the ground like a crumpled dry leaf from a tree. Kunwar Sahib though had reached unpleasantly close to the spot but he refrained from shooting: he wanted to see what Ramkali would do now. She was bleeding profusely from a number of terrible gashes. Enraged she screamed in hate and not granting any moment to the tiger trampled its head into pulp. Angry elephants are highly inventive and develop quiet individual modes of operation to deal with their aggressor. To the shock and acute discomfiture of everyone who was a witness, she placed her forelegs on the right hind leg of tiger, caught its left hindleg in her bleeding trunk and literally tore him into two parts, tossing the half cadaver into the sky. Such is the power of an enraged elephant when it takes the challenge of the super predator.

At the end Ramkali was left victorious in this amazing battle. Kippha also survived the great encounter though the loss of blood had been immense. The way he had remained mounted on the elephant despite being wounded bears eloquent testimony to his cool-headedness and presence of mind. Ramkali and he were given first aid and shifted to hospitals where both eventually recovered and happily returned to their job. Kunwar Sahib was so pleased with them that he gifted a muzzle loader each to Paeemen and Kippha.

Kippha has been described by Sir John Hewett in his book '*Jungle Trails in Northern India* as a master of every 'device and resource' required for success in tiger hunting. He had been sent to assist Nepalese authorities at the shoot given to H.R.H King George V following the Delhi Durbar in 1911. Kippha spent the later years of his life at Larti and died at ninety plus though he contended that his father had lived up to 115.

Palaver contd...
Maharaj Kumar of Vijayanagarm's Hunt

"Tiger hunting is not just the ancient disagreement of man against beast, but also the man consciously putting himself in the destructions way.

- a Tarai proverb

Post independence, in the decades of 1950s and 60s, a huge number of farmland shoots are recorded by former royalties of Tarai. Billy Arjan Singh tells, "Shooting in the forest was allocated by the system of ballot and each person who drew luck was allowed only one animal… To circumvent the restriction, one unsavoury pair of sportsmen took to going after farm tigers, on which there was no restriction."

The spot light now turns on Maharaj Kumar of Vijayanagarm.Fondly called Vizzy, he had an addiction for tiger shooting. During the 1960s, his score was approaching one short of 400 tigers when he was nominated Vice-Chairman of the State's Board of Wildlife. To celebrate the achievement, he returned to his old stamping grounds of Majhra-Singahi where the shooting season was in full swing and all the blocks were already full. Vizzy, therefore, preferred to satisfy his trigger itch in the agricultural area, where no legal complications of a shooting permit applied. By that time MajhraSingahi had been largely cultivated. The marshes and strands had given way to sugarcane but the tigers were still there.

A tigress inhabiting the cane belt was marked out by trackers and with the luxury of tiger shoot laid out on an old-fashioned scale, elephants were employed from neighboring Estates. The elephant-mounted army on the line of march reached the vista. Incidentally Vizzy was not seated in the conventional hunter's *howdah* made of a wooden box measuring2 feet X 5 feet X 3 feet with a hand rail around its perimeter. Instead, he sat on a jute seat resembling a chair, used in neighboring Nepal. It had no support or strap to bind around its occupant. The corps of beaters and *shikaar* elephants made a detour of about half a mile to get in the rear of the sugar plantation where the tigress was reported hiding. The rest of sportsmen took up their allotted position on the fringe of an open field at the edge of a water

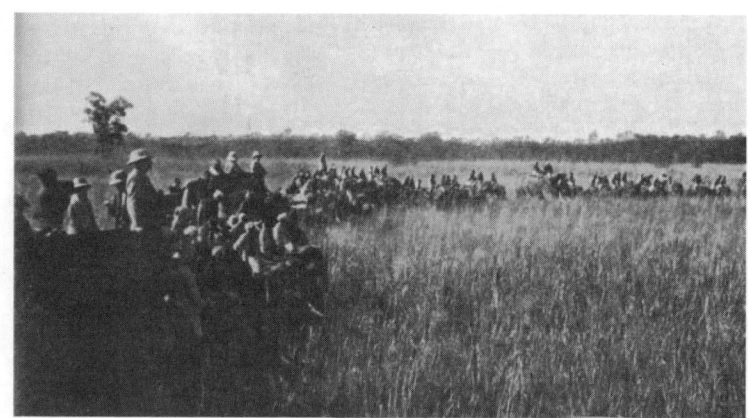

Of all the grand sights of big game shoots nothing could surpass the panorama of over 200 elephants massed together for the sport of royalties.

pond. Maharaj Kumar instructed everyone not to fire until the tigress had broken cover and driven up to his rifle. The beat started. The din created by beaters momentarily became louder and the tigress soon emerged out of sugarcrops.

Vizzy drew the bead and quickly fired. On many previous occasions, the animal had been encircled by hunting elephants but had always slipped back without the hunters getting any shot. This time also the tigress cleverly ducked back into the cover.

Vizzy's mahaut led the elephant into the crop. Vizzy stood up erect, supporting his one leg on the seat, his reloaded rifle held ready for action and eyes eagerly searching for a glimpse of the stripes, now resolutely been driven back in his direction. Other elephants had been diverted sideways to thwart the retreat of the animal.

Finally, harassed to the point of rage the encircled animal became thoroughly aroused and started moving angrily in the sugarcane, with a series of ear shattering roars. It then charged upon Maharaj Kumar's elephant while Vizzy took a hasty shot from his .375 H&H double barreled rifle at the leaping animal. The abrupt charge so terrified the elephant that he reared up trumpeting in nerve-shattering agitation. As if in confusion or in order to intimidate the tigress, it neither charged nor bolted but unexpectedly stood upright on his rear legs, high in the air, with trunk extended even higher. All the sportsmen stood spellbound watching the extraordinary spectacle as Vizzy was violently thrown off his mount into the high grass of sugarcane. The elephant then turned and bolted out of control while *shikaris* called out loudly, *Maraaj Saahib gir gaya, bhago, bachao* (The king has fallen, rush and save him.)

Vizzy's shot had broken the spine of the tigress, crippling her into absolute immobility. She lay over crushed canes with her jaws almost touching the ground as if half-crouching and half-crawling on her belly, emitting loud roars of mingled hate and anger while fallen Vizzy lay only a few yards away from her. The violent

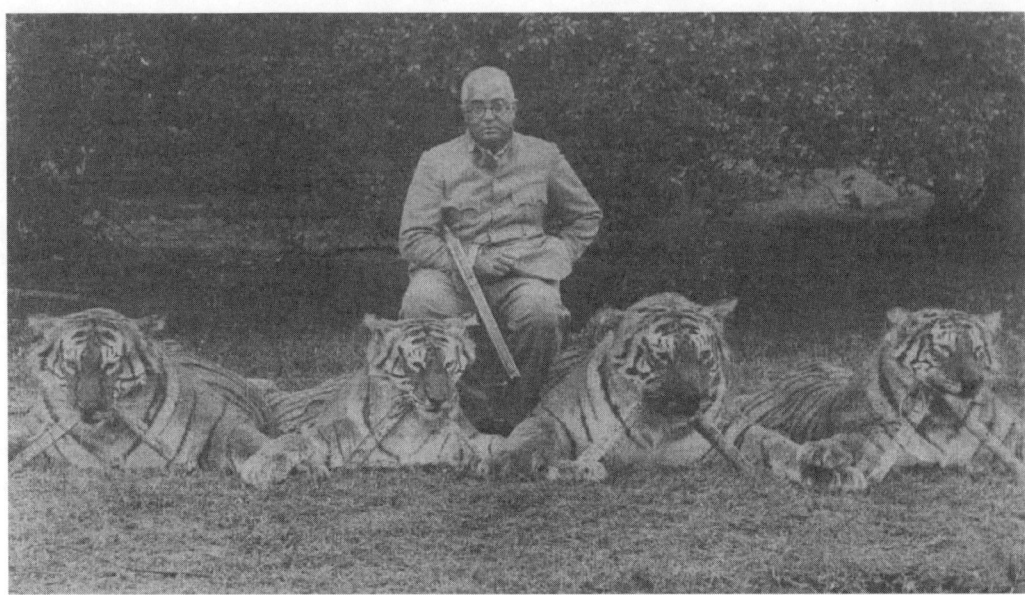

Vizzy with the four tigers he shot during one day's hunt that Chhotey had driven out for him in a beat. He is holding his favorite rifle, a .375 H&H hamerless double-barreled rifle. (Photo credit Raja Mahendra Shah Singhahi)

fall had caused internal injury to Vizzy besides seriously damaging his pelvis upon striking a hard mud pile. Hence like tigress he too was crippled into immobility.

The panicked elephants were difficult to control despite the efforts of mahouts to move them close to the scene, where Vizzy and the tigress, both submerged in a sea of high grass, lay only three meters away from each other.Both fixed at their respective positions were having full undivided attention for each other but none could do anything except to accentuate the acute sense of discomfiture into each other. Vizzy's rifle had been flung away in the fall. He called loudly for help but his voice conveying his pain was excruciatingly agonized. The tigress, in response to the calls of her assailant, roared viciously each time.

"There was plenty of fear and excitement all around, the booming of guns, the shouting beaters, along with the trumpeting of elephants combined to create a cacophony of sound which almost deafened me, we felt like in the throes of mild earthquake." recalls Raja Mahendra Shah of Singhai, an nonagenarian relative of Vizzy, who had witnessed the shoot.

He remembers Vizzy telling him that "All the while the tigress, very much alive, continued her roars, her eyes blazing at me like green emeralds and its cruel fangs bared and glittering like polished ivory. She was so close that with every growl the smelly odor of her carnivorous breath blasted me, like the dreadful fire-belching of a dragon."

For more than 20 minutes Vizzy lay helpless in the 10-feet tall sugar grass enduring the wounded tigress stout-heartedly almost upon his head. The roar of a tiger is literally the blaze of the thunder that even to the coolest sportsman is plainly paralyzing at close range. At long last, as the challenging blasts pinpointed the place where the crippled predator lay, one of Vizzy's faithful attendants brought his elephant close and a fusillade of shots was fired to finish off the tigress.

Vizzy was lifted and put atop the elephant, trusting that he shall never again find himself in a similar predicament. Unfortunately no ambulance was available. He was brought to Balrampur Hospital in Lucknow, where preliminary treatment was administered to him. Later, he was taken to England for further treatment but his injuries were so severe that he succumbed to them a few months later.

When I was a child I had seen Vizzy at a camp in Singahi Kothi. A round thickset heavy man, he was supervising the skinning of his 380th dispatch. Nine bullets had been extracted from the tiger's body and Vizzy was high-spirited. "Tigers die hard. How much lead this species can take before finally being killed"? he wondered as he fondled with a blood smeared piece of lead in his hand that had finally entered the heart of the tiger.

With Vizzy's passing the sport killing of tigers came to an end. With him died a glorious epoch of wild, fantastic adventures, perhaps an era of heartless brutality, in which the names of Jung BahadurRana, Jodha Shamsher Rana, Maharaja Ramanuj Saran Singh Deo of Sarguja, King Tribhuvan, Sawai Mansingh, Colonel Kesri Singh and Kunwar Dilpat Shah and my maternal great grandfather Pundit Chhottey Lal Dixit, gleam like changing hues on the sunset horizon. These men had all the natural amusements and power. Yet, under some baser compulsions, perhaps to ensure the ponderous dignity and integrity of their male pride, they required to prove themselves through the destruction of trophy animals – a thin edge of the wedge to justify their masculine ego. They competed for the best dimensions of a trophy, seeking citation in Rowland Ward's *'Records of Big Game'* and continued to kill, it did not matter how many animals escaped wounded in the fastness of jungles.

This set is certainly different from the constellation of hunters that hunted on foot or at the most on horseback. From looking for spoors, following them up, collecting information, inspecting water-holes, inspecting kills, selecting spots to picket baits, constructing *machan*to arranging beat and finally tracking the wounded beast, almost the entire work was done on foot. Thus, in all these exercises lay the essence of real sport that we call *'Tiger hunting on foot.'*Sanderson, Blyth, Hawkeye, Burton, Dunbar Brander, Champion, Jim Corbett, Kenneth Anderson and Kadambi qualify these tough standards. They served the human cause with no psychiatric connotations of he-manship and debased sport hunting to shine like stars in the night sky that earlier had not been so bright.

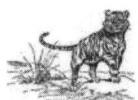

The Historicity of Sugarcane Tiger

"Farmlands appear to be natural surroundings of these tigers........"
- Anderson, Irrigation Engineer & Designer of Sharda Canal Project, 1855.

Farmlands of Tarai have historically been the harbouring grounds of wildlife where the presence of large bodied, forest and forest-edge predator like tigers and leopards was no exception. They ranged widely and preyed upon both cervids and bovids with equal efficiency. Wildlife habitats occurred even between large agricultural landscapes and remained interfaced with human settlements without creating many conflict situations. Though the biology of the species and the levels of human impact upon it decide the degrees of conflict levels, but formerly the density of human population was low. The huge extension of area that fulfilled nutritional, ecological and behavioral needs of animals exclusive of much challenge, allowed these animals to thrive.

In pre-nineteenth century India, when human population was thin and Tarai was ruled by Zamindari system, it was mandatory to demarcate large *maujas*(tracts of rural land) as *charagah*(pastoral meadows) for the village cattle. Compared to natural jungles, such areas of anthropogenic origin extended from 100 to 200 acres, as the grassy stratum was annually managed for their palatability and high nutritional value by controlled fires. It contained superior grass cover for animals. Alternative dry season forage,besides fruits also characterized the moist agricultural vista.

Human settlements were sparse and meant least harassment for wild animals. *Nilgai* and black bucks roamed freely and wherever they went the predators followed the trail to nosh on them - leopards in particular and tigers infrequently. There were small forests too with high density of trees, which were almost certain to hold a large predator.

The history data of farmland tigers is extremely scarce or almost non-existent. It is more readily available in terms of their hunting than any observation, count or description of man-animal co-existence. The widely distributed tigers were viewed as threats to expansion of agriculture and rural livelihood, at once treated as hazardous vermin and enviable trophies. Hence records of hunting expeditions are the only proven method of sampling tiger populations living within human dominated environment.

Consequently,most of the times, the *charagah* area of every village also harboured large predators. These were not meta populations living in isolation where inbreeding depression could manifest itself. Rather, these were small insular

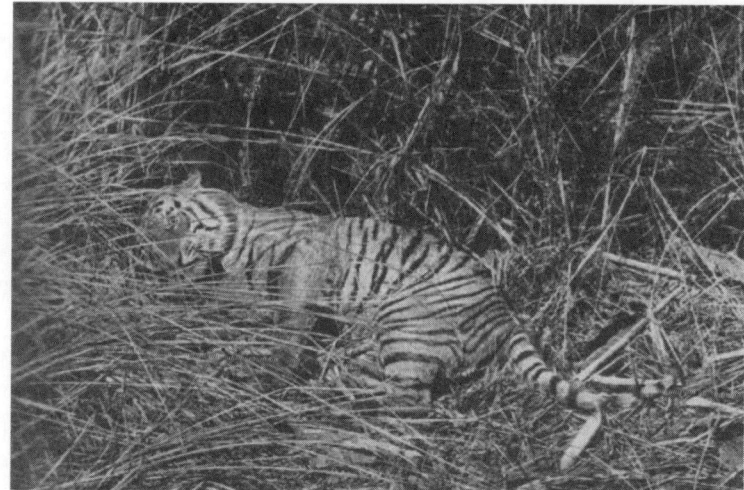

Anderson's Tiger shot in Tarai, State Archives.

populations connected to populations of other *charagah* areas where more of the con-specifics lived. Tigers were simultaneously flourishing both in jungles and farmlands that offered cover diversity of open, moderate and dense categories. In comparison to jungles, they essentially lived upon a slightly different prey composition, some preying persistently upon livestock. Perhaps they offered a somewhat different bit of gene (improved or degenerated) from jungle tigers that was, at that juncture, over represented.

In the time line, there were economic developmental projects, dams or irrigation channels, but phones, motor-vehicles and even cell torches were unknown luxuries in the faraway agricultural enclaves of Tarai where predator populations continued to thrive outside the jungle. Undoubtedly the principal killers of livestock, they were only killed in self-defence till this tide was turned by the arrival of sport guns and unsavory trophy hunters. They began to destroy wildlife in the farmlands on the ruse of protecting crops. None could hope to arrest the decline as the killing of tigers also started at an unprecedented rate and the insular populations less prone to extinction from natural catastrophe, genetic deterioration or disease went down to the fire power of the guns.

There is a car load of royals that scored between 500 and 1000 with Maharaj of Sarguja topping the score with over 1100 tigers. Thus the bulk of the annual loss of tigers went to hunting mortalities. Lindsey et al, working on breeding potential of cougars suggest that the cat can sustain annual removal of 15 to 20 % of all animals over one year of age. Bradley M. Smith suggests that these rates might be relevant to tigers, until hunting mortality is completely added to background mortalities. The sport hunting continued, reaching a point where tiger numbers visibly shrank and faltered and finally the animal disappeared from farmlands. As regards Tarai, the great hunter Vizzy's statement to Raja Hemendra Shah of Singahi

Estate, as late as 1960s is worth quoting: "Each big farmer's and great landholder's tiger space outside jungle is still fully stuffed, and I can shoot to my fill anywhere without permit."

Old style natural history dating to only a century ago forms the backbone of modern wildlife science and is a key to the riddle of present-day sugarcane tiger. The accounts of these animals, though relatively poorly served in hunting literature, are found in Sanskrit and Awadhi literature of Uttar Pradesh state, as well as in the Old Persian and Urdu memoirs of Awadh court. Becoming important in this context are Nawab Siraj-ud-Daulah's hunting escapades, who mowed down quite a few of these beasts on the outskirts of Lucknow city, near a place called Dilkusha garden. Later a Victorian Englishman Daniel Johnson, a surgeon in the East India Company who published *Indian Field Sports* in 1823, described random presence of tigers in sugar farms who were shot by NawabVazir of Oudh between Lucknow and Sitapur. It meant that the intermixing of wildlife with human landscape was a natural hazard. Apparently the presence of tigers in tall crop plantations was not an uncommon phenomenon and small insular populations did exist at several points.

Lieutenant Anderson, the Engineer and surveyor of Sharda Irrigation Canal who in 1852 charted the Southern Tarai region then recorded as Gogra-Gomti Doaba region (Gogra denotes present-day Ghaghra river) from Banbasa of Nainital plains to Lucknow, writes: "We have left the jungles far behind but as the survey work continues we are surprised to find tigers pug marks in the farmlands of Sitapur and Lucknow. In fact, farmers of these districts appear used to tigers and often report about their peripatetic vocalizations in the surrounding tracts."

His successor Captain Forbes renewed the project in 1871 post-armed forces' mutiny of 1857 in which all charted records were destroyed. He finally completed the construction of the 12,368-km canal in 1928, spanning 12 district and adds that "Croplands of Jaunpur and Pratapgarh district appear to be natural surroundings for leopards and wolves... tigers are also heard dwelling in reed beds of water bodies..."

Incidentally Captain Forbes' assistant, Lieutenant Michael Lancaster, came to a sorry end when he was killed by a potentially aberrant tiger in Jaunpur croplands while planning the further course of canal now known as Sharda Sahayak. He further adds that "Farmlands appear to be natural surroundings of these tigers...the important contributory factor to their survival is the presence of deer and antelope population that occurs in abundance in farmlands and privately owned patches of forests."

This writing indirectly demarcates the difference between high quality and poor quality habitat of great jungles and farmlands. It also offers a sort of phenomenological explanation to wildlife in farmlands, with a punch sentence that "Farmlands appear to be natural surroundings of these tigers." Despite incompatible land use, a small breeding population of striped cats had always lived here, which

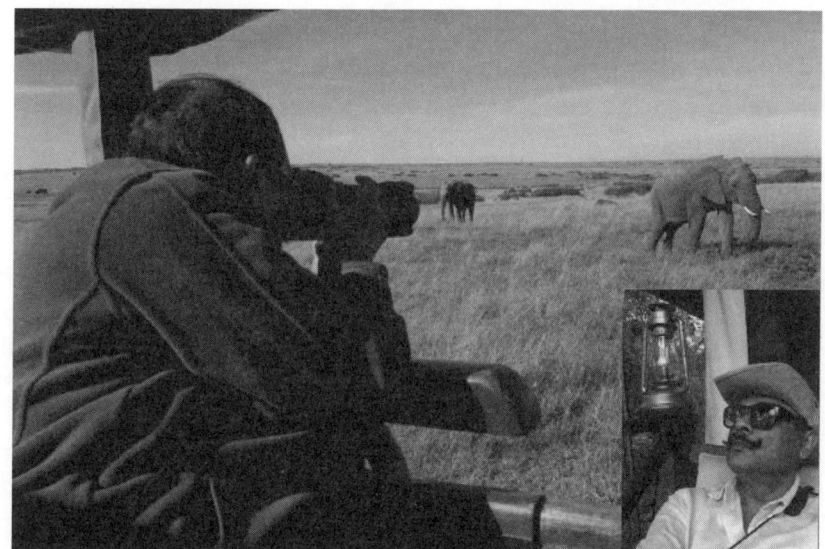

Maharaj
Balrampur
Dharmendra
Prasad Singh
photographing at
Masai-Mara,
Kenya.

was also perhaps tenuously connected and the inferior terrain was not much conflict prone. Incidentally the reports collected by Michael Bright, a naturalist and former director of British Broadcasting Corporation (BBC) estimate that during the same century in 1822 some 500 people were killed by tigers near the metropolis of modern-day Mumbai whereas a half a century earlier over 400 people were killed in similar manner by several tigers near the city of Nagpur in Central India.

The Gazette of Bombay Presidency tells how tigers which had steadily expanded their territory into agricultural lands near growing cities triggered direct conflict with man and were compelled to recede by systematic eradication with bounty instituted on their heads. This substantiates that the majority of farmland tigers were considered havoc wreckers and a form of vermin.

The nineteenth century Indian farmlands were a wonderful place for a rifleman. The diary of Mr Okeden, judge of Moradabad that his family gave to Sir John Hewitt, mentions of tigers being found in Moradabad district. The sporting record generated between 1821 and 1841 tells of several camps and tiger parties in the agrarian areas of the district, besides mentioning a fierce hailstorm that killed 400 humans and some 7000 heads of cattle in the same district. There was no way to dispose of so much of flesh, on which jackals and hyenas fed for days and tigers and leopards too were no exceptions.

Even Dunbar Brander mentions of such tigers that lived outside jungles in non-tiger like localities. "Nevertheless tigers have vanished from the comparatively open *nalas* in which our ancestors found it so easy to kill them, and even in my time they have disappeared, or at the most are only occasional visitors in many of the outlying jungles." He mentions of a tiger that remained near some villages for 15 years on cattle diet.

He also mentions of isolated tracts, amidst heavy agrarian areas that held small tiger populations of their own, where tigers were shot out and the forest isolated. No others wandered in and the surrounding villages were overrun with pigs and *nilgai* and many fields had gone out of cultivation. In ecology predation is the simplest mechanism of population control; hence the great cat is not without its functional-response in the humble villager's economy. As an observant forester Brander wrote that, "To enlarge a couple of tigers in this forest will be a great boon to people... extermination of tigers in such places should not be permitted." Baker mentions of a tiger that lived in agrarian areas for 14 years entirely on cattle, killing some 500 heads. This clearly shows that some tigers were used to living in farmlands; and in absence of wild game or in their fondness for cattle they survived on their redundant lot without harming people.

The situation is still no different. Even modern scientists believe that wherever tiger populations thrive and border with human landscape they may pose a threat by preying on livestock but rarely go for humans. This was the matrix of co-existence then which is still relevant in the present times.

James Inglis of *'Tent Life in Tiger Land'* was a planter in three Tarai areas – along the Kosi in North Bihar, on the Indian side of Chitwan in Nepal, and finally in Dudhwa area of Awadh. He describes lots of commonalities in areas where the tigers lived, especially along the Kosi river as a part of a semi-human dominated landscape, and survived in large numbers. This landscape was also not always wilderness – over the past few thousand years it has oscillated between wilderness and agriculture. Here, interfaced with hard-edged agriculture areas, many tigers were addicted to live entirely on cattle.

Big game hunts were a popular way for Indian princes to extend hospitality to visiting dignitaries and guests, and those were held on an enormous scale. Maharaja D.P. Singh, the chieftain of Balrampur Estate, recalls the past, "Jungles were more than ten miles away from our palace. When the callers came and there wasn't much time for a proper shoot in the jungles we preferred to take them a mile away into farmlands where some tigers essentially lived. These were less elegant hunts without much of ceremony but guests would have a happy time. I remember three tigers were shot by British dignitaries in 1942 and they were all full grown."

An old treatise of hunting *Mrigaya-Mayank* (The Hunter's Moon) is preserved in his library. Written in Awadhi, it deals exhaustively with behavioral aspects of Tarai wildlife including man-eaters.It tells as how natural history changes are not natural at all when wildlife faces firearms and how "*Nahar* (the tigers) began taking long leave from Tarai farmlands as other quadrupeds drifted into acquiescence of their own extermination. *Chital*, hog deer, wild boar and black buck sought cover miles away to save themselves from this new urban atrocity. Smiling sourly at this desertion, now it is their despised juniors that supersede the absentee seniors – foxes, pigs, jackals, porcupine, shrews, rats and snakes; all glorify the law of compensation that they are too insignificant to merit extinction from farmlands."

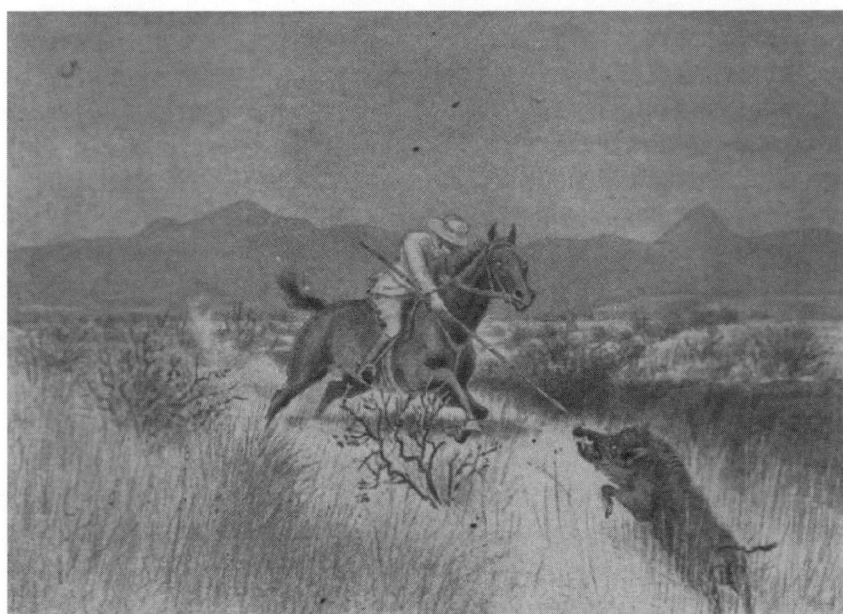

Pig sticking was the king of sport and sport of kings.

This passage underlines that distinction only invites extinction. An *Awadhi* proverb says that "the taller the tree the more it must meet the blast of the storm." Thus *nahar* qualified this status more than any animal.

"Just a century back there were pockets in my Estate where man was among the animals that flourished in the rich environment, until he finally out-competed the tiger. This loss, brutally expensive in biological terms, is now just a part of tiger history," says the Maharaja. Many hunting episodes of Balrampur royals are jotted in the book as their scenes are impressed upon Maharaja D.P. Singh's memory. However, such restricted references provide a glimpse into the window of the past permitting inferences only about three-dimensional variation in tiger abundance within prey-rich farmlands.

Tigers lived in farmlands via random and natural process. Interestingly in old *shikaar* books words like farm tigers are not found but their mention clearly takes place as the tigers living outside the jungle. Champion mentions of such tigers telling that "some 25 of these are shot every year outside the jungles."

Despite having a plethora of hunters and native trappers after their blood, tigers remained relatively numerous. An Anglo Indian Irrigation officer Walter Mendel mentions in *The Pioneer* of November 1920, about tigers shot at Barabanki district along the banks of Gomti river. He also tells a large herd of swamp deer, having over 500 heads venturing near a pilgrimage place called Mahadeva. They often walked down just behind the temple to eat leftovers from a *bhandara* (community feast) arranged for sadhus and saints. In 1944 the same author wrote about tigers:

"...I understand that they are no longer found in this tract," though the remnants of the swamp deer herd are known to have survived in Mahadeva till 1980s.

Pig sticking was an adventurous sport, constantly sorted out in open harvested farmlands. Another article in *The Pioneer* in 1950 by the same author mentions as how tigers were adapted to farmlands in Puwayan area of Shajahanpur district, which was a famous grant belonging to the descendents of a mutiny hero..."Regular patches of sugarcanes and irregular patches of bushes and grasses, where pigs are found, are no doubt habitat of predacious beasts including tigers, which seem timid and inoffensive in wild state... Even when disturbed at any rate, they show no ferocity but move away. Perhaps the knowledge that it is dangerous to confront man is hereditary in their blood; they therefore take good care to avoid this danger."

The old man of Dudhwa, Billy Arjan Singh also cites about such local beasts. He writes in *'The Legend of the Man-eater'*, "It should be realized that vast areas of grassland were claimed for agriculture and the displaced tigers, which could not be accommodated in adjoining forest areas remained in these cane areas." The old doyen reveals of a man named Agha, who had taken to shooting tigers in farmlands, where there was no restriction on numbers and a neighbour Boaz whose gun had been taken away by dacoits. Boaz had been sniping farmland tigers "so perhaps this was poetic justice."

On page number 60 of his book *Tiger! Tiger!* Billy makes the following observation: "The shooting in the forest was allocated by a system of ballot...to circumvent this restriction, one unsavory pair of sportsmen took to going after farm tigers, on which there was then no limit. After they had shot a few...the chief wildlife warden worked up a case against them... although it failed but had the salutary effect of putting an end to that particular form of shooting and gave the local tigers a respite." However, the sketchy picture drawn by Billy provides only half information about the phenomenon while the better half is provided by villagers and farmers who faced the perilous appearance of cane tigers at their very doorstep.

Over the last century the tiger landscape has changed dramatically. An expanding human population has put increased pressure on the tigers' habitat, its prey and on tigers itself. *Charagah* and grasslands in rural areas have been lost and degraded, and small pockets of high density tress, called Banukiyas, have been fragmented as the ungulate populations inhabiting them have declined precipitously both in number and in distribution.

All wildlife experts including Scheller and Sankhla unanimously agree that in India hunting has been a recognized factor in historical decline of wildlife. Brander mentions that when he searched for innumerable herds of water buffalo mentioned by Forsyth as frequenting the zamindaris in north of Bilaspur, he found none. He writes "so far I was able to ascertain not one single animal remained."

As vermin and hunters' trophy, farmland tigers were more vulnerable than jungle tigers who had enough space to hide and dissuade their pursuers. Hunting can render any species vulnerable to extinction. Biological traits of tigers, such as intrinsically low densities, protracted rates of body growth and maturity, smaller litters, long life span and requirement of obligate meat-eating, make them vulnerable to disappearance from stochastic factors related to demography and environment. This must have turned the survival of farmland tigers very hard. As hunting declined the tiger numbers inside principal jungles and almost all the remaining populations in distant farmlands became small and isolated and then slowly and utterly shrank into jungles. In last fifty years since Sikh refuges displaced from Pakistan's Punjab colonized Tarai, the change process has accelerated, adding to the concern for the continued existence of farmland wildlife.

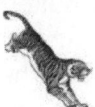

In Search of Eco-type Tigers

"In its very essence, sugarcane tiger is an adventure and an expression of summation of my life's experience. It is an attempt to question the world of conservation practitioners who take rigid and logo-centric scientific dogmas as the final truth and ignore the complex patterning of reality. Tigers are flexible enough to adopt new environmental changes including anthropogenic pressures of farmlands. The whole story of my observations is an acceptance of this chaos that encourages a play of nature with meaning, and makes my theorizing of tiger's existence in sugarcanes, an attempt to find a new and more truthful version of changing facts about tigers in their farm range based existence."

\- Author in a meeting of State Wildlife Advisory Board, U.P. Government, Lucknow, 1997.

Tarai farmlands cover approximately one quarter of the land mass of Uttar Pradesh state, and have historically provided a wide range of habitats for wildlife. Many indigenous species are adapted to living in agricultural landscapes, and so are some tigers. Next to jungles, the sugarcane farms have long afforded conditions ideal for the breeding of big cats. Thus, while contemplating the problem we have to conceptualize it in its totality and discuss it from two perspectives—historical and contextual. From natural history point of view, the problem revolves round one fundamental question: is it a chance based non-systemic phenomenon, or a systematic matter-based (or matter-specific) phenomenon such as behavioral adaptableness of tigers to seasonal crops?

Post-independence records show that there was not only a wide variety of game in farmlands but the phenomenon of farmland tigers also roughly dealt with territory of nine districts of Tarai, namely, Nainital(plains), Udham Singh Nagar, Pilibhit, Kheri, Shajahanpur, Bahraich, Gonda, Basti and Balrampur. All these districts are contiguous to principal forest trails that run along Indo-Nepalese border. The feature occurred where human population density was low and agrarian and livestock practices with cheap, free ranging native breeds of cattle were in favour of predators. The feature was a boon for hunters who shot them with intensity in any season without government license on the subterfuge of preventing human-carnivore conflict.

But nobody was scientifically conscious of this biologically meaningful feature. None cared to think seriously how demographically viable populations of carnivores could inhabit farmlands though they were sensitive enough to register their significant population decline. A rational approach to this problem compelled me to acquiesce with analysis and theorize the happenings. I postulated some inscrutable course of natural history that had led to the foundation of farm tigers with their irreplaceable territorial organization patterns that sustained them well for long – even against deterministic factors such as hunting.

The root cause of sugarcane tiger phenomenon naturally goes down in the depths of history. Theorizing the cause we presume that through eons of time, there must have been tigers whose ancestors, under the pressure of their own powerful kin, had left their essential and stable jungles. They had intruded into human zones, adopting unstable farms as their night-time home. These cliquey beasts were the ones who had never accepted barriers of zones between jungles and human habitat and habitually violated their ecosystems. They had actively occupied farms under the demands of their own escalating population. By the same token, aggravated by selected and enforced biological requirements, they had developed a penchant for a different prey composition.

Because of the adverse impact of wildlife on human interests, farmlands do not carry numerically abundant wildlife as the jungles, and overstocking of cattle also often leads to ungulate prey being out-competed. But farmlands do carry large animals weighing up to 1000 pounds like pregnant feral cows and buffalos, including blue bulls and this is different biomass of prey assemblage, not found in the Tarai jungles.

Most of these facts are of untraceable origin. Their value in terms of survival of farmland tigers therefore is an issue. Hence assuming a safe line of reasoning, it can be deduced that when jungles were filled to their brim, the peripheral tigers adapted to agrarian expansion by modifying their hunting pattern and technique to kill prey differing enormously in size, in order to make best of the conditions, whether for camouflage, or for attack and defense. When tigers can live in a diversity of habitats, put up with a wide range of temperature from 45 degrees Celsius or more, heavy rainfall, produce large litters up to eight cubs, quickly salvage the loss of a litter with short inter-birth intervals and go without food for weeks, then shifting into agrarian lands where even larger home ranges could be maintained was not a big challenge. Eventually these physiognomies are the hallmarks of a resilient species.

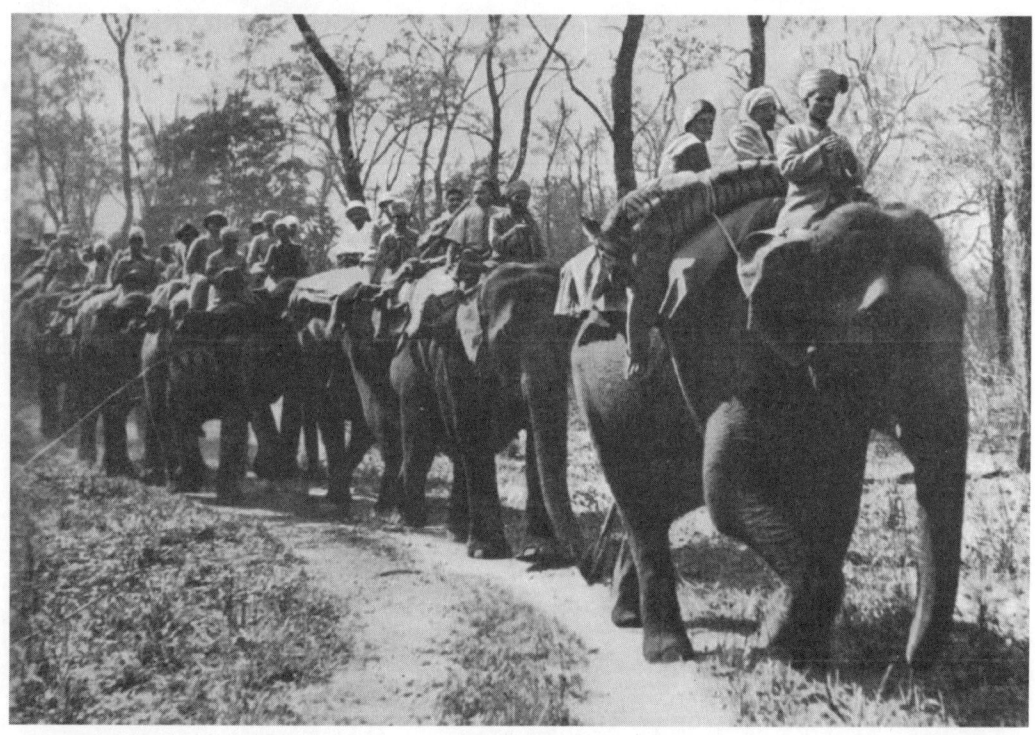

Grand procession of elephants for the benefit of Royalties, assisting in their sport for the Big Cats.

An improved understanding of carnivore behavioral ecology shows that wherever tigers are dispersed they are alike in general characteristics but in their interaction with man, individuals differ in character and habits. One may behave as being bold and fearless against humans, addicted to preying on cattle in village neighborhood. The other may continue to live in the same landscape but depend mainly on wild animals. Some tigers may challenge shepherds and may not easily leave the cattle they attack while others may retreat before the shouts or mere presence of a cowherd boy. One may confine his operations to a comparatively small area while another may wander far and wide at his will and this may not be connected with the distribution of animals for food or their abundance or scarcity. Similarly some tigers prefer to stay put in the jungles while others, owing to their large scale seasonal movements, develop personal predilection for farmlands and continue to stay there for longish times.

On scientific scales of time and space, all populations of one species separated in specific spaces of true ecological variations, tend to become distinct in one to two generations and acquire a different behavior to meet the demands of new environment. This acquired behavior is gradually transmitted culturally across generations of animals, making that subtle finesse genetically hard-wired and transforms into a strain. Ipso facto driven by harsh environmental factors of terrain and prey composition the gene hardens and turns the particular segment of species into an ecotype animal. So there was no denial to the fact that it is heritably an altered tiger, the plodding progression of which had remained undiscovered for long so that very little was actually known about their hardcore segment. They are a representative reminder of history's tangled webs, of the many strange ways in which the fates of people and wild animals intersect and what happens when man interferes with nature.

Prior to Sikh settlers when grasslands were intact, there appeared to be minimal conflict between humans and tigers. Game was abundant and human population was exceptionally low. As a result there was plenty of room for both animals and man. But when the grasslands were cleared and large sugarcane farms came up, the ecological opportunities for tigers to expand their ranges opened up again.

This behavioral adaptation to sugar-farms, led by a perplexing dilemma of circumstances,heralded an absolutely original chapter in the history of nature. Here, the combination of both natural and anthropogenic factors supported large carnivores.Interestingly the fearsome animals guarded farmers' crops and even provided him with meat of crop raiders and also a great meaning to their life where occasional human predation appeared to be of ancillary value, until this prehistoric understanding was disrupted by the arrival of sport guns. Thus the history is trapped in these tigers – a few remaining pure species of tiger from their farmland habitats– as much as they are trapped in the history.

The ancestry of some of these cats in question might not be suspected. It is reasonable to suppose that a teensy genetic component of ancestors had made a selected group of tigers to adopt sugarcanes as their basic home, which later became their natural home. It was neither deviation from basics for them nor any evolutionary stake to have put most of their bets on the abundance of a particular habitat of sugar crop. British conservationist John Aspinal, once during an online conversation with me, described these tigers as ecological freaks. "Yes they are no doubt grounded in history, but with so much of human population all around them, these have now become ecological freaks because their survival is on different scales." 'Ecological freaks' sounds uncomplimentary, but it may be true. Adaptations usually occur because a gene mutates or changes by accident! Some mutations, physical, mental or behavioral can help an animal survive better than others in the species without mutation.

On the same line,hard sugar tigers might be 'ecological freaks'. For ecological freaks like genetic freaks do not evolve according to the age-old laws of nature. They evolve abruptly and revolutionarily. Like tusk-less elephants that live to breed and pass on their genetic propensity for tusk-lessness, the ecological freaks do the same and create a category of their own. It is something like handedness in

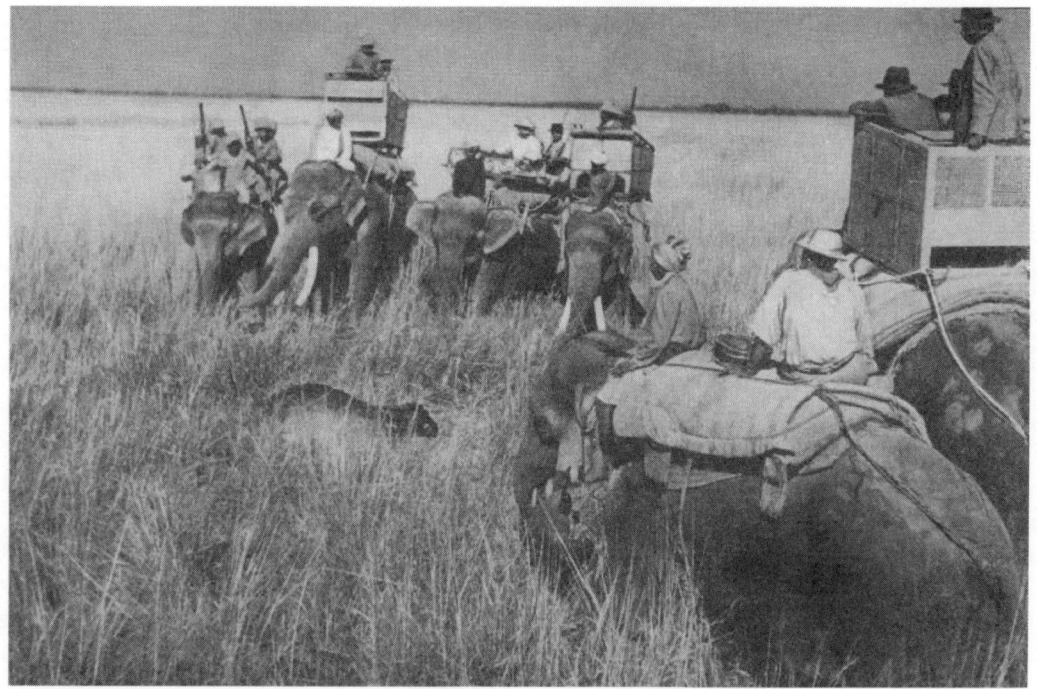

A killed bait in grassands being examined by hunters, family archives.

the human beings where left-handed people are not considered normal only in the sense that there are more right-handed people in the world.

Keeping this context in mind, my conjecture of a possible putative strain endorsed that the natural selection does not create anything new; it only selects from the accessible genetic information. (It is the theory of the 'survival of the fittest' and not the 'arrival of the fittest.') The two strains – the behavioral strain that is coded in the brain and the biological strain that is reflected in the body – create eco-types. With this judicious prudence in mind, the existence of sugarcane tiger appears no mystery. It was old imprecise natural history that remained undiscovered for long and was now viewed through skeptical eyes as new natural history (Neuro-biologists consider behavioral strain as hard as a biological strain, for example in Sunderbans, the endemicity and persistence of man-eating tigers suggests that it is an acquired behavior turned into a putative behavioral strain, which evolution has done in millenniums).

There is nothing like bewildering pseudoscientific mish-mash of presumed subspecies, subclasses and types. To my mind these tigers are the compelling evidence of their former continuity – the progenies of genetic aberrations of positive 'eco-types' – whose gamble to change their habitat proved to be of advantage to them and consequently their life style was hereditarily altered. They had been using the farm ranges, adapting to ever-altering crop dynamics and land use change for hundreds of years, and that their numbers with minor variations had never multiplied to such an extent that they could seriously interfere with the environment. Their potential was only realized when sugarcane took over as a major crop in the Tarai and their so called ad hoc populations and it's so called ad hoc turnover transformed into continuous turnover, maintaining a viable gene pool in perpetuity. Their slender population then suddenly swelled and became detectable. Unfortunately whenever the problem of conflict arose, then without any prior identification of guilty or innocent individual in a population many were eliminated that made it extremely easy to deal with man-eaters.

❖

It could possibly be a putative strain, like ecological adaptation of the frost-resistant tiger of Siberia, which is now extinct. When in harsh winters most of the tigers migrated to southern fringes of Siberia, as they presently do by descending on Muraviov-Amurskii Peninsula and Vladivostok area, this tiger easily operated all through dead of winters in the northern expanses of Siberian Taiga within Arctic Circle One. It was a behavioral strain that later transformed into morphological strain, more adapted to habitat conditions for extremely valid reasons that created a frost-defiant category of tiger. It could live in sub-zero winters and would not lose its toes in frost bite nor would its nails go black and blue with blood coagulating.

VladimirTroinin records that the last 'frost-resistant' tiger was killed in1905 on the Aldan Plateau of Sakhalin Mountains.

This frost defiant predator, I firmly believe, should be acknowledged as a well-qualified example of putative strain. It exhibited how by separation in land terrain ecology or just by staying put into harsh winters, this animal developed into an eco-type —reflecting modified characteristics from other tigers, while others migrated. My hypothesis about possible putative strain, of course no more thanbehavioral, developing into hard core sugarcane tigers was no different from that. Indeed this simple postulation needed no endorsement from so called acknowledged authorities on tigers.

THE LEGEND OF SUGARCANE TIGERS

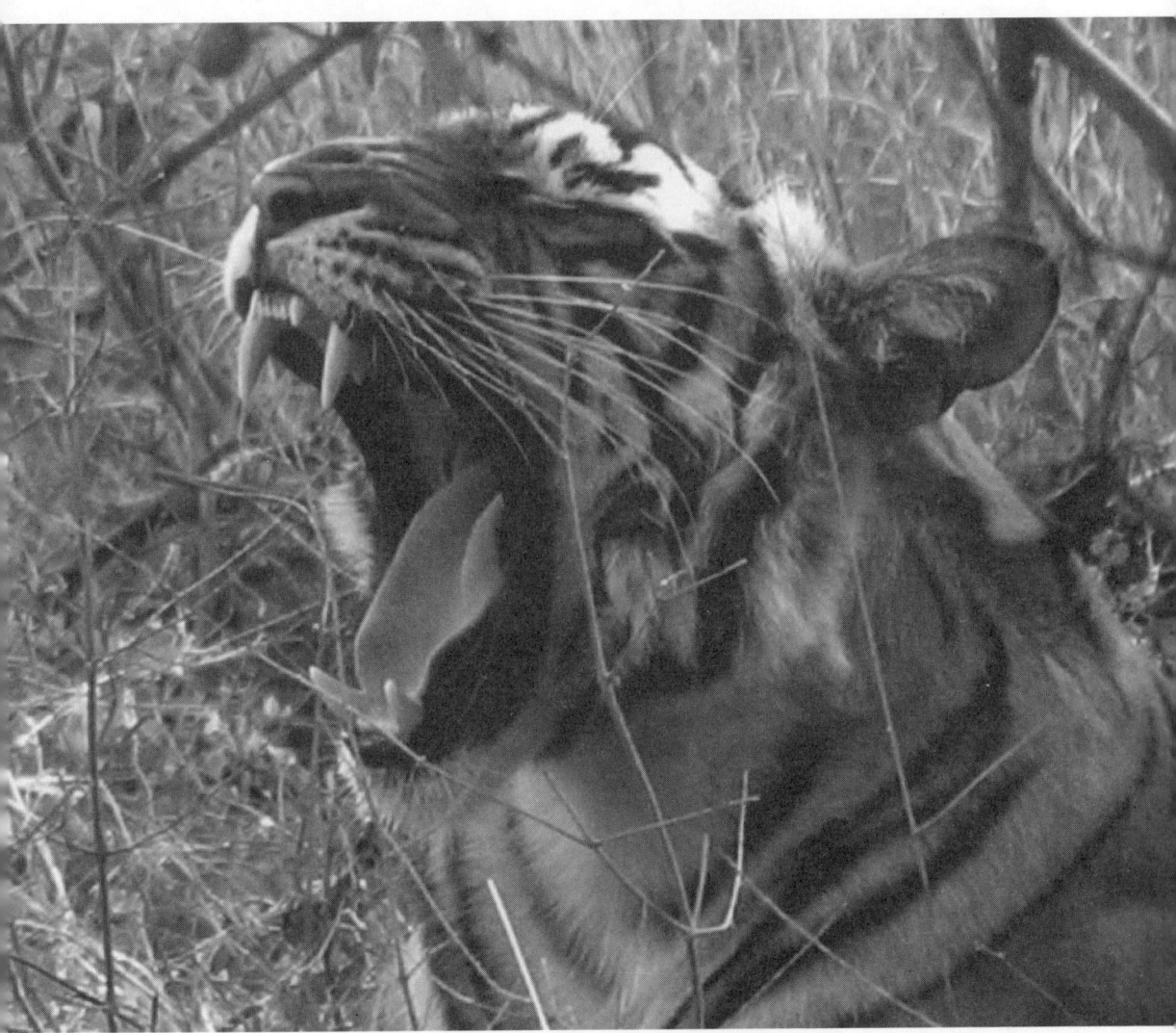

CHAPTER 4
FARMLANDS: WHERE THE TIGERS ROAR

Chapter 4
Farmlands: where the Tigers Roar
(Genesis of Sugarcane Tiger Environmental Factors & Tiger Population Dynamics in Sugarcane Farms)

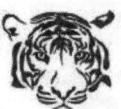

Conservation of tiger in a constantly changing, human-altered landscape requires that we have a clear understanding of the animal's limits and capabilities.

- Mel Sunquist

THE HIMALAYAN NATION OF NEPAL, THE ERSTWHILE HINDU KINGDOM, where the king was once the divinity abuts the northern boundary of India for its entire length of 900 kilometres. A hundred miles in width, it lies between 80 and 88 degrees longitude and 26 and 30 degrees latitude. It is hemmed in by two huge countries – by China on the north, and by India in its south. It is bountifully endowed by nature. The great Himalayan mountain system runs almost parallel to its entire length, comprising the highest peaks in the world. This great chain of Himalayan high hills and low hill regions register a heavy rainfall of 100 inches annually that irrigates the land profusely. It nourishes towering trees and creeper-clad undergrowth on the lower terrain, making it the ultimate breeding ground for tigers. The rainfall naturally generates an immensely strong stream system that creates a *Bhabhar* zone, consisting of detritus wash down from hills. Overlaid with pebbles, sand and boulders, it stretches up to 10 kilometers.

The great river systems of Tarai emerge from these hills. To the east is the basin of seven Kosies; drained by its tributaries. To the centre is the tract drained by seven Gandaks, including Narayani and its tributaries, while in the west Karnali (called Ghagra in India) and Mahakali (called Sharda in India) flow with great force, creating great floods in rainy season and giving way to the landscape of the Tarai, which follows the vast expanse of forests. Formed millennia ago by the shifting courses of flooded rivers, it is an excellent habitat for predators with a full canopy of creeper-clad forest, immense grasses and its diversity of luxuriance.

The belt of principal Tarai jungles that runs along Indo-Nepalese border in Uttar Pradesh is some 500 kilometers long. On an average, on the Indian side, it is 15 to 20 kilometers in width, at points it shrinks to just 6 kilometers in width while at

Dudhwa area in Kheri district the width suddenly increases and stretches up to 60 kilometers southwards; extending up its *sal* forests up to Khutar range in Shajahanpur district. This great tiger span is caught between burgeoning human population from both sides of Nepal and India. The immensity of sugarcane farms that outspread around pristine jungles needs to be seen to be believed. Stretching for miles unabated, on thousands of acres with death like stillness, the exuberant crops present a picturesque feature of wild and savage grandeur. The stretch as a whole demonstrates the phenomenon introduced by sugar farmers as a kind of new eco-imperialism that has replaced the old grassed terrain for the sake of new agrarian practices but has not changed the essence of environment that still remains the grassland.

The view is eminently characteristic of an endless savannah. It is a luxuriant forest of grasslands, and a kind of canopied and monotonous ecosystem. It creates an artificial biome because sugarcane has no doubt destroyed most of the biodiversity of the Tarai. For that matter it has done so worldwide, wiping out several agricultural species. In scientific definition if any large area is identified by a climax vegetation type it would qualify to be biome; though in this case the biome is entirely manmade. This not only offers shelter to a range of wildlife but also offers ecological opportunities for the large carnivores to expand their range. Hence sugar plantations sustain a good number of big cats because of its proximity to tiger range jungles.

An interesting paradox is that whereas the pressures from farming, animal husbandry and forest product collection, including large developmental projects, degrade the physical quality of many tiger habitats, sugarcane plantations stand as a contradiction. They provide quality habitat to tigers. The croplands carry all the specific elements of wildness such as water, cover, shade, sunlight and food. When this man-managed wildness is at its bloom, it is a particularly good tiger habitat which is in no way inferior to dense grasslands that work to the advantage of tigers as their natural home.

The formula is simple. Sugarcane is the principal field crop of the Tarai. The unbroken extent of sugar grassland offers a complete situation of wilderness, having qualities of tigerine wilderness that last for good four months. It also makes good biological sense for tigers to inhabit it and use it to cross over to other jungles. The plantations also sometimes achieve extraordinary higher tiger densities because the prey densities are also high at this point of time. The grassed-crop until harvested, remains in a first-rate condition for months and there is no physical degradation in its thick reed-like stems. In fact there is a constant improvement in the quality of grass habitat.

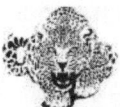

Snapshots in Time

"The sub adults-and for that matter any adult transients-can be thought of as a population reserve. It is wrong to consider them as surplus population; in situation in which, the residents are bound to suffer recurrent loses; these tigers on the waiting list may be viewed as delayed increment".

- Charls Mac Dougal

After the great human tragedy brought about by the partition of the sub-continent into India and Pakistan, a large number of displaced Sikh farmers from Punjab came looking for land in Tarai to start life afresh. The feudal landowners of the area already faced the abolition of their feudal rights and appropriation of their surplus land. Therefore they hastily began to lease land blocks to new arrivals, rather than wait for the Central Government to take over land for a nominal amount as per the *Zamindari* abolition regulations.

The newcomers found it tough to adapt to their new environment. They had exchanged the dry heat of their homeland for the humid and enervating climate of the Tarai. The native community, rendered ambitionless by its hardships such as crop raiding animals, dacoits, water-logged forests, flash-floods, virulent malaria, typhoid and endemic dysentery etc, had always lived at a minimum subsistence level. Having nowhere to go, the colonizing refugees hinged to the minimum and latched on grimly as hardships of Tarai took a great toll of their lives. Clouds of mosquitoes rose in the evening and the refugees covered their bodies with cow dung leaving space only for eye and nose. All this while, their tractors continued to open up the pristine grasslands and marshlands. Once the optimum habitats of wild pigs and swamp deer herds besides conventional breeding grounds for tigers paved way for large sugarcane farms; it slowly turned the virgin Tarai into prosperous land.

However, sugarcane plantations, seemingly a replacement of *Saccharum munja* or the tall grasses, did not bring much change in the mood and environment of wildlife. The protein rich farms, shimmering with 20 per cent multicolored agricultural crops and 80 per cent sugarcane, were still an ideal ground, inviting and sheltering wild animals. Swamp deer, pigs and tigers again returned to them – their original homeland – and this feature gradually created a buildup of prey base in addition to large carnivore community in farmlands. Though wild animals were depredated by native *shikaris* - trappers, snarers and shooters - but tigers were still real sport hunters' game, spared for people like Vizzy and his friend D.R. Jardine, the MCC captain that accomplished their unlicensed hunts in Tarai farmlands.

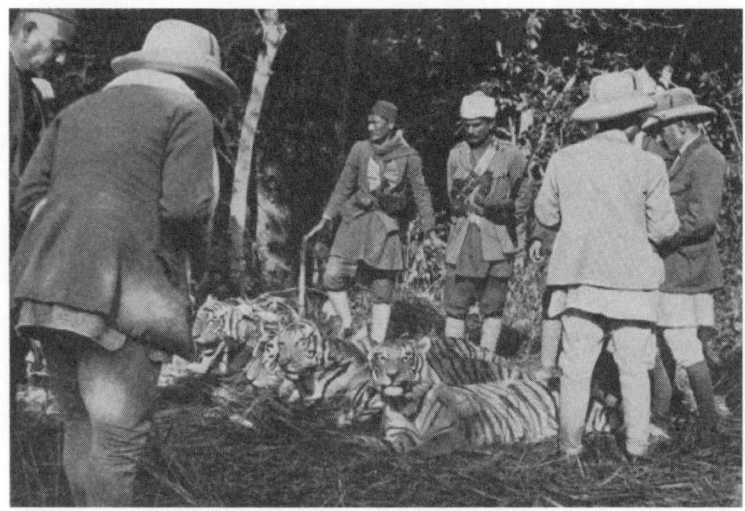

In the plantitude that was Tarai, animal trophies were realized almost throughout the year by hunters.

Incidentally in an extended colonization of left-out grasslands, some local politicians tried to settle landless labor from Eastern U.P. and fresh clashes between tigers and people erupted. By an amazing coincidence, half a dozen tigers killed around a dozen people. However, as sport hunting was very much in vogue, so no restraint was advocated. Jardine shot five troublesome tigers in Majhra Singahi sugar fields, while Billy also dispatched three man-killer tigers, solving the problem with simpler and irresponsible solution of destruction because of the vulnerability of these lonely animals in sugarcane.

In 1970 post the blanket-ban on tiger shooting, elaborate rules for conservation were established and the tiger population increased slowly, both in jungles and farmlands. Around this time the cane field tiger phenomenon was first registered which soon transformed into a kind of new signature of Tarai. This was no extra population but through means of communication between far-flung kin it was well-connected with jungle population. For many experts it was a puzzle as to from where such a plethora of large cats had come to live close to human settlements. It was this time when I happened to enter actively into this scenario to solve this riddle in small ways of a newspaper correspondent. In 1976, I had been given a contract assignment by Charles Baptista, the then Resident editor of *The Pioneer*, an esteemed newspaper of Lucknow. While reporting on these tigers and analyzing the phenomenon closely, I was compelled to think outside the box that this was definitely no new bastion of tigers. Farmlands had been among favourite tiger beats and the event had a long history in rural areas. Occurring invariably outside the boundaries of conventional jungles, where known habitat niches had been occupied by tigers. I was already well acquainted with it but now it needed to be understood better in a systematic way.

As per the terms decided by the paper, I submitted six write-ups to *The Pioneer*, reporting man-tiger casualties, tiger poaching, their poisoning, electrocution and trapping in baited cages. However, by the time my assignment finished, my investigations had assumed the shape of a research project and my concern for these tigers had intensified. To start with I already had with me the rather lengthy reports that I had prepared for the newspaper, so I decided to carry on this research with my personal resources. In nature's scheme of things there appeared some grand purpose in extracting and compiling these queer facts in one place, which could bring a gradual paradigm shift in conventional thinking of experts. However, this emotion existed only in my mind while for people cane tigers were ravening monsters who had sinned against man-made laws.

Scientific data is the most powerful and reliable evidence, so potent that rational people don't hesitate to sacrifice even their most tried perceptions in face of contradictory scientific evidence. In fact the tigers that had learned their lessons during shooting days had slowly given up their shyness and had come out in the open. Big cats have massive powers of 'ecologically surplus ability' that is the capacity to crack problems outside their specific adaptations to their environmental niche. Such abilities permit cats to cope with rapid or unexpected change in the environment, which are often very significant and make them accept changes with remarkable aplomb. Hence it was no irony that nature had decided that tigers must reside in sugar plantations.

The tigers' flexibility to modify the rules of their predatory behavior was based on changing local environments and circumstances in face of biophysical conditions. Anthropogenic disturbances had never been taken into account. No expert had ever sought to explore the question as to what life style large carnivores might adopt to eventually share living space with man without being at odds.

I firmly believe that for years despite their ingrained abhorrence of human race, attributable to lethal lessons that taught tigers to give men as wide a leeway as possible, they had lived moderately sheltered lives in the neighborhood of man because only 30 years ago the very fertile land on which the sugar plantations stood had been their historical breeding ground. And big cats demonstrate a great fondness for their ranges that they don't leave easily – their 'ecologically surplus ability.'

Breeding activity is closely linked with extended movements of large predators. When the activity level exceeds a location-specific threshold, it is probable to see tigers coming out in selected farmlands. But now the activity had actually reached a 'red' level, and they were breeding like proverbial rabbits and humans were coming across them at many sites, precisely in the time and space continuum of the central Tarai farmlands.

British conservationist John Aspinall who had visited Tarai as Billy's guest some time in 1970s, once told me during an online conversation in 1998 that he had witnessed the phenomenon first hand. "It was so truly raging then, that I couldn't say whether tigers were trespassers in human territory or humans were trespassers in tiger territory." However, to my mind to believe that these tigers were trespassers was a futile self-deception. There was nothing wrong in acknowledging that it was their old legitimate home and these were in fact living in mega grasslands of sugarcane, utilizing their 'ecologically surplus abilities' to their best.

By early 1970s, the northern area of the Tarai forests falling within the Himalayan Kingdom of Nepal had unfortunately ceased to be a prime tiger habitat. The unbridled deforestation in Nepal to settle ex-army officers' families gave rise to hundreds of new villages. These Nepalese veterans from Gorkha Regiment of Indian army whose pensions were and still are maintained by Indian Government at par with Indian nationals had settled down in Nepal post retirement. Incidentally as per 1953 treaty with Nepal, their army chief is still designated as Honorary Chief of Indian Army and vice versa. In 2014, Indian Prime Minister Narendra Modi's statement that if someone says he doesn't fear death, he is either a liar or a Gorkha was an example of how Nepal is present in the Indian cultural loop.

Being an academician and professor of history, I take the opportunity to add that during early 1947 when the date of India's independence was drawing near, Vinayak Damodar Savarkar, a Brahman leader from present-day Maharashtra felt insecure about the fate of India's Hindu community under extremist secularism of Mahatma Gandhi. He felt the majority community was sure to be marginalized in future as majority of Muslims that had supported the idea of Pakistan were requested by Mahatma to stay on in India. Savarkar was elected president of the All India Hindu Mahasabha in 1937 and continued to be re-elected for the next seven years. He had thought of building Hinduism into an organized system, devoid of untouchability and other related practices. He was instrumental in getting the Ganesh Utsav open to all Hindu communities. His idea of reforms was based much on the archetypal template of Christianity and Islam. Islam, besides divided in many schools and seats of scholarship, also presents the King of Saudi Arabia as King of the world's Muslim population and so is the Pope of Vatican Estate, the worldwide king and the chieftain of Christians.And both of these are designated as the representatives of the divinity.

Worried, Savarkar wrote a letter to the Maharaja of Nepal, the only Hindu Kingdom at that time as against 43 Islamic and over 40 Christian countries, urging him to declare himself as the King of worldwide Hindu community. But the idea could not materialize under the impact of neo-Leftist and emerging Nehruvian thinkers. They ridiculed the thought and opposed it in discussions and media outpourings, and the Nepalese King was advised to refrain from such an engineered declaration. The prevention of this declaration is still taken by a majority of learned Hindus as a great loss for India, causing a permanent recurring deficit in political, cultural integration and brotherhood of the Hindu community between India and Nepal as well as protection of Hindu minority in core Islamic countries like Pakistan and Bangladesh.

Incidentally under the impact of leftists Nepal has now also 'become a fundamentalist secular nation while in Afghanistan the last Hindu temple was demolished in 2010 and there is no Hindu community left out there; and after the demolition of 70 meter tall statues of Bamiyaan Buddhas, similar has happened with the Buddhists.

❖

However, the increasing human pressure on the Nepalese side affected the Indian side as well. Illegal intrusion by men and women, unbridled collection of fuel wood and cattle grazing rendered huge tracts of forests waste, resulting in shift of major tiger populations towards the south.

Billy Arjan Singh's argument was that "The immigrant tigers found favorable niches already occupied by residents and were obliged to settle for the occupation of ersatz and temporary cover in sugarcane plantations." The wholesale destruction of grassland in Nepal, especially of Churia range, a prime home of tigers and a source of graduated supply to Indian forests, had triggered the sugarcane tiger problem and unmitigated immigration had compounded the crisis. This was a conspicuously misleading statement as all tigers in sugarcane were not of Nepalese origin; *ipso facto* their immigration had unremittingly nourished the sugarcane tiger population on the Indian side.

All logic is about one single truth that grasslands are critical components in the wildlife matrix. This was the conventional knowledge of old *shikaris* that tigers breed largely in grassland and not in *sal* forests. Thus the reclamation of grasslands was also a cause of decline in Indian tigers' population. But my argument is: Whether the grasslands were really gone or in fact they had increased manifold in volume and size in form of sugarcane grass? This not only accommodated the foreign population but also gave it opportunity to multiply and develop in human-led environs. This so called ad hoc base of agricultural land was now the steady holding ground of tigers.

The great stretches of *ikra*, reed, *narkul*, *phanta* and *zhaoo* had been replaced by vast plantations of sugar. For wildlife, it was a larger extension of their habitat with many additional advantages which their previous natural grassland home never had. For instance, the edible value of this new grass for wild prey species was much higher than natural forage, and constant irrigation meant constant availability of water even in dry season. Though the environment is man-made and not isolated from human endeavor, its habitat value is definitely much higher than previous grasslands. That is why tigers used it so profusely. Moreover as stated earlier, the prime season of sugarcane also corresponds with the breeding season of tigresses and they use it as a ready nursery.

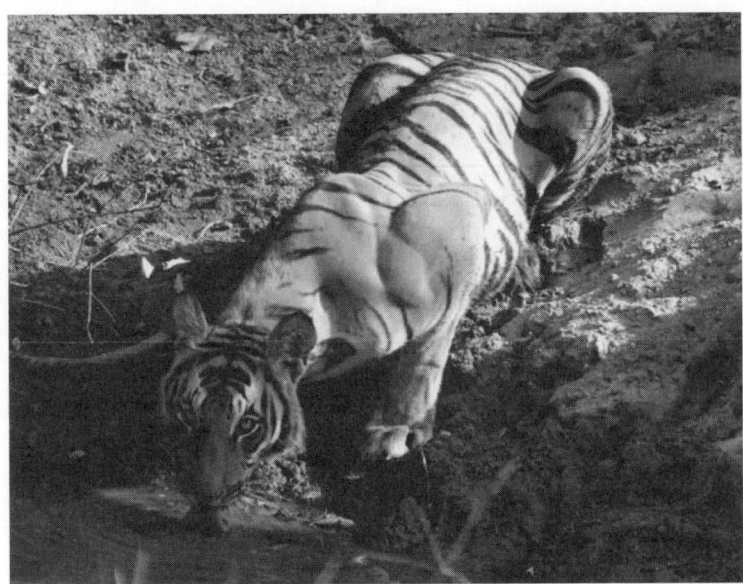

A tiger at a water pond

One has to be extremely circumspect in issuing statements on matters of tiger populations. This was no sudden increase due to habitat attrition in Nepal but was a slow and gradual development that became really noticeable with the arrival of Nepalese population. Moreover, Churia was a small range hardly 100 sq km in size that could at the most hold 8 to 10 tigers. Thus Billy's contention was not palatable on scientific scales. The farmland tiger population did not comprise traumatized refugees caught in limbo between human and animal worlds, but was very much an Indian material, living comfortably in canes. It was the result of some kind of pre-programmed ancestral logic in their mind because their ancestors had also lived and bred in sugar farms. And they were themselves born here to mothers who had sought birthing dens in these very thickets.

Deforestation of Churia might have made some additions to this soap opera but it was no dust that needed to settle down with time. It was indeed a midpoint phenomenon happening for years till the unfortunate human-tiger conflict turned that midpoint a death zone, resulting in a sharp plunge in cane tiger population.

During early 1980s, the official tiger count of Dudhwa as declared in Park's pamphlets was 122. It revealed 80 tigers occupying the park while 42, excluding cubs occupied farmlands outside the Park. The subject was worthy of constant monitoring and re-evaluation because the issue of tiger territories is a complicated one. They can be small and big, temporary or permanent, depending on priorities whether females are to be attracted or food resources are to be scraped together on a stable basis. These vary in size and purpose, when other related members of clan accommodate each other, creating flexible boundaries without generating any dispute. However, the then Field Director of Dudhwa, Dr R.L. Singh, later Director

Project Tiger Government of India, stated in his official capacity that growth of farmland tigers was resource-based expansion. He felt that this was least an overcrowding and despite so many pressures built up against their survival, tigers were indeed, evenly distributed throughout the available farmlands falling between North and South Kheri forest ranges.

Three years later another count yielded a steady upward trend with exquisitely reassuring precision; 83 tigers were found inside the park while 45 were residing outside its boundaries. Despite competitive existence and occasional fatal encounters amongst individuals, which is the mechanics of cat behavior, including the pressure of poaching and poisoning by natives, the loss through which was estimated between 15 to 20% the great cat population seemed to have stabilized. To put in plain words, it was a biologically meaningful super population, no longer an unknown fraction of carnivores that could be safely called as farm dweller.

Breeding generously, is key demographic trait of tigers when four conditions are fulfilled. First the terrain should be as little disrupted as possible. Secondly there should be sufficient number of worthy adults from both sexes with in connecting distance of each other. Thirdly there should be established male residents and as little row as possible between them, and lastly there must be a constant supply of water, shade and food that must be accessible to females from their nurseries, where they rear cubs.

To the amazement of foresters there were some half a dozen breeding males, with preponderance of females reaching up to 30 in number. This had turned the sugar fields into an absolute kindergarten of cubs as quite a few nuclear families were also recorded. Perhaps by some antithetical quirk of nature, great stretches of sugar farms, perennial in nature, seemingly nurtured all the basic requirements for tigers to breed. Hence so many tigers had dispersed into sugar plantations that had become a serious tiger habitat – a range of grass savannah.

Tigers can live with a good deal of tolerance and range intrusions, without much conspecific aggression when plenty of prey is available. Male tiger territories are larger. Starting from 50 sq km these may go up to 150 sq km that helps him secure access to all the receptive females within that area. Biologically the species necessitates smaller number of males to breed, which may be just one fourth in proportion, about 25% or even fewer to the number of females available. On this line of reasoning if we allocate a precise area of 30 sq km to a breeding female, it would mean that some 900 sq km of farmlands were occupied by these tigers which naturally included the separated ranges of the resident males within them. Some males were also coming from jungle to mate with farm tigresses, while juvenile transients were shunting here and there with no territories.

Importantly the biology of the species and the levels of human bearings on wildlife determine the degree of encounter levels, therefore, conflict is biologically normal, particularly when crop harvesting pressures on land intensify. But conflicts, in proportion to tiger populace recovery were relatively low, much within socially acceptable limits meaning thereby there was adequate nourishment for tigers, or else there could be no ecological explanation to defend this super population in farmlands. And finally when for last three years, tigers were clumped peacefully in limbo of human-dominated ecosystem, supported by history of endemicity as previously extirpated carnivores then what their re-colonization in farmlands should be called in scientific lingo. They had lived here facing foremost challenge of keeping peaceful coexistence with humans and had done it moderately well with the goodwill of farmers. Now when the probabilities of their population persistence in future seemed reasonably high, then what appellation this successful tiger population could acquire except Sugarcane Tigers.

It was a singularly qualified data but Billy Arjan Singh was haunted by this claim. He called it a "dismaying, euphoric statistics." In his opinion in a Third World country like India, successful tiger management had become a status symbol where managers were ever increasing the numbers of tigers on papers. This maneuver necessarily needed a cool, impartial reappraisal by some international agency to find real status of tigers. But one thing was certain – sugar farms encompassed more legroom and elbowroom to accommodate tigers than jungles had, as here the sanctity of a solitary individual's space was better ensured.

Geographically after the end of Himalayan mountain ranges, the hill zone starts that slowly gives way to Shivaliks that stretches up to 15 km in width and then gradually paves way to Tarai Dooars, much of which naturally falls within the boundaries of neighbouring country of Nepal. But in context of India's political boundaries, the demarcation of Tarai zone is differently opinionated. Here the very farmlands swathed between two immense tiger range jungles of South and North Kheri had come to serve as the real Central Tarai Area (CTA). There was plenty of game for tigers had they wanted it, if not there, right on the spot then not far away too.

Sugar farms were stretched far and wide with glens and moorlands in between. It was not possible to increase the area of reserves even at the expense of cutting down on some smaller and less viable wilderness area. This included buffers where tigers shift out when they fill the given spatial area, as their populations cannot increase beyond a limit in a fixed area. This was large rural terrain. Incidentally, human population of the section earmarked as habitat of 45 tigers had increased by 6% in three years but tiger population had never expanded much. The favourite niches of both habitats of jungle and farmlands had maintained a status quo or remained full. No expert called it artificial surplus or overcrowding as these tigers were evenly dispersed in time and space and through linking cane corridors were affecting genetic exchanges on their own.

This declaration of the forest department, with an annual rate of increase at 2% was hailed as rock-bottom figure. It gave the segment of farmland tiger a scientific credibility which they would have lacked otherwise. Moreover the problem that the 500-sq km park was full and there was no accommodation for added tigers was being amplified by the unique situation of the Tarai's farmland tigers better than any other animal.

Incidentally Hemanta Mishra, a Paul Getty Wildlife Conservation Prize winner from Nepal and writer of *Bones of the Tiger*, cites Billy reporting about retaliation killing of tigers in 1986, against a stray incident of three men killed inside Dudhwa jungles. "He counted 23 tigers brutally butchered by booby traps, guns and snares in an attempt to punish one tiger suspected to be man-eater." In absence of data, I am not sure about this huge number of retaliation deaths but that year I personally remember seeing many dead jackals and vultures that had fed upon poisoned cattle (laced with pesticides and insecticides), including 14 tigers in farmlands of Kheri. It was enough proof that a huge segment of tigers was seeking their living in the pervasive environment of sugar fields as good neighbours to humans. And the relationship, at least from their side, was not antagonistic but symbiotic. But man, in his diffidence and self-doubt had broken the ecological principle.

The mishmash of crop raiding ungulates and livestock raiding predators is the greatest nuisance that creates adverse impact of wildlife on humans. But some tigers' presence on farmlands was not all conflict, they existed on friendly terms with humans and the Palnapur tiger stands as important example, whose activities were exceedingly partial to humans.

This animal inhabited farmlands of South Kheri between March 1985 and September 1986. He killed around 66 feral cattle and was never harmed by villagers, because he was actually ridding them of the menace. A gentle tiger otherwise, he used to kill his prey with a rare technique of biting on the nose so that the animal was asphyxiated to death – a special adaptation for dealing with large prey so that it falls quickly due to the lack of breath. Shaped by his own ability to co-exist with man, this tiger was considered a prudent benefactor and a regulator of natural equilibrium.

The young fellow's exclusive fondness for killing feral cattle was simply because of the ease with which they could be stalked and handled. Once in a night he had killed four cattle in a gram field and left them uneaten. Such feasts are normally partaken by young tigers that still have to understand the economics of prey base that is based on eating the interest and not on eating the capital. Incidentally, Sanderson had several times noted four to five and once fourteen cattle on the ground after a prolonged attack. Locke also reports of a robust male which killed 23 cattle over a period of seven weeks without eating them.

Wild ungulates are wary and controllable. They have small appetite therefore they graze on the move while voracious feral cattle devastate overnight a crop ready to be harvested. The presence of Palnapur tiger had virtually altered this structure and functioning of the ecosystem within 60-sq km area by regulating and limiting the numbers of feral cattle. I remember seeing this tiger's pugmarks along the banks of Ull River up to Katna catchment area. The white bones of many cattle were in the grass around, beside the gleaming crop that had clearly come to life in that winter.

The impact of predation on the number of prey can never be expected to be constant. It changes from season to season and also from species to species. It is reasonable to accept that if this so-called temporary aberration of singular feeding adaptation becomes a regular feature in a predator's life, then this is in fact an eco-system approach of a predator. This presents an extraordinary model of prudent predation and it temporarily plays a temporal keystone species. This apparent intelligence, flexibility and ability to adopt new situations and often an interim role of keystone species are born out of the need to survive in extraneous environs. Thus, predators increase the biodiversity of communities by preventing a single species from becoming dominant.

Then one day an increasingly hostile tigress appeared in the area. She was injured and half her tail was missing. She always lumbered towards the tiger to claim a share in his kills. Despite his impressive size and robust health, the male would retreat in face of her formidable opposition. She first forced the tiger away then disappeared from the area.

Though living in human dominated terrain this tiger did his best to avoid the proximity of man. An ironmonger Behari Lohar told me that "There are quite a few *Bangailey Gaiyan,* that wear small tin bells round their necks, as a reminiscent of their domesticated days. This tiger never kills them. Perhaps he still associates them with human livestock". Indeed there seems to be an inviolable line of control -which has steadily matured over timeless generations of inter-relations between man and tiger- he never crossed that, while simultaneously presenting an extreme example of specialization in cropping an initial resource of the environment.

At Laghauri and Lalpur village near Nighasan, natives claimed of a big tiger in the Sharda riverbed area who had been there for years, just in the backyard of Madnapur village. A confirmed bachelor for his trails have never been recorded along with any female, he made round of many villages fields fairly regularly, helping enormously to thin out populations of pigs and blue bulls that came raiding. "He has never killed our cattle and never interferes with man," claimed Sugreeva, a native. "We often hear his sing-song roar after he has eaten a pig but before the day breaks he makes his way back to the grass belt along the river". Such is the friendly manner in which tigers had lived constantly in Tarai farmlands and there was nothing surprising about it. Indeed the queer factor was freshly emerging man-tiger conflict.

Once a tiger acquires a definite taste for any kind of flesh - whether cattle, wild pig or human flesh in case it turns into a man-eater, it will go to the most amazing lengths to satisfy its craving. Liv Karpinove, a Russian tiger biologist tells about

Primorye tigers that kill and eat brown bears on fair and square basis. This is shocking because ordinarily no predator weighing on average some 600 pounds, would consider another predator like a brown bear weighing more than him, as prey. Brown bears belong to same species as American grizzlies and can weigh as much as 1000 pounds. Their ferociousness and potential for destruction is legendary and so are their canines and paws. Yet, they are no match for a tiger and what causes a tiger to pick up fight with such a dangerous antagonist is the taste of his flesh. This also satisfies his two discrete itches - neutralizing the threat of a competitor on his homeland and getting a quantum of meal that will sustain him for weeks.

In those early years having dedicated a decade to field research with many findings and a store of data at my disposal, I still had no proper infrastructure to document the complex matrix of big cats in the sugarcane that the experts address as quantitative index. Like snapshots in time, my knowledge about tigers was restricted to a single season study in a particular pocket, and there were many pockets where stripes were reported that I could not reach. However, all this permitted inferences only about abundant distribution of animals in farmlands was least useful in probing time-based subtleties of their populations. I was sure a focused research was desperately needed to figure out as to what special adaptations had come to exist in these tigers.

My questions, for instance, were: What was the composition of their prey in sugarcane environment; the dependence of variety of life forms on this environment in certain situations and conditions; factors which generated differences in behavioral responses of tigers that live close to humans as opposed to further away in the jungle, and their pattern of predation. There seemed to be no study of this kind yet in the country. There were studies related to predation of livestock by carnivores focused on economic losses of locals and their vengeful reprisals. But no study had been conducted which might help us understand as how dangerous animals like tigers and leopards live among high densities of people without causing any harm. And eventually what animal communities inhabit sugar farms in high numbers and what measures of protection were to be implemented if the tigers were to survive in the ersatz surroundings.

Sugarcane crop is a managed wilderness which must always work to the advantage of animals. The term 'management' involves coordinated solicitation of specific agents and methodologies for the sake of prompting a desired result, in which the managers meddle with nature to do so. Interestingly till seventies, when tigers were managed up to the brink of extinction by Indian foresters, it was again international conservationists' intervention which revived their population by changing the agents and methodologies of their management. Conversely it is better not to meddle with nature if it means troubling the animals. But even in jungles starvation follows when tigers injure themselves in fighting, which leads to

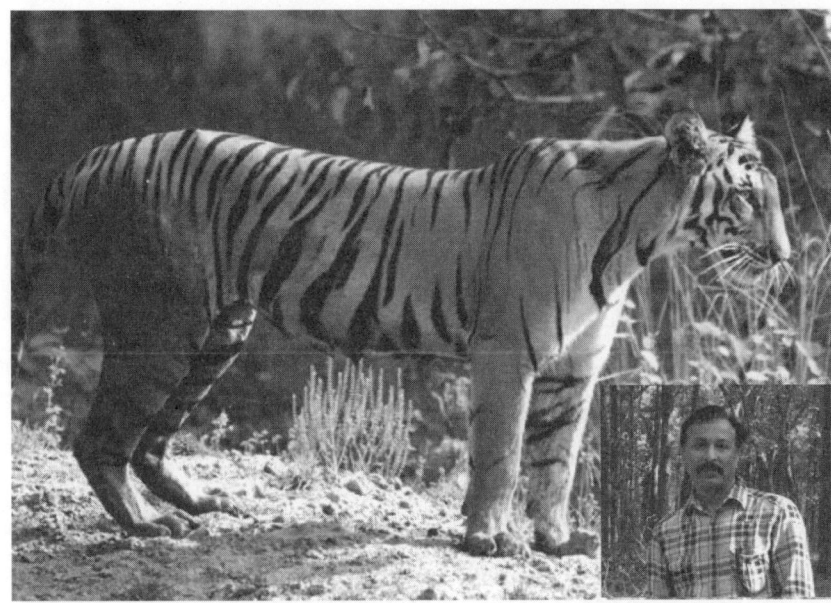

A majestic young male with its rear half covered in slush came out dolefully from the cover. (Inset Photographer Sanjay Singh, IFS, Field Director, Dudhwa National Park)

infections and lingering agonizing deaths. In such situations sugarcane farms of Tarai indubitably enriched their living with more food and played a great role in their survival.

Tigers apparently looked upon sugar farms as a sanctuary, for nobody was deliberately hunting them and possibly their new generation had not heard the rifle speak for years, much less had they ever been shot or wounded. It seemed that long years of immunity had been responsible for some of the inhabitants of the sanctuary losing their natural healthy respect for humans, the future consequences of which were bound to be bad.

In 1988 I made my first project proposal on sugar tigers and submitted it to Worldwide Fund for Nature (WWF). I could not have been more adroit in stating the facts and demanding radio-coloring of four tigers that were seemingly living only in sugarcane plantations between Nighasan and Puch-Peri Ghat area. The project was rejected with a comment that I was thinking outside the box, which was more vague than scientific. Moreover radio-colouring was not possible as the high cost and logistical difficulties severely limit the use of radio telemetry to monitor big cat moments.

In 1993, I re-shaped my old project and submitted it again to Project Tiger office in New Delhi. This entire story, expectedly, seemed strangely romantic to the elite mandarins. And stranger was the fact that they asked for more evidence to prove my contention. But I could only vouch for the facts which had often also puzzled me greatly. On the basic foundation of these facts I asked for a grant of Rs 2.50 lakh (about USD 3500) to weigh my qualitative study on quantitative lines. The officer concerned looked at me ruefully; extremely suspicious of things as if in my over-ambitious attempt I was trying to cheat the organization by providing false information.

It was a long haranguing discussion with the officer. He could not understand as how villagers tolerated presence of tigers by their side, which nature has most selectively evolved as predator with extraordinary size exceeding 9 feet. Despite this an ordinary villager's coexistence with dangerous predators has always been a cultural expression of Indian society. The evolutionary forces might have shaped the tiger into an alpha predator with all his faculties directed towards catching live prey; so much so that they sometimes develop a taste for human flesh. But the ancient Hindu traditions of *Vanaprastha* and *Aranyak* provided people with a code of conduct to follow, and as long as people stick to them they are safe, regardless of the enterprise they are engaged in.

I lectured the man well and proper, telling him that such a way of life, rooted in seemingly arcane ideas, expressed by ancient Indian sages, is a subject of paramount study for sociologists, anthropologists and wildlife experts. Anybody associated even tangentially with tigers understands their worthy significance. In *Aranyak* tradition the pantheon of Hindu gods is associated with wild animals where people often feel responsible for the well-being of animals that live around them. The Bishnois of Rajasthan protect black buck, Brajbasis protect peacocks and even *nilgai* is often spared, considered to be a relative of the sacred cow simply by its name (*gai* means cow.) This also includes the eventual energy of nature. Tigers are treated like honorable neighbours by natives. Though death of humans by dangerous animals has been a co-existent hazard, but this threat is miniscule when compared to the death from dog bites, electrical equipments and road accidents. Do we ever realize that far more deaths take place by traffic accidents in cities than in the real wilds? But we never give the traffic a second thought because we have been accustomed to it all our life. And the same exactly applies to the Tarai native who spends his life in the domain of the tiger.

This is the yardstick by which villagers have always lived in the neighborhood of big predators. Perhaps this tolerance for each other was initially built into the evolutionary system in nature. More I toyed with the knotty problem of evolutionary improvement, adaptation to new niches and co-existence, acceptance and tolerance appeared to be the keywords. In the face of conventional wisdom, this important point had its own yard-stick approach. Finally it was sad to realize that my detailed sermon could not change the mandarin's stand and my dream of getting some economic assistance was shattered.

However, all through this time the Tarai had passed through some really bad phases. As per available data, largely responsible for the impending catastrophe were the juvenile tigers whose period of transience, an extremely risky part of a tiger's life, had landed them in trouble. Being smaller and less skilled than the resident adults they lose fights and die from wounds. The survivors generally disperse out from jungles near human settlements and get stranded in hostile landscapes where they are quickly branded as problem tigers and punished through poisoning or trapping.

Such simmering of man-tiger conflict not only substantiated my gloomy apprehensions about the future of farmland tigers but raised a question: For how long the 'unfortunate reality' could be ignored by the forest department? A rational decision had to be taken when nearly 20% population of Tarai tigers, as well as their prey population found in jungles, had made residence in farmlands. Some of these valuable cultural icons of the country were rendered lame from traps they had fallen into, some limped from bullet wounds, and some were mangy from eating bad food, while many more were missing and I was crestfallen with not much financial resources at my command, spending a substantial portion of my income to continue my studies.

Sometimes it was extremely dangerous to travel in areas infested with pro-Khalistan elements. These were actually terrorists demanding Punjab to be declared a Sikh homeland separate from India. It may be mentioned that the Sikh farmers had so thoroughly taken over agriculture in this part of U.P and their sturdy husbandmen had so smoothly integrated with this land that the separatist politician's also claimed the area as an extension of Khalistan. During eighties their new homeland map had also begun to include the Tarai areas of Nanital,Pilibhit and Kheri in it. In June 1984 the Indian Army was constrained to take action in the Golden Temple at Amritsar, and as its aftermath many terror groups escaped from Punjab and sought refuge in the Tarai. These terrorist' settlers occupied small hamlets and operated out of grid and outside the law. Living incognito and undercover they were occasionally known to use deadly insurgency weapons to massacre wildlife.

One late evening in the spring of 1988, I was camping near Barotha at Grant Number 10, studying a matrilineal colony of three jackal-eating tigresses when just before dinner I heard a clear, metallic rattling of gunshots arising from far away farmlands. It continued rhythmicly like a fusillade for about 20 seconds then abruptly stopped, restarting again for a few seconds. We sat silently looking towards the direction of the sound that once again emanated for a split second and then finally died down. It seemed no less than three AK-47 assault rifles were being fired simultaneously. Some insanely dangerous militants were ensuring a bit of target shooting or something else.

Next day news arrived that a group of five militants had a party at a *bhatta* (an illicit liquor brewing distillery) and were returning inebriated when they confronted a sounder of wild boars in the wheat crop and riddled them with bullets. With their all-powerful twentieth–century artifacts they perforated some 22 wild boars with complete disregard for sex and age. The entire sounder was found dead within

100 meters of both sides of a dirt road. The terrorists did not lug even a pound of flesh and left it all there as a testimony of their dreaded presence.

It may be said that wild boars are the most incorrigible creatures, destructive for every type of crop at any stage of growth. At nightfall they regularly come out of their hideouts and show such a fondness for wheat, barley, maze, potato and yams that even the yelling cries of natives cannot scare them away. Night after night they dig the potato tubers up with their tushes, consuming hundreds of kilograms in a very short time. Hence people don't sympathize with them. The case was never reported to police, for natives were more than happy to get a massive supply of flesh free of cost.

Shortly afterwards 29 people, mostly petty grazers, were killed by same group, near Jugrajpur area.

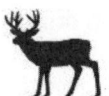

Dictates of Mother Nature

The real voyage of discovery does not consist in seeking new landscapes, but in having new eyes.

- Marcel Proust

There was an eerie reciprocity energizing the scenario of man-tiger conflict. Poachers were putting holes in tigers with their illegal guns and weak loads. The tigers, instead of retreating to safer zones, were answering their attackers with spontaneous retaliation. There was a phase in early eighties when I encountered more injured tigers in Kheri farmlands than normal ones. In 1992, I reported to Forest Department about no less than six wounded tigers operating in Kheri and Shajahanpur farmlands. One tigress inhabited a farmland near Khutar range of south Shajahanpur and was found having a 20-kg iron trap stuck in her right paw, and she was moving with it, killing cattle and living on them. Villagers admired her grit for, despite her physical inadequacy she was a devoted eliminator of feral cattle.

Although opinions may differ about the role that tigers play in sugarcane plantations with regard to natural selection of prey but it may be assumed that they have an important function in maintaining a natural equilibrium in farmlands. Besides blue bulls that are dispersed throughout Tarai areas, several ungulate species on which tigers prey find refuge in farmlands and deserted cattle are undoubtedly a big menace. They exert great pressure on crops and are easily tackled by a tiger that wields a profound influence on this community and other biological communities through predation. Agrarian environments of Tarai are suitable for wildlife hence suitable for tigers as well, since these offer favourable conditions for a change of

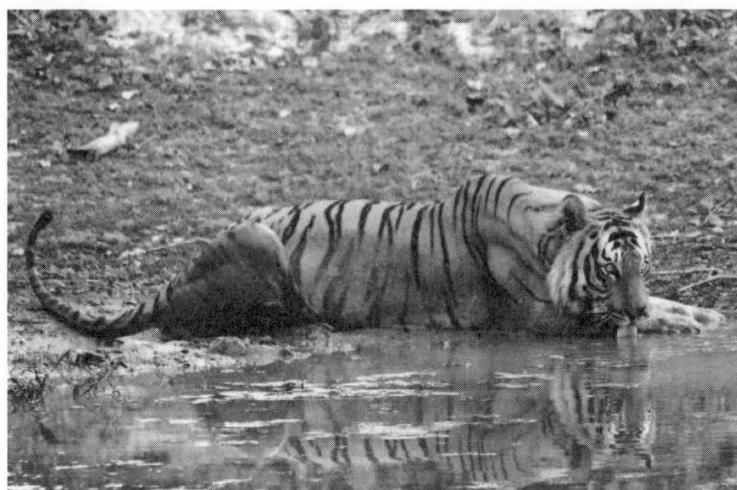

Relaxing in a swampy
wallow

taste for big cats. There is abundance of nonproductive feral cattle, which of course offers a changed composition of prey.

The state Government, however, seemed to have adopted a step-motherly attitude towards sugarcane tigers. There was no tiger management plan outside reserve areas and there was no sensitivity to take into consideration the plight and concerns of the people living around the reserve. Those relatively high densities of tigers were characteristic in the past as well, when good tiger habitats were far more extensive and continuous. There was less pressure from surrounding human populations. Now as humans had carved out farms from jungles, the tigers had spilled onto farms. Their densities had again increased with a major difference – it was a human-dominated landscape and not their jungle any more, even though the land was the same. Thus, it was still a part of their territory.

Carnivores like bears and members of the dog family often supplement their diet with fruit and other vegetable material, but a tiger's body system is not adapted to such things. It can only deal with meat, skins and bones. So they must kill continuously and their specialization enables them to do it ruthlessly and efficiently. And, like a proverbial elephant in the drawing room which cannot be ignored, this trait poses a real problem when tigers come to inhabit agrarian areas.

I was saddened to see that the Forest Department was doing nothing to prevent human or tiger deaths in farmlands. There was a kind of policy paralysis and lack of proper vision to combat the menace. Seeking to cushion the impact of the killings, the Department argued that preying on humans was not at all typical of any predator species and the official figures of killing were much too low to cause panic. In fact, there was no area in the Tarai which had not recorded a degree of man-eating and little was being understood about why these killings had started and how the change of diet had changed the killers' *modus vivendi*.

For many experts, screwballs and chest-beaters, the occurrence of tigers on sugar farms meant ecological chaos. Any endeavour to pump money in a project to support this chaos appeared no different from supporting some monumental klepto-capitalism that dictionary defines as 'injecting money into the bloated carcass that might revive the old trollop, eliciting those watery coughs and glazed blinks seen in drowning victims."

However, in my project the tiger was the bellwether, indicating a trend. But nobody seemed mature enough to understand that the micro populations of one of the highly vulnerable species were dwelling in the farmlands by the dictates of Mother Nature, which is neither our enemy nor our slave.

Dr P.L. Punia summed it up knowledgeably at a meeting of foresters: "Tiger is not a fragile species (that is) dependent upon some highly specified biotope. It has proved that it is made of hard stuff by adopting a wide range of habitats and recovering against persecution of hunting days. The scientific rational presented by Shukla makes sugarcane tiger a weighty concept, which one as the whole is observed less in theory and more in the field."

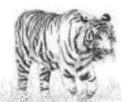

The Spurt of Man-eating

Conflict with humans becomes an inevitable consequence of successful tiger population recoveries... there usually is a lengthy edge where wildlife habitats interface with human settlements.

— K. Ullas Karanth

It is not as if tigers' presence in sugar farms was all smooth sailing. They are the brawniest of all beasts of prey that the prudence of Nature has selectively evolved. Their sheer style of functioning accelerates man-tiger conflict which goes against the complex rules of survival. In Kheri district alone, records show that between 1978 and 1984, the mortality figures due to man-tiger conflict had rocketed to 1586 domestic animals (not including dogs and feral cattle) and more disastrously, 169 human beings. How much more the figure could have been in this eternal war raged by tigers is anybody's guess.

The worst phase of unrelenting man-eating lasted till the early nineties. Time and again man-eaters were shot providing respite to people. But invariably there would soon issue another SOS from the same unfortunate area that a new tiger had commenced his fresh reign of terror. The problem seemed insoluble. This continued happening off and on and on a fairly sustained basis for over ten or fifteen years. It was the highest number of man-eaters that post-independent India ever had to tackle in a small pocket of land, in which fifty-plus prime tigers and tigress having cubs were removed from the scene. When tigers could have easily lived on eating feral cattle, pigs and *nilgai*, why they were choosing humans was the unsolved riddle.

It was this phase that brought the greatest compliment to my specialized knowledge of farmland tiger. One day, in the summers of 1984, Girish Mehra, the then Chief Secretary of Uttar Pradesh, introduced me to C.B. Singh, the state's Chief Wildlife Warden. He offered that I join the official hunting team constituted to control the new outbreak of man-eating. "Your research will be of much use to us in this context. We would be able to analyze as what is going on with some degree of expertise," said he. It was a compliment not because the high-ups knew me personally but because I was well acquainted with the Tarai with firsthand experience of its aberrant tigers. Besides, I also had some reputation as handler of firearms that could be relied upon in tricky situations.

A lot of Tarai gets into your blood than its hooch and cane wine when you travel it on foot. And this fact about me was apparently known to many.

The lethal control of a carnivore is an abhorrent practice but unfortunately it is the only practical option available to mandarins in intense cases of man-tiger conflict. The tiger is a conflict-prone species and its biological requirements can easily tilt the levels of conflict towards the worst. When they are around, their conflicts with humans are biologically inevitable, much because the dilution of fear of humans in tigers incrementally induces some of them to become man-eaters. Tarai was then the epicenter of man-eating and I joined the hunt with a flush of euphoria to humble the mighty carnivore and foster the image of masculinity to capture the imagination of my friends.

But the expedition turned into a complete flop. The three tigers that we pursued in north Kheri farmlands escaped from our hunting team but were comfortably collected by poachers. This apparently showed their better expertise about farmland wildlife pattern, for they monitored the movements of man-eaters on the mend more than the Tiger Watch team and succeeded.

The expedition, however, helped me understand the man-eating phenomenon both colloquially and scientifically. It was caused by more tigresses finding breeding cover in the sugarcane crops on the borders of Tarai jungles as prey animals had been shot by agriculturists in the forest areas. Consequently human causalities were increasing. The social mechanisms to address people's grievances were insufficient and almost non-existent in many areas. Many instances had gone unreported and in some cases the affected local people were not compensated adequately. This had caused widespread panic and distress. Villagers had lost their confidence in their normal environment. Perhaps the most consistent danger crop was sugarcane; the cause of all this menace.

It won't be out of context to mention that in grasslands of Tanzania, Mozambique as well as Malawi, man-eating activities among lions rises to a crescendo when high grasses hold normal hunting prey animals. This behavior is definitely exceptional but its matrix needs to be cracked to understand the causes of man-eating among healthy lions. Among them, man-eating and often man-killing is not sporadic but temporary yet widely prevalent.

It seemed the same pattern of seasonal man-killing or man-eating could also be applied to tigers in Tarai sugarcane areas. During the winters of eighties man-eating was prevalent in Majhgai, Bhera, Bela, Ghola and North Kheri's Naugawan, Paraspur and along irrigation barrage of Soheli. Locals believed that man-eating had started because the number of tigers had increased dangerously. Actually, however, it was animal aberration only in a limited sense since all this had started with harvesting of sugar crops, perhaps as a natural reaction of tiger to exploitation of post-harvest habitat. If such animals accounted for one or two human souls they were quickly weaned by foresters. The odds were high and they were never given any chance to return to normal lives. The argument of foresters was that the man-eaters' depredations would probably spread and assume far greater dimensions if an early end was not brought to their career. This was agreeable to the liking of people also.

To my mind, both opinions had their exponents and the entire gamut of their theories hovered somewhere in between. This is no question that the farmlands inhabited by tigers are a perilous place at the ground level, where there was apparently no chance for any long-term study of this queer man-eating cycle. It would be madness – which could realistically not be allowed – to make any effort to understand a tiger's natural disinclination to eat humans and a human corpse as a deterrent to his so-called aberrant behavior. Throughout this phase deaths from snake bites in the area numbered five times more than deaths caused by tigers, but people were still walking around the fields with country-made guns and pistols as if they were hunting a criminal.

To analyze the causes of this ecological problem, it is crucial to acknowledge that tigers living in sugarcane zone come across a different assortment of prey. Under all circumstances they have to select their prey within the medley of their own prey range, though their food choice may show different priorities. Well-nourished tigers demonstrate their preferences and kill selectively but rarely this selectivity extends to unnatural prey species like man, to which they are driven by stressful circumstances. I wonder if there is some identified biological explanation for this fatal predilection of tigers.

Aberrant behavior ensues from various factors like ill-health, injury, ageing and stressful existence. Yet, basically it is starvation caused by prey scarcity, where they are seldom able to get what they like and even unable to feed on regular basis. Then they start picking and choosing their quarry randomly, often regardless of normal constraints like too large or too small size of the prey species. This also extends, willy-nilly, to *Homo Sapiens*; a phenomenon which cannot be equated

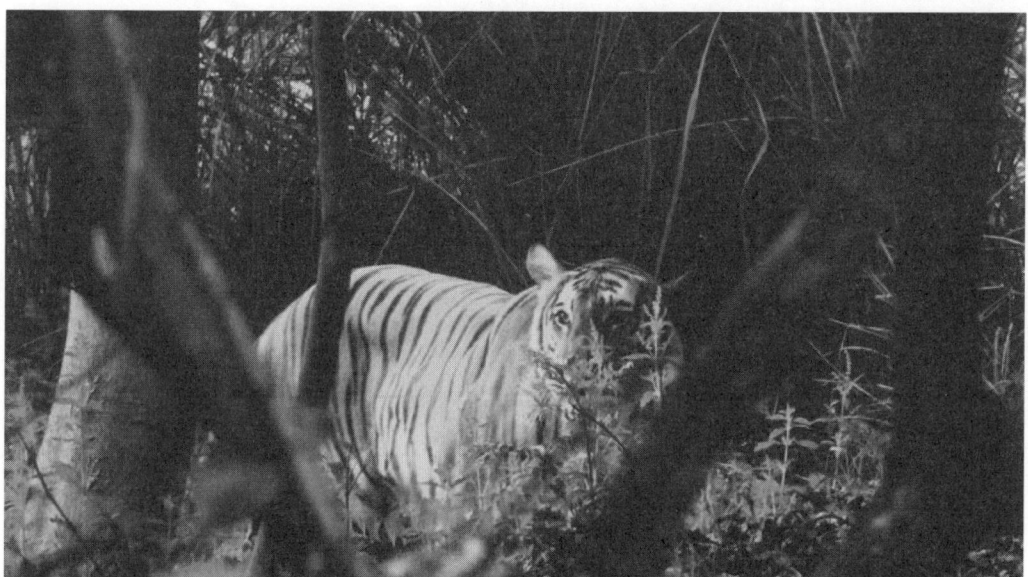

A sugarcane tiger in pinch period, in the local forest of Sonasar in Shahjahanpur district (1993)

with compulsive and selective preying on humans as described by Patterson in *The Man-eaters of Tsavo* and also in Jim Corbett's various works.

While Tsavo man-eaters were young and healthy, many of Corbett's man-eaters were old and decrepit; affected by the scarcity of proper prey base and constrained to starve. They were compelled to catch pathetic prey of rodents like porcupine. A worthless animal from a large predator's point of view, weighing at the most three kilograms, thus of ineffectual food value; it serves inadequate purpose to appease a tiger's appetite. Yet the starving predator seized the rodent and got their paws and mouth struck with quills, which subsequently incapacitated them to meet the challenges of their proper prey and turned them aberrant.

However, the situation was different here; like Tsavo man-eaters all the man-eaters shot in Tarai were found to be strong and healthy. Billy ascribed the feature to the paucity of their principal prey that had been shot away by agriculturists and becoming the cause of starvation amongst tiger had prompted them to go for humans. It is quite probable that in former days, when natural prey was abundant in farmlands, tigers roamed about human-dominated areas without harming humans. In old times native *shikaris* were limited and poorly armed with muzzle-loaders and other primitive weapons. But now the modern guns leading to increased destruction of wildlife in farmlands, perhaps had caused a proportionate increase in the number of man-eaters, whose taste for human flesh exceeded the occasional opportunism demonstrated by injured, old or confused tigers.

I did not agree with Billy's answer that singular eradication of wild animals from agriculture zone was the cause of this havoc. This was not an acceptable explanation. My experience told me that in the first place all the farmlands of Tarai, adjacent to the jungle, essentially held respectable amount of prey for tigers and there is no native method of hunting, including old water-pipe guns, which will easily wipe out immense population of wild pigs and *nilgai*. Furthermore, when wild animals are scarce, there always are abundant numbers of domesticated animals gone feral in their old age, and they are available as cushion. In such situation, tigers are known to go after domestic cattle and feral animals. Then, why the tigers had directly come upon humans was a puzzle that needed an answer from the emerging quarter of sugarcane tigers.

My question was: why a healthy tiger will carry off a herdsman in preference to his cattle? Or, leaving a sleeping dog untouched, seize its master? Billy's answer to this was that "the causes of this propensity are often obscure." But since cause and effect should be properly related it was safe to infer that this rampant man-eating by healthy tigers was an epidemic generated by cub rearing accountabilities of tiger families, specially the mothers. To my mind some cane-dwelling tigresses, by design or by accident must have brought up their cubs on mixed food of wild, domestic and human prey and these tigers when grown up had taken to bad habits making the situation widely prevalent and not sporadic.

Just like dogs, wolves and jackals exhibit no aversion to eating human flesh and vultures feed indiscriminately on all carrion, the obligate meat eaters like tigers when brought up on mixed flesh would not be disinclined to include humans in their prey list.

Besides normal tigers, there are two categories of recluse animals. One is the raven aberrant and other is a potential man-eater. Though both are essentially starved and disoriented in their depredations, there is wide variation in their attitudes that can better be described as confused and intransigent. The line dividing the two is very thin but nonetheless important. It needs to rationalize the nuances of the incorrigible man-eater, who knows that human is the easiest prey of all and an aberrant, who is generally a non-conforming accidental man-killer. It might even have resorted to this under dire and prolonged hunger, but would have certainly abandoned its kill with a morsel or two. I am sure that there is no enigma about these two types.

For example, during 1998, I recorded a transient tiger in a sugar farm at Tulsipur, Pilibhit district. It was known to strike down men in one blow of a paw and stand near the victim for some time and then walk haughtily away without attempting to kill it. Was he not an aberrant, having done this to some half a-dozen people? And what had made him commit these purposeful daring assaults on his human neighbors is not known.

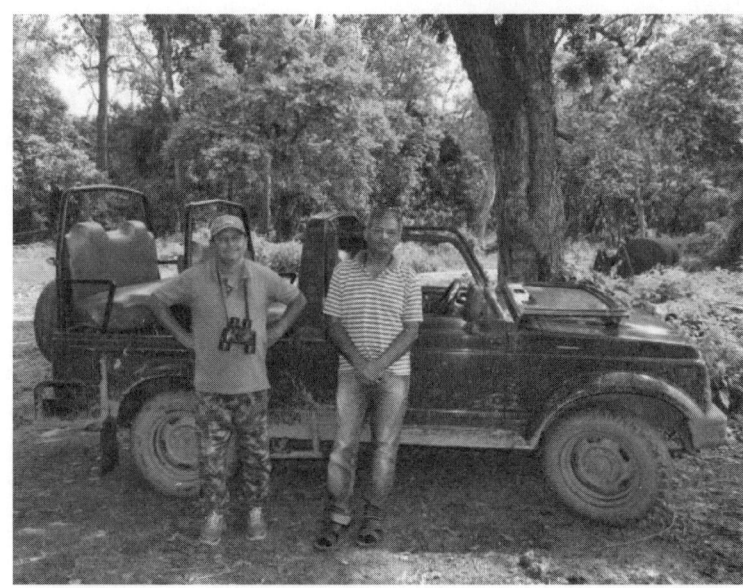

Author with Naseem, the famed tracker of Dudhwa, who underwent a nasty experience when he was surrounded by a family of 5 tigers; a male and female with three half grown cubs. Facing the trauma and swinging his bag, for over good ten minutes he escaped being ripped open by inches. (Photo credit : Vijay Kumar, IPS, Addl. Director General of Police, UP)

The animal lived in the area for about a month, creating terror among brick kiln workers and farm labors. Then one day, alarmed by the excessive hullabaloo of men, he disappeared into the blue. To this day he has not been heard of since.

Reviewing tiger attacks with scientific reasoning, I find that capriciousness of tiger is the key to his powerful reputation. In many cases we fail to recognize the value of their natural peaceful temperament with which they come to adopt their lives in human landscapes without creating problems. If we understand their 'this very' nature properly it is only then that we would be able to understand the aberrations. However, to my mind such so-called crimes of an animal are in fact his temporary strategies to live peacefully.

During long years of my tiger time in Tarai, only once in 1986 I come across a tiger of most destructive manifestation in the fields in Pilibhit district. The tiger was in an unfamiliar territory of Sultanpur village and it is not confirmed whether he was injured or not but he had already killed a donkey. When the owner tried to recover the corpse, the tiger first hid in the sugar field but when stone pelter's continued to disturb him, he came out with combustive energy and struck the group of kill retrievers for little over a minute, only to retire back in the crops. In such a short span of anger, overcome by the inexorable impact of the prizefighter, three out of eight men were left writhing on the ground in mortal agony. They were pounced upon one by one, bounded in short wrestler like embrace, bitten through shoulder, legs and stomach and slashed and torn to shreds in wild wantonness. Two of them whose heads were crushed like walnuts died on the spot and one later in the hospital. The donkey owner and his son recovered but the tiger's handwriting remains carved deeply in their shoulders and chests. Surprisingly the tiger never tasted human flesh. It simply pulled the donkey inside the crop, finished it and went away.

Vast majority of human mauling and deaths under hunting circumstances are logically from wounded tigers. But under normal circumstances irritated tigers, whatever the reason, are often threatening enough to cause serious damage. Their behavior is inspired simply by bad temper, or a desire to demonstrate their strength and contempt. A deliberate killing, impelled by hunger is sufficient inducement for a predator to feed upon that carcass.

Parenthetically, the professional predator does not kill more than needed and a killed human is disincentive to appease hunger. So, what had happened was an unfortunate accident that is certainly chalked up to human error of provocation. In fact such reactions are illustrations of abstract thinking that tigers develop to answer back direct physical attacks from other animals.

This is as Shrivridhi articulates: "Never underestimate a tiger, in a marked degree it is a thinking animal. There is an incalculable strain on some tiger's mentality, which defies logical analysis on the part of naturalists. Perhaps their sudden and violent change of mood reflects all too clearly their wounded psyche and state of terror they often feel in trauma of competitive existence with man."

In the meantime tremendous hatred was built up against tigers. The big animal, which the early settlers claimed to be friend and unpaid watchman, was labeled as an enemy. People forgot that no graminivorous animals attempted to raid the crop where a tigress had laid cubs and no herbivores trespassed when the great cat travelled through the field. Even its feces lying in the crop were enough to keep the crop destroyers away.

In the first place all this had started just when the tigers were beginning to trust humans, and humans had turned out to be as bad as they had always been to them. These most debated and least understood tigers had spelled a notorious phase of terror in the region, making Tarai a profoundly unhealthy place. The endemic of man-eating, not by perforated tigers but healthy ones with abnormal proclivities would eventually earn Tarai an ignominious nickname of hell and make its tiny map prominent like Chernobyl, a perverse monument of Russian catastrophe.

Sugar farms were infested with such brutes. Over the years, nearly thirty tigers were held directly responsible for this chaos and all were done away by officials. Many more recorded just as 'found dead' were actually done away by the natives.

Newspapers had taken a pro-people stance and were repeatedly grumbling at the laxity and negligence of the forest department for having indirectly caused death of so many people. Though it was keeping the problem in focus but unfortunately the media was also indirectly promoting the death sentence for them, as more man-eaters were being declared. The easiest solution to solve this ecological problem was to kill them. While sugar farms, now considered wicked, continued long to maintain their evil reputation for the ferocity of its wild beasts.

The conservation of tigers in farmlands had indubitably turned into a formidable business. Confusions and complexities were too many that needed be tackled on a large scale. It was even argued that tall crops, including sugarcanes were a potentially dangerous innovation for they make tigers too tolerant of human presence and increased chances of clashes between two species. Hence these should not be cultivated up to ten kilometers from the jungles and farmers should be given compensation for not sawing the crop. However to my mind, this proposed cure seemed worse than the disease. Sugar farms are an important zone for mixing up of mammals, reptiles, birds and amphibian species. The permanent removal of this crop would thereby mean taking away the tiger's new lease of life as the species would lose a substantial chance of sustaining itself on the buffer-less borders of jungle.

Much of the confusion stemmed from the lack of adequate and relevant knowledge about these tigers. I wondered at the human scale of values regarding wildlife. The tiger is a national animal, a glamorous and newsworthy subject whose plight arouses immediate public interest – but there was no outcry on his behalf. Some so-called experts in their ignorance juggled to annihilate these masterpieces of evolution. And above all, there was no attempt to acknowledge the sugarcane tigers when as the very clique of experts admitted that tigers faced imminent threat of extinction even inside the protected wilds in absence of enduring action and sustained financial backing from rich donor countries. A case worth mentioning is that of Sariska, a tiger reserve in Rajasthan, where in 2004, a network of poachers made tigers disappear with alacrity. When poachers could outwit law enforcement in jungles then why they could not tap economic potential of defenseless sugarcane tigers? With no mechanism to prevent poaching in farmlands they were destined to be the first casualty.

Keys to Survival; Curious Features of Sugarcane Biome

Surviving carnivores that avoid humans and their domesticates may gain a relative advantage and pass on their learned genes or genetic avoidance to future generations.
— Jorgensen *et al*

One may say that sugarcane crops are an artificial habitat as the crops are not constant for a tiger's requirements. But it is biologically meaningful to understand that since the crops are constant from June to January, then what could be the reason that creates the abundance of all kind of wildlife within this biome that stays there for good seven months? In Tarai, sugarcane crop are planted earliest by mid-February to March and lately by mid-April to May. The early crop is harvested by November while the late crop is taken by February. Thus save for four months from February to May, the crops do stand but are not worth to sustain wildlife. This period is counted as secondary or pinch period. However, the crops are constant and perennial because the ratooning ensures that harvested must regrow on the very place.

Sugar farms seem sensitive to wildlife needs, for water and fodder is abundant along with an exploded number of ubiquitous feral cattle that make the pyramid of life bottom-heavy, which can easily afford the large predator's way of life. I didn't know if there was any noticeable or steady yearly rate of change in tiger population which, if compared with scientifically generated data for two years in a sample area, would have reflected the real tiger population dynamics in the sugarcane during primary and secondary periods. It would have indicated as to which tigers or tigresses repeatedly return to inhabit and breed in the study area. However, my feedback revealed that tigers, both male and female, had a solid penchant for sugarcane crops and since humans ventured in the terrain harvesting agricultural resources, it multiplied opportunities for tigers to encounter humans. Despite this fact there were many selective reasons for which tigers had adopted the sugar-savannah and these were common to all areas of the Tarai.

The physiognomy of sugarcane matches with the exact characteristics of *narkul* or reed grass habitat that provides an excellent stretching cover for tigers to relax and move through. The thick heavy growth of vegetation at all levels, with flowering fronds at the top prevents the direct penetration of sunlight inside the crop. Thus the shadow-mottled foliage of the crop along with cool and damp environment gratifies the extra needs of a big cat's thermo-regulations.

Tolerance to water-logging and deficiency of moisture are the chief characteristics of sugarcane crops. Because of the dampness of the soil, the thin film of water that floats over it, makes it an ideal home for a tiger.

Tiger is both a crepuscular (active in half-light) and nocturnal (active in pitch darkness). The retina of its eyes has an abundance of receptor cells known as 'rods'. These cells are sensitive to low light levels, which enhance its ability to see even in pitch darkness. A hazy twilight permeating the inner recess of the crop gives an extremely soothing effect to nocturnal animals. It works as a light shaded sunglass for the eyes of a tiger.

Because it is a carnivore, the tigers' face, nails and body have small particles of flesh adhered to it. This constantly attracts flies and they hover around its forequarters and nostrils. The thickness of the crop deters the repetitive circling movement of all kinds of flies, especially the 'scarlet dragonflies', mango flies, blowflies and blue–bottle flies, they do not enter the crop due to bad light conditions; this keeps the animal free from the pest.

Sugarcane also offers a perfect camouflage. The pattern of a tiger's stripes almost dissolves in the pattern of crop, enhancing the tiger's ability to remain

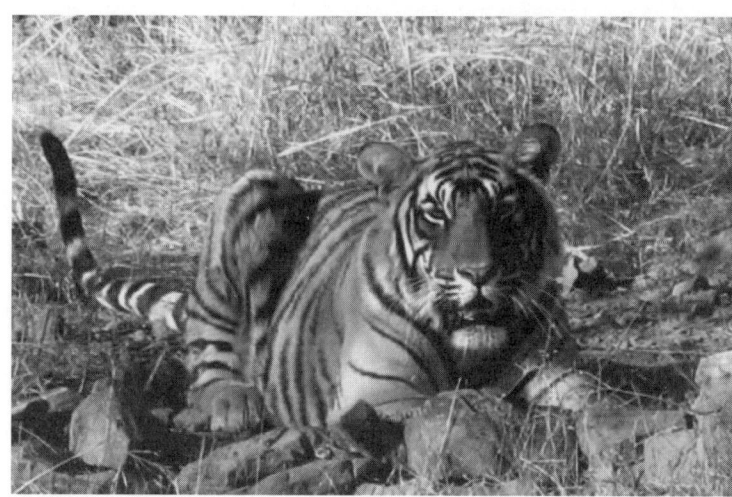

A snarling tiger showing displeasure at intruders.

unseen while pursuing its prey. The complimentary habitat provides constant cover to a large, solitary, 'stalk and ambush' predator to easily get close to their circumspect prey.

Farmlands of the Tarai are compatible to the needs of wildlife. Wheat, pulses, paddy and *chana* (gram) etc grow simultaneously with the cane crops, besides potato, peanuts, and cabbage. All kinds of herbivores and graminivores are attracted by this staple food. Wild boars, porcupines, chital, hog deer and swamp deer visit these fields and tigers having no option but to follow their prey wherever it may lead them, arrive in cane fields.

Besides, livestock like cows, buffalos, horses, donkeys, goats and pigs roam about the vista. Wild boars and domestic pigs are the same genus *Sus scrofa*, and genetically the same animals. They mix up easily and interbreed very well. I have seen village sows going feral and associating with wild pigs, even feeding selectively on roots and sugarcane. One domesticated sow at Larti had bred in an igloo constructed beforehand by some previous occupant. An old male assisted her as long as she stayed in sugar crop. Unfortunately when she refused to return to her owner she and her partner were worsted and hunted down by natives. Inter-breeding is indicated by striped piglets, which are often seen in a villager's piggery. Moreover they feed selectively on a wide range of plant and animal food including carrion and dead cattle. This additional factor makes pigs attain highest densities in sugar plantations, often ranging from 5 to 8 in one square kilometer. This means that a hundred sq km area would contain some 500 to 800 adult pigs, which is geometrically a super-population of a single prey species that is enough to sustain at least four tigers in 100 sq km round the year.

However, pigs comprise the routine prey list of the tiger and are definitely slain by him with little effort in comparison to what they put up in the jungle. Assuming

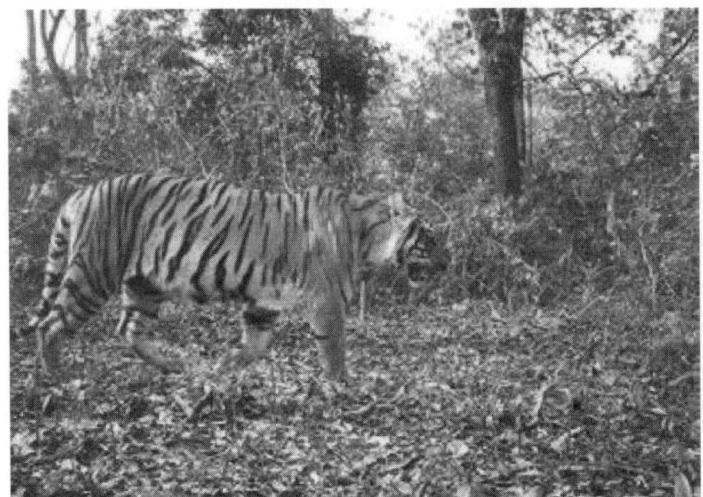

Young tigers sufficiently adapt to survive are able to generate a good network with their abandoned family and dispersed kens. They carve out some sort of range terrain for themselves as soon they are ready to breed. *(Camera Trap Shot- Royal Bardia Nation Park, Tarai of Nepal)*

that a tiger kills pigs weighing 50 kg at a rate of one every 4 to 5 days, it needs less than 100 individuals per year from this large population. It is thus more than sufficient to feed a large predator. Pigs are super-breeders, their extra large litters carry over 20 piglets at one time and they breed no less than thrice a year, which makes their population scientifically surplus. That is why pigs can sustain heavy cropping rate and despite a substantial percentage lost to netting and trapping they thrive well all over Tarai. The tiger's propensity to scavenging on dead cattle also ensures its survival.

Furthermore Prof Carl Berret, an expert on prey and predator dynamics, describes the prey's benefit as the "anywhere but here" principle. It means that what the entire prey community needs to do is to be anywhere where the predator is not present. Berret explains that it is immaterial whether the predator is a yard or a mile away, but what matters is that the prey needs to be smart enough to avoid the predator, to live another day in time. Similarly the predator has to be smart enough to subdue the prey so that it must not starve. A predator like tiger always has a better chance of survival where its prey base of ungulate population is bottom heavy, having more opportunities not to starve. Farmlands of Tarai support this pattern of survival where a predator's mastery of time and space, land pattern and behavior of man-reared feral animals give him the edge. The sense of self-defence of domesticated animals is much diluted and it naturally holds tigers in farmlands despite enormous odds. Parenthetically while jungle animals are exquisitely sensitive to the presence of predators, farmland animals are not.

Sugarcane farms are healthy eco-systems and the food chain it sustains is in no way inferior to the food chain of jungle animals. Sugar farms are more exposed to sunlight than canopy jungles. The electromagnetic energy flows through light and heat and travels in the form of radiation, which the earth receives in enhanced quantum than jungles. Plants convert this electromagnetic energy into chemical energy and the flow of its extra dose in normal diet makes the ungulates of the open plains, such as *nilgai* and blackbucks much more prolific breeders than jungle dwellers.

SR Chaudhery's hypothesis is that females living in sugarcane plantations easily come in estrus and the breeding activity of young tigers is more pronounced since the trouncing big daddy's are back there in the jungles. With strong healthier genes of young tigers; the chances of baby boom, as well as of their survival to maturity are relatively high.

The health and productivity of tigers living in sugarcane demonstrates how a small increase of the incident solar irradiation on the biosphere can lead to enormous beneficial increase in the energy available in the food chain. To my mind this is also a reason why the reproductive dynamics in farm tigers is much more prolific in comparison to jungle tigers.

In the world of tigers, females compete for suitable habitat that contains sufficient prey and other resources, in order to maintain themselves and to raise their offspring successfully. The male tigers compete for females. The presence of cub-rearing females draws male tigers from the jungles and often also accelerates the process of their adoption to canes.

Tiger mating in the Tarai is more pronounced after the rains and a majority of young ones are born in November or December. Thus the prime season of sugarcane also corresponds with the breeding season of tigresses. As the parturition date approaches, the movement and the range of a tigress becomes restricted. A long period of gestation – 103 to 110 days – and a large fetus make it difficult for mothers to secure food. The danger of accidents and miscarriages is great. Such parturient tigresses, more pre-occupied with finding a safe home, readily take to sugarcane and spend most of the time in the vicinity of the den, familiarize themselves with the movement of prey and water supply. Hunting upon a complex community of ungulate prey, they spend their last weeks of pregnancy there. This also seems a reason as why females should preponderate sugar farms.

A tigress naturally searches for a dense patch of cover to make a nursery that should be well concealed with dark interiors. The spot should also be located in a position from where it can be readily defended. These preconditions are instinctively sought by tigress, for cubs are born blind and helpless. They are highly vulnerable to predation by the second and third order predators such as scavengers. The predation risk decreases with the density of vegetation because greater foliage density prevents transmission of visual, chemical, or auditory cues by cubs. From August to February cane crops are at their best and provide the mother with a perfect hideout to breed.

During litter the tigresses are most localized. Their movements become restricted and their home range also shrinks to a fraction of its usual size, often to a minimum of 4 sq km and easy availability of prey becomes an important factor. This is a time of great risk for the nascent cubs. Their eyes open one to two weeks later but clear vision comes only after a month. The newly-born demand constant attention from their mother and her body odor plays an essential role in this. For the first few days, she helps them to find her teats to provide them with vital nourishment.

The tigress is alone, without a mate to help her. While she is away hunting, the random food searchers like jackals and foxes, and also infanticidal males of her own species, may find and kill the little ones. This makes the mother remain with them constantly. She can't afford to be away in search of food. In the event of disturbance she keeps shifting them to new hideouts by carrying them in her mouth.

The principal cause of mortality of cubs in the wild is starvation caused by the mother's failure to hunt enough prey. Such times are tough for a tigress in the jungle. But in cane fields big cats have feral cattle as alternative prey. Livestock, dogs, goats and even chicken provide an answer in emergency situations. But this is a ludicrous state of affairs which is apparently dangerous and cannot be allowed to continue for long. Such tigresses with sucklings must keep hunting on their own twice as hard because they have cubs to feed. The tiger's huge appetite needs at least one animal weighing about 55 kg per week which comes down to 50 animals a year. On the other hand, as the cubs grow the tigress needs nearly 70 animals a year to feed them which is not an easy task for super predator in jungle but which is easily met in farmland living off feral cattle and blue bulls. But it may also wrongly drive a tigress to accept humans as prey.

Sub-adult tigers steadily leave the area where they are born and raised. The reason for this deliberate dispersal is increased intolerance towards them by the resident adults. The father stops tolerating the actions of the young male and the mother acts the same way towards her female offspring. As a result, a segment of sub-adult population usually builds up on the periphery of prime jungle. Through con-specific competition, this segment is continuously enlarged as cubs grow up and begin an independent life. These emigrants to buffer zones later infiltrate into sugar-farms.

It is unfortunate that human intrusions in forests have dramatically lowered their wildlife carrying capacity and water logging impacts have turned many Tarai forest ranges into poor secondary forests. Madrahia-Sathiana area is a glaring specimen of this crisis where high flood levels manipulated by the closure of the barrage outlets, ensures 2 to 3 feet water logging inside the tenements of wildlife. In contrast, seasonal refugium of large sugarcane farms (that is of a long-term nature) offer a much better and wholesome breeding landscape for wildlife. For example, the annual migration of hundreds of swamp deer from Sathiana-Dudhwa into adjacent sugar fields of Ghola village to deliver their fawns continues to be a notable feature for years. This dramatic wildlife carrying capacity of sugar farms provide tigers with enough food and cover.

Proposals under the ambitious Project Tiger to create corridors between forest blocks involve major decisions like land acquisition, compensation, people's resettlement and elimination of developmental programs. It is time-taking. However, in the intervening time, sugar crops continue to serve as temporary corridors for tigers to move from one place to another. Sizeable breaks in forest continuity caused by heavily populated human settlements have cut off the connectivity between tiger populations. For instance there is a distance of 30 kilometers between Katarnia ghat and Bilrayan, and between South and North Kheri forest divisions respectively, but they get connected through uninterrupted cane corridors during the season.

The extensive stretches of dense crops enhance the landscape connectivity and scope for tiger movements. Like far thicker and more continuous areas of grass cover for tigers, the plantations serve as a corridor between fragmented forest ranges. This feature essentially improves the interlinking of populations and the status of sporadic meta-populations of the species that are effectively cut off from the forests and live in isolated spaces. Perhaps under pressure of creating post dispersal ranges, male tigers disperse further than females do. This way, often the unstable meta-population of one or two females otherwise destined to fade away, may well resuscitate and breed.

Tigers also relish sugarcane the way they like the soil and grass. I could discover this important factor towards grand finale of my research when to my astonishment in 1997; some villagers from Chaltua informed me that they had noticed a tigress with a pair of cubs eating sugarcane, after she had finished off a wild boar. She pulled out soft stems, and sitting in a squirrel like posture munched them with the support of her forepaws. Presumably, sugarcane juices aid the tiger's digestive system. Frank Simpson, in *Sport in Eastern Bengal* (1886) writes that "they catch fish, turtles, crocodiles, and large lizards. I believe they will occasionally eat sugarcane and maize."

I may add that eating grass is not of any nutritional value. Grass is mainly fiber and is pretty indigestible to cats and also low in nourishment. Carnivores eat grass, maze or soil specifically as an emetic substance that induces vomiting when administered orally. It is meant to discharge the toxic contents of their upset stomach. Intestines of obligate hyper-carnivores like tigers intestines lack the micro flora and bacteria designed to absorb carbohydrates and break high cellulose diet. I do not think they can ever transform into facultative-carnivores and munch through a quantum produce of sugarcane, such as a meso-carnivore or hypo-carnivore like jackals and foxes do in emergencies. But still in view of their diverse diet, this may be an 'out of the ordinary reason' that prompts the tiger's adaptation to farmlands.

Joseph G. Brand of the Monell Chemical Senses Center in Philadelphia, US, believes that cats have no ability to taste sweet as they harbor a genetic mutation that renders the sugar detectors on their taste buds inoperative. But still they need some sugar in form of glucose to transport cellular energy. It seems that such exceedingly subtle adaptations are not only temporarily revitalizing to a tiger in sugarcane plantations but are more practical in their final consumption.

It may be also partially true for grass. Although mainly an indigestible fiber lacking almost everything the cat needs in its diet, grass does have a lot of moisture, some trace minerals, vitamins A, D and folic acid, a required nutrient. Grass also contains chlorophyll, which before the discovery of antibiotics, was a remedy for pain, infection, ulcers, skin diseases and anemia. Tigers, like most other animals, are very skilled in controlling their needs for particular nutrients and finding healthy diet supplements, some of which can come from grass.

An American zoologist George Schaller, in his study of the scats of emaciated tigers discovered the presence of grass along with tapeworms wrapped in it, concluding that tigers eat grass in order to rid of their intestines of parasites. The same may be the role of sugarcane in a tigers self cure therapy.

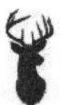

Riverbed Cultivation

"Tigers were living in sugar fields, and unbelievingly, my every bit of knowledge about them, whatever I had read, heard or known was proving wrong, biting dust but it implied that they had enough food to subsist on and enough cover to go about their business without hampering the routine of their human neighbors; perhaps after much toil and trouble, a symbiotic relationship had been reached for co-existence."
— Author at a meeting of Wildlife Advisory Board, U.P. Government, Lucknow, 1998.

Sugarcane grows well in the rich silt of the river. In Kheri district, the illegal cultivation of crop along the river bed of Sharda is massive. I remember till the decade of the 1970s, though being partly claimed by colonizers, the tamarisk brushwood lining the Sharda riverbed was still there and often in monsoon season the area echoed to pounding of swamp deer that came to breed there. During the decade of early seventies when my feelings towards wildlife were of ambivalence I had found two male deer locked in fighting on this very bed near Nau-gava and saved them by separating them. However in the present date, every inch of agricultural land falling under *gram sabhas* (village committees) has gone in allotment to landless people and the tamarisk brushwood and reed stretches have been completely reclaimed by powerful interest groups. Land-grabbers and their musclemen had also joined the fray and every square yard of arable land appears to have been made useful with a vengeance – scraped off, ploughed up and altered in one way or the other for the benefit of illegal cultivation. Hence this problem has acquired political nature with commercial overtones.

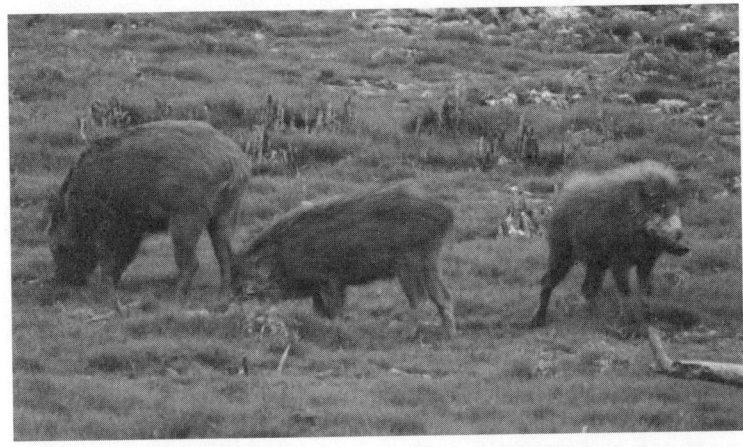

Wildboars in the grassed
ravines of Sharda.

During summers the river bed extends 2-3 km on each side of the river that covers nearly 2600 sq km of the tract only in Kheri district. It is free land for everyone to grab where a free crop on low investment and without irrigation and without fertilizer can be sowed and a substantial profit can easily be made. There is no system of issuing contract permit for this land or giving it on lease. Consequently, it involves a commercial nexus of revenue, police and forest department staff. The lower-level employees take their subvention cuts from private agencies, the money is divided on pro rata system and illegal cultivation is encouraged. The crops are sowed before the break of monsoon season and as the area slowly gets flooded the crops keep attaining heights. The flood level often rises by over a meter which essentially degrades the forest, but the logging does not affect the crops. The nature of sugarcane is such that if the primary leaves of fronds are above the water it does not take the impact of water logging and does not degenerate, but keeps growing healthy.

The devastating floods caused by insensate exploitation of timber in catchment areas is an ecological problem which in monsoon season alters the course of river and often washes away entire villages rendering thousands of natives destitute and homeless. This can only be controlled by creating dams or launching vast forestation schemes to prevent further erosion of land soil. However on a micro level, the mega encroachment of sugarcane cultivation on erosion-prone banks helps contain the silting and washing away of the precious soil which no doubt seeks to remedy the situation from getting bad to worse.

By mid-September the flood situation worsens dramatically when bordering country of Nepal releases hundreds of thousands of cusecs of water into Indian rivers and the entire tiger habitat in Pilibhit, Kheri and Bahraich districts periodically gets submerged sometimes under two meters of water. Generally when most of the tribes of cats are averse from entering water, villagers report that tigers often swim for miles and may frequently be seen crossing large rivers like Sharda and

Ghaghra, when no object appears to be in view. Water-logging disturbs the ecology of jungles and more tigers leave them seeking refuge on high grounds and even enter the sugar farmlands in neighborhood, where their prey has already reached. The site becomes the vortex of wildlife activity.

By October, the monsoons transform the landscape into a verdant paradise. The steady inundation of sugar farms also makes it an even better swampy habitat; the sunshades formed by the fronds give the plantations a character of canopy forests that becomes more welcoming to tigers. As the feel of the closed environment becomes much stronger and more overwhelming, there is a marked increase in the density of prey animals and tigers too arrive to prey upon them, delighting in thickets, for they are addicted to lying in water.

While there is considerable disturbance in other agricultural areas, this river bed savannah of sugar is still absolutely free form human interference. No operation of any kind takes place and the crop furnishes an undisturbed breeding cover for carnivorous animals, becoming their real holding ground.

Despite monsoon being over, the riverbed continues to remain partly flooded, offering a squelchy and muddy habitat to wildlife. The lingering water level of one or two feet makes the area totally inaccessible to humans. Foresters do not patrol here nor do the farmers go inside it, no tractor with ploughs or crawlers enters the dense thick set crops that are left to them in the care of nature.

The unflustered conditions remain conducive not only to wild life but sometimes also for poachers who indulge in their nefarious activities till the lands hold the water. This is a remote area where tigers invariably linger on.

Incidentally the concept of preservation of the habitat does not apply on sugarcane plantations which go against the ecological parameters of a sound habitat. Scheller says, "without strictly protected sites, it is nearly impossible to conduct longitudinal studies of carnivores that are critical to scientific management and shaping positive public attitudes towards wildlife." But this unreal habitat is biologically an exceptionally endowed terrain and despite the human use of resources can still be declared as Sites of Special Scientific Interests (SSSIs). The wide swath still holds many biologically meaningful and unanswered questions for experts, including the causes of seasonal time-specific tiger abundance that reaches up to 4 to 5 tigers, besides some leopards that also use the same riverbed and share middle and small size of prey. Why do so many animals live here is not known. This is a point where cold analysis falters.

Fortunately in 2016, WWF field activists installed both active and passive camera traps (active contraption reacts to an animal interrupting an electronic beam while passive contraption is activated by animal's body heat) in this uniquely important biological laboratory to sample tiger populations on spatial and temporal scales. By capturing and recapturing protocol we might learn the potential pattern of tigers' periodical occupation of the crops – of course on landscape and terrain scales -

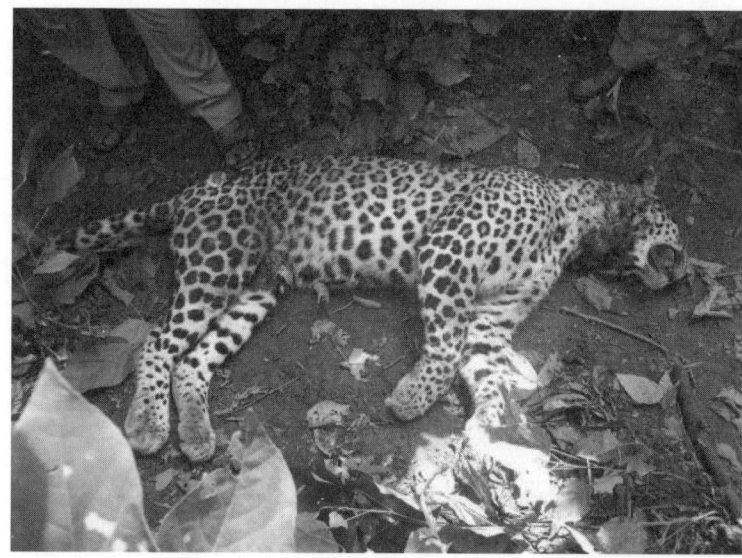

A male leopard killed and partly eaten by a tiger in Bankeyganj area. 2014 (Photo credit : Abhishek Verma)

and also ascertain whether the same or any of these return to inhabit the belt every year. Ecological investigations may also answer as to where do these cats settle down during secondary period or in absence of crops, and also what happens to a relatively high proportion of transients in search of territories, scientifically held as condemned or doomed surplus. Do they also come back or never, including prey disposal in standings of ungulate population rather than the great biomass?

Though this cultivation is illegal, a solution to this is difficult since laws are set to naught and local influence or collision with underpaid subordinate employees of Government, including sugar factories and crushers are among the involved interests. But the Geo Information Systems utilized by Japanese Information Cooperation Agency (JICA) maps the extent of this almost unbroken cultivation swath as stretching on more than 200 sq km of land.

The historical record of tiger colonization shows that in many regions tiger distribution was dendritic associated with watercourses and river basins. Studies of Herptner and Sludskii reveal that even where watercourses penetrated deep into desert, suitable wild boar and tiger habitat was often linear, only a few kilometers wide at most. This land is a petite model of this theory where two kilometers either side of the river, tigers inhabit sugar crops with sparse reed beds and numerically dominant ungulates that are *nilgai* and wild boars.

However, as this attribute of land terrains and same land use pattern is maintained truthfully for many years, it is worth understanding for research in context of tigers' population dynamics and multi-year trend estimates of tiger population size and prey community structure, that supports their living in the crop. Moreover this great moist landscape, is an ecologically representative site of Tarai as old tiger and swamp deer habitat, lies in critical tiger recovery area. It is a varied and complex biotope of central Tarai, encompassed by immense ranges of reserve forests and Dudhwa National Park (DNP) one of India's most important tiger conservation landscapes. In a sense the presence of tiger in this bed in his quest to meet basic needs represents an enormous canary of biological mine; because for a certain phase of time this river bed enriches tigers environment to the hilt and a micro population of 2 to 4 animals essentially comes here to make their livings in legal ways.

The full treatment of the subject is beyond the scope of this chapter. But I can candidly say that when even DNP is being used as a political crowbar by some radical factions, seeking to protect local land claims and Tharu culture, advocating allotment of more land for agriculture purposes to support their families inside parks; by comparison this illegal cultivation on otherwise desolate river borders is a petty issue. It can even entail a fair and transparent participatory process and be properly legitimized for it is not that human activity is expanding into the habitat of highly endangered animal but it is actually the other way.

It is human activity on the river bed that has sufficiently enabled the peripheral population of an endangered animal to secure another segment of extensive habitat ensuring a higher carrying capacity to breed and survive. I have even found *sambhar* pellets in this area. There is no study underway as how this illegitimate human intervention supports a plethora of wildlife. But on my part, having spent four months every year for five consecutive years in this terrain, I can safely say that I have gained extraordinary exposure to big cats in this riverbed forest of sugarcane.

In the absence of serious barrier maintenance – which is practically not possible and ecologically also not desirable – much is voiced against human-carnivore conflict. But as Corbett declared long back, committed predators of livestock and humans don't acknowledge barriers and they have never been encumbered by most barriers for long. Studies by Thomson and Shelton proved that "Given time some individuals learn to penetrate any barrier." Their findings not only put the debate aside but also dilute its contents. But my observations for six continuous seasons between 2002 and 2008 show that these tigers, despite being in human zone prefer to remain isolated and even the presence of domestic prey populations all around is not inducement enough for them to transgress their self-imposed barrier.

It is not before December that the water really dries out and the low investment crops that were left to themselves are healthy and full of juice, ready to be harvested by their illegal owners, sent to factories and money shared.

In regular agricultural enclaves the situation is similar save for advantage of natural irrigation by flooding; here the diesel pumps irrigate the farms. Wild boars are first to arrive in big numbers. They create leafy igloos and breed and then scatter everywhere, wandering without restraint as the water and cove is sufficient.

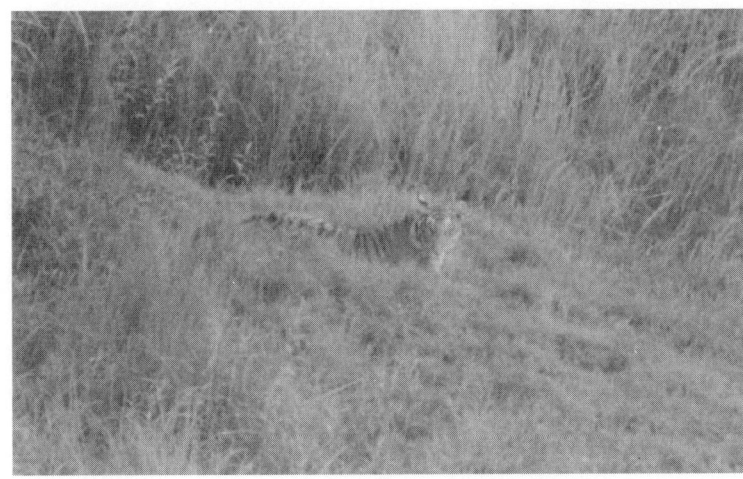

He sat watching us intently with unwavering attention.

Sloth bears also come to feed upon juicy canes causing much destruction in their manner of dining. While jackals pull down the single sugarcanes by nibbling at their base, the large sloth bears stand seven feet tall on hind legs. They seize a big bunch in both hands and pulling it back tightly endeavor to lie down on the ground, thus uprooting the entire cluster in this process. They eat few and leave the rest. Then hog deer and monitor lizard arrive to bear their young, followed by swamp deer that come to breed here from jungle, showing sharp numerical changes when they return and as all these are important ingredient in a tiger's menu hence they also follow them.

Moreover, on regular farmlands composite agriculture is practiced. There are fine stretches of intermittent gram, rice, wheat, mustard and lentil fields that attract herbivores for protein rich nourishment. These short crops, in forms of clearings and grassy glades, provide a sense of space and long view of the landscape. In the midst of tall dense savannah of sugarcane the staple fields of cereal and other foodstuff, pale green in the evening sun and charming to the eyes, serve the purpose of meadows that contain browsing food. Here, prey animals that subsist on farm crops congregate in the moonlight and tigers usually hover around looking for them. That is why both legal and illegal sugarcanes plantations encompass quite a few micro populations of tigers while there are a lot of jungle areas which have no tigers.

Inside jungles the habitat deterioration is extremely subtle in its impact and therefore more destructive in its final consummation. However as this template doesn't apply to farmlands, it is also important to understand the pinch period matrix of tigers, which is shaped by the harvesting of the crop, when the multicolored crops along with sugarcane grass stratum are consumed and the fields lie barren for miles without cover.

Sugarcane plantations, like perennial grasslands, are extremely productive habitats for general range of wildlife. In the jungle, the geology and topography, rainfall and evaporation, animal feasts in the form of regular grazing, and controlled fire by foresters are factors that control or limit the form of vegetation. In agriculture fields, crop harvesting creates the same effect and controls the existence of this extremely productive habitat.

The bio-network of sugarcane crop and its agricultural cycle takes a quarter of a year to grow to maturity before it withers away, quite like disproportionate annual grasses. Tall coarse grasses have little food value once they have grown past the young palatable stage. By the time they have flowered and die, most of the food has been transferred to their roots for storage – an evolutionary adaptation designed to cope with the oncoming dry season. The controlled fire is judiciously employed in phases so that the wildlife is not harmed, and it later creates a more suitable habitat for the ungulates that rapidly move into recently burned patches to feed on succulent and nutritious new shoots.

Very similar to the disproportionate annual grasses in the jungle, the sugarcane attains full growth in nine months. Once the maximum protein/fiber, glucose and cellulose ratio is achieved, the crop sustains it for a couple of months and then starts declining and its edible value significantly reduces. The skin becomes thicker and harder, and the small stomas in the nodes, called eyes, sprout out petite green root like shoots that indicate that the ageing of sugarcane has begun.

This is the season when the harvesting starts in phases. From a tiger's point of view, it is a habitat reclamation for human use for they don't know the meaning of crop and its usages in human lifestyle. However, the main importance of a dead or dying sugar crop appears to be that it affords cover and shelter; but sugarcane grows perennially from the root system known as ratoon rhizomes that remain in the ground and re-sprout from each stalk. Ratoon crops grow faster than the primary crop plants because the cutting blade is placed to a height of three inches to prevent the loss of roots. This speedy regeneration restores the habitat within months. Moreover the entire crop is not harvested simultaneously; it is taken in installments, thus the wildlife gets ample time to seek refuge in other patches, which are often of considerable size.

It has been established that the grasslands produce a greater animal biomass than the monotypic forests. Harvesting temporarily retards the habitat and also works as a check on the population of farm tigers as well as of ungulates. This significant feature indicates that the exclusive harvesting of sugarcane crop, like the spring season grass burning in the open plain after frost has made it inflammable, is a natural and ecologically sound exercise. It later improves the habitat and allows it to meet the food shelter requirements of most of the ungulates.

It may be noted that grass fire doesn't increase the number of nutrients in the soil – it just releases them from dry grass making them available for nutrition of plants. Similarly the stripped-off leaves of sugarcane, left in the fields in mountainous loads, are later disposed by burning, leaving plenty of nitric compounds and organic matter to enrich the soil. The opportunistic grasses and lentil seeds also germinate simultaneously within all type of crop plots and the natural young growth easily attracts grazers. The function that the annual grasses perform for the wildlife in the jungle is achieved to some extent by the sugarcane in the fields.

Different insights arise from difference in perceptions. It may seem strange, but the impact of harvesting is not very tangible on mainstream tigers, for it is just a part of their adaptive cycle that goes with crop rotation patterns. Yet as the impact of habitat degradation is considered lethal in its outcome, the animal might come into head-on conflict with the livelihood requirements of people and the cases of man-tiger conflict and even man-eating might increase at such times. This illustrates that inanimate patterns determine the animate patterns we encounter in the environment. Such interactions between flora and fauna, and people living next to them, keep the sequence of the environment in motion and trigger a new resilience in life systems. It does not matter how and when man-animal conflict triggers but the factors supporting tigers' long-term stay in the crops remain relevant for tigers year after year and they return to it without a hitch. Finally these ecological parameters coupled with interesting animal communities shape the unique animal that is called 'The Sugarcane Tiger.'

By the end of February, the jungles thin out, days become longer and hot but the nights are cool until the middle of March. Sugarcane is almost harvested by this time but the river beds still hold irregular patches of tamarisk, clusters of *jamun* trees and *narkul* where tigers prefer to shift while the crop is speedily harvested. However, there is no complete absence of sugarcane plots, a few plantations stand here and there. It so happens that due to oversupply of crop sugar factories stop issuing indent slips to planters who keep postponing the harvesting of the crop. If despite a long wait the mill slip is not issued they leave their product abandoned. The harvesting is not economically viable for it can't meet the cost of labor and transportation involved. In course of time the crop grows yellow and falls on its own and in absence of water and frond canopy it turns into a very hot spot, which the tigers reject altogether as habitat and go several miles to a more suitable place.

"Habitat fragmentation," as John Seidensticker says, "is the single largest driver of the ecological change because it disrupts foraging movements, dispersal, migrations and colonizing abilities of animals. Fragmentation disrupts demographic and genetic functioning of populations and drastically reduces long term population viability." It does not seem to apply much on these farmlands for it is a temporary period in which the land rejuvenates to produce more cover and protein-rich food in future and the hard-core dwellers of the land comprehend this fact thoroughly. During this interim period they disperse here and there in small pockets of cool shaded marshlands and glitches. A fraction may permanently move out of the area, waiting for the cultivated land, their new discerning breeding ground, to breathe life again. This makes the life-style of some tigers compulsively altered for they know the basic character of land use pattern remains the same and its ecological harmony is never fragmented, thus it is not entirely inimical to peripheral tigers' survival.

It can be said that Tarai is a land of violent contrasts with the heat of the tropics and the cold of the north. Here the drought and the floods of the rainy season intersect one another as though following the lines drawn by an architect's ruler. Yet the animals make at home everywhere. The fauna merges itself in its surroundings and regulates its minor needs and its way of life accordingly with an incredible pliability.

Though much water dries up with the arrival of summers the habitat seems fully fragmented or even eliminated of many biological communities. These include itinerant ducks, swamp deer and *chital* and their niches are engaged by other species like pea fowls, pangolins, porcupines, occasional black bucks and hog deer, snakes waking from hibernation, packs of jackals, feral cattle and *nilgai* staying put like all season compatriots. Leopards come to the delight of farmers with their sawing musical grunts. Black and brown partridges also arrive to breed in dry scrub of lower regions and among exposed tree roots and grasses of high banks, while passing elephants and blue bull herds seek salts on the knolls that stand in the neighborhood of the river.

As summers build up villagers often report tigers roaming about the beds of attenuated rivers. They relax in its pools and glitches, sometimes in genuine caverns on the side of large mounds, which form suitable retreats for the accouchement or for the habitation of a cub rearing tigresses, also entailing an accurate knowledge of the season and its impact on their food supply.

This does not bring much change in the pattern of a tiger's life, save for sub-adults that split up and move away. A fraction of dispossessed residents goes to regular jungles in north or south and permanently emigrates out of the area. Some sub-adults become transients, while others linger about the area in irregular grass and swamps that extend from 100 to 200 acres in size. Vegetation maps acquired from satellite shots show some of these patches as suboptimal and some as excellent quality habitat adjoining cultivation but away from human habitation. There, like evicted occupants, the tigers live with compensatory shifts as if waiting for their under-construction home to come up soon.

Reflex action and conditioned learning are a part of normal behavior. But a different type of learning is required for more flexible behavior, one which enables the cat to predict the consequences of its own actions, especially in their relations with human beings, and modify its actions based on failures. I believe that such tigers know their terrain well. They know the spots from where they can watch the daily routine of village flock. They know the habit of their prey animals, they know

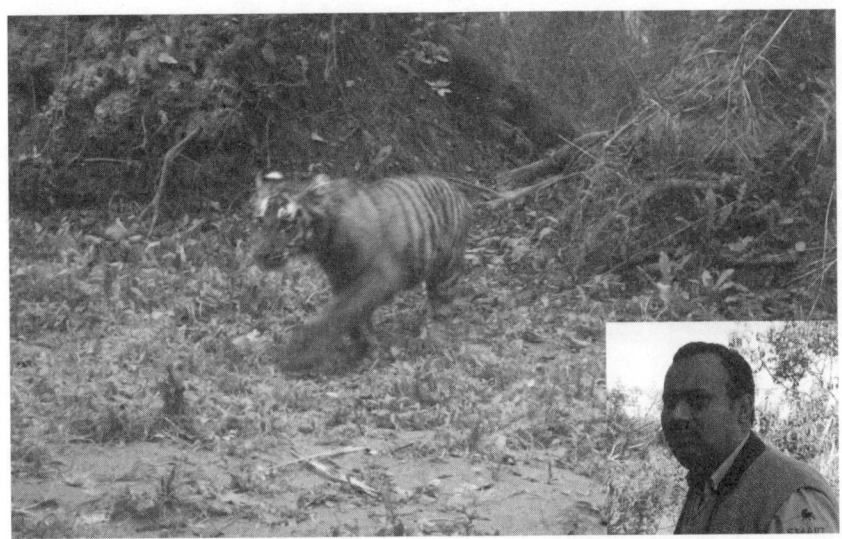

A tiger cub in the glitches of Sharda river. (Inset Photographer Mudit Gupta, Field Officer, WWF, UP Chapter)

when the people are occupied in their own affairs and when they are likely to go poking around in their coverts, they know when it is not wise to disturb them. I maintain that tigers that belong to farmlands hereditarily possess the natural etiquettes of living in human environments.

Survival is measured by successful adaptation to changing circumstances. Countless ancestors of such multi-generational beings have lived in these farmlands and their neuron conditioning has evolved, predisposing them to interact with their environment in a certain way. They nurture instinctive orientation as how to live here safely. Otherwise, what could have made them stay back in the crops for so long? However, this is not to say that they become house cats; they are still completely wild and potentially dangerous predators, yet their conditioning hardly makes them confront the villagers.

These are hardcore, unremitting cane tigers, content to stay within their prime farmland boundaries, and feeling no urge whatsoever to leave their own little chosen acreage. Some of these also evolve a symbiotic relationship with humans. It is two species doing more or less what they would do in any event but tolerating the close presence of one and other while they do it. Toleration is the key which costs virtually nothing in terms of energy, but increases the chances of survival in human environs. Scientists call it the innate grasp of primordial relationship, which is a genetic legacy based on millions of years of hard-won experience of each other and this is how different species adjust peacefully. Such behavior allows them to go about their daily regime on autopilot mode and free up more of the brain for confronting other challenges. On the other hand some experts suggest that tigers nurture a fear complex with regard to man as it has been passed down over timeless generations. It emerges from a feeling that a relationship between man and tiger is not favorable relationship, synergy or symbiosis but the relationship is of covert nature based more on avoiding man than meeting him. It is artificial symbiosis but even this situation has certain norms. Unfortunately it is again the man who is main deterrent to it.

By March the river bed of Sharda becomes a key human use area, much prone to illegal hunting when the second crop of summer season is planted. Sandy river banks are conducive to *kakri* (cucumber), watermelon and musk melon. A creeper crop locally called *palash* is not left abandoned like sugarcane owing to large scale flooding. But in summers the river bed is largely dry and water levels are very low, hence farmers construct their temporary hutments and reside upon the very banks protecting their crops from innumerable *nilgai* and black bucks that arrive to demolish fruiting *palash* in dark nights (Sadly black bucks are now extinct in the area. The last I saw was in 1996).

By this time water ponds in the jungle start drying up and thirsty herds of *chital* and others walk long distances in the night to drink at the river. *Palash* creepers are low in height, a foot above ground and lack cover hence animal's profile is easily silhouetted against the horizon and a lot of poaching takes place. Members of the nomadic *kanjar*, a hunter-gatherer tribe arrive, and their trap settings, nettings and crudely fashioned leg-hold snares become devices of everyday choice. Active searching and shooting with the help of domestic dogs increases, and predation on fawns and small wildlife grows. Traditional techniques which proceed silently in contrast to gun hunting take a heavy toll of wildlife, which often makes the biomass of prey species fall drastically. The area remains prone to illegal hunting and even wild tigers, the flagships of this ecosystem, turn vulnerable.

Incidentally during the eighties the tiger count outside Dudhwa's protected area had included this terrain as important habitat holding a substantial segment of matured tiger population, ranging around ten in all. Since a large course of river runs through mainland Tarai or central Tarai area outside the jurisdiction of forest department, no proper mechanism to control poaching appears effective. Gun-hunting with a "sit-and-wait in a pit" approach is recurrently practiced by natives in the neighborhood of fruiting *palash* (like sugarcane *palash* is also a conflict-prone farming practice though much less in degrees of severity.)

The anti-poaching patrols are legally empowered to eliminate dogs in wildlife areas and fire back on poachers in self-defence. During my tenure as Honorary Wildlife Warden of the Park, out of 48 individual poachers that I caught in all, thirty-odd men were picked up along this riverbed; some of which surrendered after a cross firing. They were embodiment of rampant native wildlife consumerism with brutality and callousness for it did not matter to them how many animals escaped wounded in the dark nights.

Surprisingly upon interrogation none of these men ever remembered encountering any official forces, police or foresters patrolling in the area but for

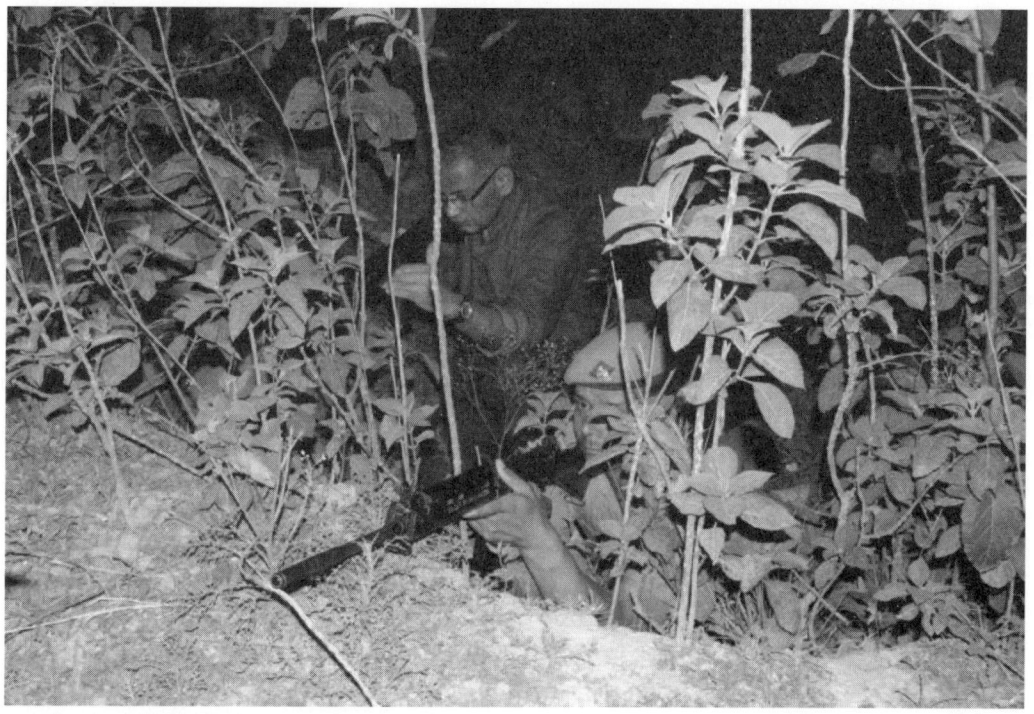

Author on an anti-poaching operation, April 2016. As I stroked my gun, I remember thinking - I should have better listened to my wife and gone to Paris to cuddle my new born grandson - than to come on this business (*Photo credit : Abhishek Verma*)

their first ever encounter with me. They were aghast when I and Ravi Prakash Verma, the then Member of Parliament from the constituency of Dudhwa and at present a member of Rajya Sabha (Upper House of Parliament) confiscated their nets and traps with illegal firearms. They took this hunting as recreational and normal occupation with complete disregard for any rules and told us that when the officials ignore us it means their silent consent is there. They agreed that law implementation efforts were ineffectual in restraining poaching as none were ever caught or prosecuted.

The factor responsible for higher degree of hunting is the absence of jungle patrols along the riverbed and absence of permanent anti-poaching camps with enough force to dissuade hunters from targeting wildlife that already thinned due to summers. Interestingly there are Hindu hunters that kill *nilgai* and sell it and Muslim hunters that kill wild boar and do the same. But when this hunting-prone site got some anti-hunting protection during 1998 to 2003 it showed a salutary effect on the populations of target animals and the numbers of pea fowls, wild boars, porcupine and hog deer were reported to have increased.

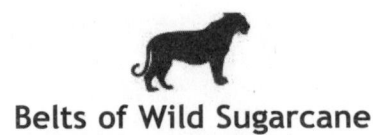

Belts of Wild Sugarcane

"Tigers fall especially vulnerable to the building of roads. They are known to use manmade routes to patrol their territories rather than to blaze through the bush themselves."
- Dale Miquelle, Hornocker Institute.

Approximately 1200-plus sq km of Dudhwa National Park triangle, including Katarnia and Kishanpur, is surrounded by about 5000 sq km of sugarcane fields. And when such a tall crop is all around, exactly when the landscape animals like tigers cross the real ecological line is not known. The contention that the adjustment of tiger population would be contained by construction of available habitat, does not seem to hold much meaning in this boundless habitat of sugar forests In spite of everything, tigers have a tendency of transgressing their eco-systems and ranging beyond protected areas.

In northern Pilibhit and Kheri districts, the river bed area also contains some solid blocks of wild sugarcane attributed to anthropogenic origin. When due to non-consumption of surplus produce, the plantations are left unharvested, they turn into rough plots of crop, and with declining food value they don't sustain much wildlife. However jackals, wild boars and sloth bear continue to reside in them while the ghostly silent figures of tigers also pass through them in the nights looking for their food. Such chunks slowly take up to wild cycle, receding in summers and regenerating again in rains and by the coming of next season turn into fully wild sugarcane. Cultivation furrows disappear and transform the sward into a forbidden low-lying grassy swamp, a dense secondary forest that is more solid than previous yield.

These plots are often left abandoned for quite a few seasons because it is no one's land and nobody is ready to take the burden of clearing it. But the tigers reject these crops as its solid density badly hampers their passage, though they use it to relax in seclusion. Their chief desideratum is any spot along which they can proceed silently and which affords a fair vision. This wild sugar-grassland is devoid of both.

It is important to understand that cultivated sugarcane and wild sugarcane plots are tracts of different nature. Cultivated tracts are planted meticulously in furrows with a standard distance of 2 to1½ feet which allow free movement to animals between clear-cut lanes into deeper interiors, providing uninterrupted corridors for scores of miles to support their crossover to other jungles. Tigers are mercurial animals and their free movement is important. Wild tracts of thick tall cane are very difficult stuff for heavy-bodied animals like tiger through which they have to try to

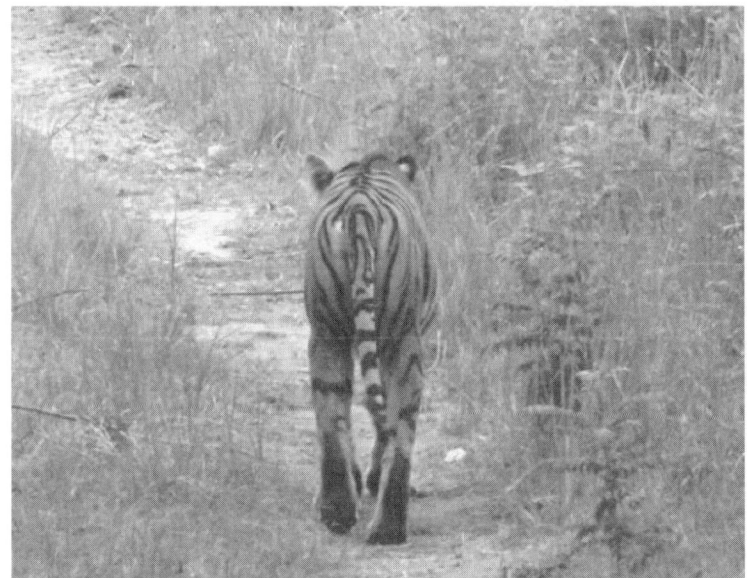

Tiger moving on the dry
mud-path

force their way. Compact stems, with circumference of 2-3 inches, are not idly suited to function within. These grow close together and as some animal forces its way through them they clash and rattle against one another and don't allow the animal to move freely. Such growths are in fact inedible hiding covers of prey, a protection against predators and do not largely support large-sizes animals' movement patterns whether of prey or predators. However, such pockets naturally serve as mother 'caches' for both the species of prey and predators for their earlier phase of litter-rearing, as long as newborn are semi-immobile and need concealment. Tigers enter them in search of prey animals, to hide their kill and also use these to sleep in seclusion.

When not hunting, the large animal prefers relatively open spaces for movement with reasonably clear vision at least in one direction. That is why in dense *sal* forests they are much more liable to be encountered wandering about during the day time. They are often tracked along an open forest road for miles, travelling great distances by night. These paths beaten out by bare feet of countless natives throughout centuries offer far less likelihood to either man or tiger picking up thorns in their feet when walking along them.

As I have already said that when residing in cultivated sugarcane, tigers prefer using furrows to get from one place to another rather than cutting straight through the cane. Moreover owing to the variation in the density of cane in different places, from plot to plot they are unable to maintain a straight line. Hence when not under pressure of humans the soft footed animals are more likely to select mud paths in disapproval of furrows. I have several times encountered them on the pathways flanked by canes.

Tiger pugmarks inside the cane crops can easily be traced between furrows. They only zigzag when they search for prey, while mud paths running between tall flanking crop plots are selected for longer perambulations. This proves that it is human intervention factor that actually facilitate the daily schedule activity of large predators in sugar farms with comfort and fair vision that no wild grass habitat can provide. WWF India Field Officer Dr Mudit Gupta reports from ground zero: "Cultivated sugarcane is like grassland-wilderness restored with furrows. It allows them easy movement for miles which the wild plot of any species of grass and especially sugarcane grass would not allow."

Precisely, from a tiger's point of view, wild patches of sugarcane, without paths and furrows are actually secondary status habitats. These are much too impenetrable and making a long journey through them does not fit into their routine patrolling. Tigers enter deep inside unbroken stretches of cultivated sugarcane while in wild sugarcane they confine to outer limits thus using the swath least as a habitat.

It was in this area that once searching for gin traps with Wung Longwa, the Field Director of Dudhwa that we came across several beautifully painted cardinal bats. These bats are usually found in heavy elephant grasses, flitting from cover to cover and looking like gorgeous butterflies. That year their flock had come to inhabit the wild canes freely. Sloth bears also show a predilection for matted growth. Cowherds tell that when bears are chased by dogs they are not deterred by difficulties of ground from making straight to the center of the jumbled sugarcane and even barbed wire entanglements of thorn and scrub, often seeking refuge in utterly inaccessible places where dogs don't dare to enter.

It may be paradoxical to argue that perhaps farmland tigers are unable to meet harsh compulsive demands of the forest because of the constant pressure of the resident tigers and their adjustment with local population getting difficult to achieve. Therefore they prefer these optimum conditions where at least there is some easy food and water. Though competitive interactions among tigers operating in cane zones do generate selective pressures, especially when during secondary period, they adjust downwards with human induced depression of prey, but these pressures are definitely of different type than those inside the jungles.

These are no transients for the transient parameterization does not necessarily correspond to what tiger biologists Sunquist and Karanth term as transience. Their model of photographic sampling to access tiger population specifies that transients are tigers caught for only one time. These have virtually no chance being captured again, because these do not reside in a particular area and are viewed as individuals. But the tigers in question were not passing through the cane wilderness, while possibly trying to become residents elsewhere they were actually living here as individuals.

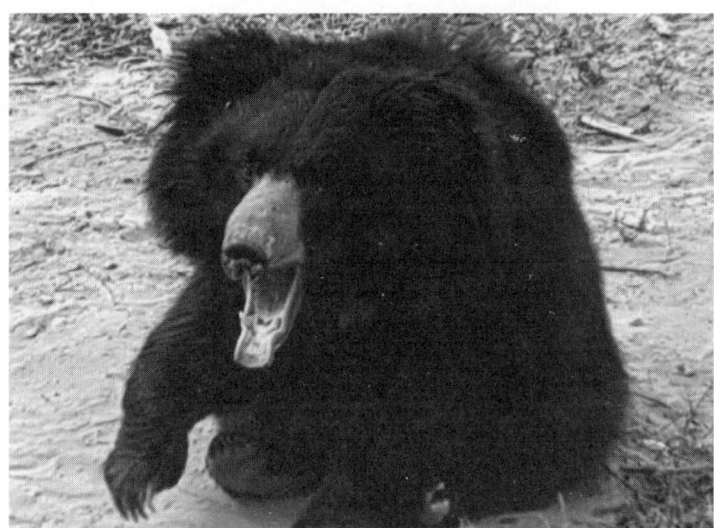

In Tarai farmlands sloth bear are rigidly nocturnal. Their food mainly consists of sugarcane, fruits and insects but in hunger they have been seen eating carrion near villages. *(Photo Credit : Sanjay Narain)*

The solitary nature and territorial spacing mechanism of tigers contributes to their relatively low densities. Owing to their wide-ranging nature, estimates of demographic facts are extremely difficult to obtain. Moreover in sugarcane farms the ecosystem these tigers represent is not inviolate like jungles though there are many wildlife niches outside protected areas that they rationalize to live in, as these are separate from human pollution. And once this compromise is accepted it is the beginning of the process of rationalizing their existence for living outside the jungle. Perhaps this is the cutting edge on which the proposal of Project Tiger to have multiple use areas, occupied both by man and tiger was based; a least regressive thinking that opens a great debate for co-existence.

Forest Department data reveals that for four consecutive years between 1992 and 1995, a micro tiger population comprising three females and one male inhabited a rural stretch along the course of Sharda's riverbed up to Nighasan. At every 15 km or so, prolonged stay of at least one tiger was recorded. This tiger count made from individual identifications of tracks showed a stable trajectory that met the needs of three important characteristics of the species - isolation, extensive range and secretiveness. These were maintained for good three years till the tigers disappeared. There were also some single populations and interrelated meta-populations operating on a wider scale, far off on the very riverbed, and the prey level for the single population was still sufficient. Significantly in this area *sambhar* pellets were found and their sightings were also reported.

To what extent tigers drifted southwards I did not know but the unfortunate and unavoidable, man-carnivore conflict was not concentrated at the edges of principal forest ranges. The distribution of livestock attack sites showed that a larger segment of tigers was clearly restricted to within 10-15 miles of the nearest jungle and not spread all across the area. A substantial proportion of kills (over 60 per cent) was from tigers and 30 per cent was from leopards while in remaining 10 per cent kills that were found in dilapidated conditions, the identity of the killer was uncertain. The households sampled on this basis did not report any depredation by tigers from further-off lands, though leopard areas extended further and stray attack of tiger overthrowing a pony was also heard from far-off places that could not be timely verified.

The events helped me conclude that the sugarcane tiger phenomenon starts from the periphery of the jungle and gradually extends southwards, up to a maximum width of 15-20 km in agricultural land. The extension or contraction of area depends on the number of tigers inhabiting different pockets, which involuntarily regulate their space requirements according to seasonal needs.

This also indicated that any beast floating down further south could be treated as having strayed. Such free-floaters transgress their eco-system, cross unacceptable terrain, and emerge in the most unanticipated places. Scientifically this lot is identified as a doomed surplus of youngsters and transients that die as a result of intra-specific aggressions including hunting-related injuries, starvation and deaths during attempted dispersal. Though such an individual scrutiny of tigers is simply not possible yet learning their size and weight from their spoors, as of over one year in age, I included them in my study for they seemed to be born in sugar farms. As a doomed surplus their long-term survivability was seemingly not possible but for me it was premature to issue any potential statement on this natural crisis. I needed to be cautious and aware of every aspect of managing and coping with this phenomenon or from a different viewpoint, the crisis situation of sugarcane tigers, which permitted no generalizations of tiger's ways.

Tiger movements are intensely linked to fraternizing with their own kind. The range expansion of a tiger, as to how far a tiger has to move in sugarcane in search of a prey or to avoid inter or intra-species tensions and then get back into his natal range, depends on the constraints of ecological factors and also the maintenance of chemical communication with neighborhood tigers, especially females. A tiger advancing in a sugar zone might continue to exploit the rich prey base of feral cattle and domestic livestock, but a complete breakdown of the social communication network with other tigers is a critical determinant in the straying of lonely tigers.

Influx of dispersing animals from jungle into population and vice-versa the influx of animals retreating from it is the factor that affects the size and dynamics of sugar tiger population.

Unfortunately several alien species of plants have invaded the ecosystem of Tarai forests, posing a threat to its biodiversity. Inedible vegetation like lantana, congress grass (*Parthenium*), carrot grass, *Saccharum munja*, *ban maura*, castor and water hyacinth have drastically exacerbated the forest. Their aromatic oils

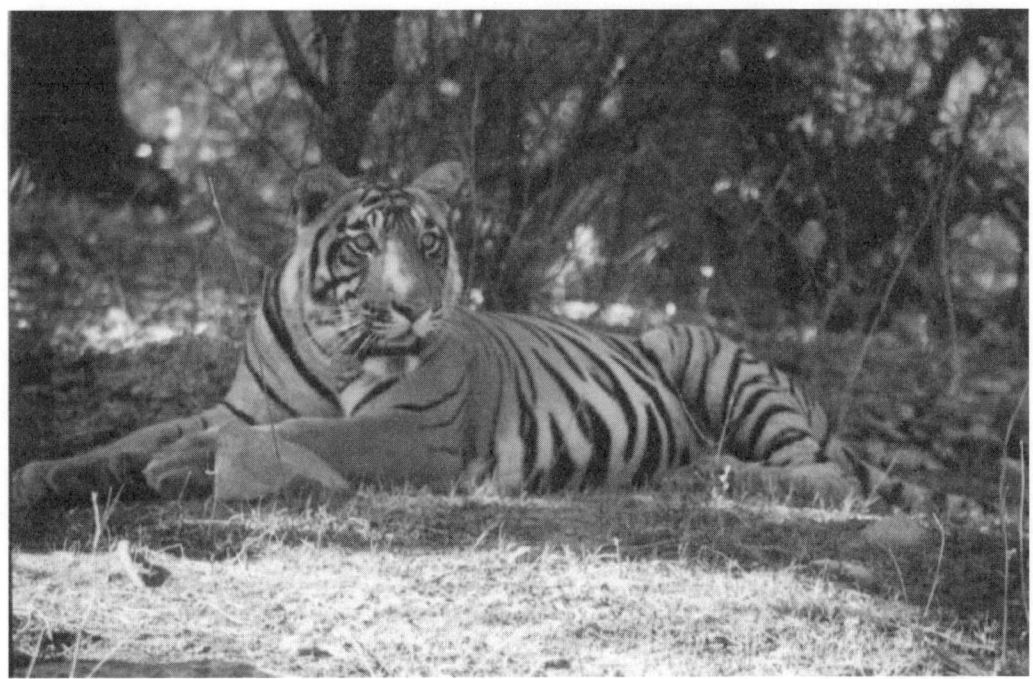

The regal tiger was too relaxed being full of cattle meal

and exudates of leaves and roots have an anti-biotic effect on natural edible species. It retards the growth of edible species suffocates and prevents their seedlings from germination and finally eradicates them from the area. Moreover, indigenous coarse grasses are unpalatable and nutritionally poor which reduce the carrying capacity of herbivores within jungle and they run out to agricultural fields where tigers follow them, accelerating the progression of the sugarcane tiger phenomena.

Sugar harvesting does not seem to produce an acute forbidding impact on tigers. The crop is harvested smoothly without causing much damage to wildlife, save partial poaching. But in the jungles the erosions of grasslands, through fire or inundations are prone to be catastrophic; resulting in colossal loss of bird eggs and the near wipe-out of reptilian life. For example when Kaziranga grasslands are annually battered by excessive flooding, a great number of ungulates drown and die, including rhino calves and tiger cubs. But no such big toll of life is sacrificed in erosion of sugar habitat; harvesting is the mildest method of habitat erosion which the tigers and their prey easily endure.

The dual characteristics of sugar crop - cool in summers and warm in winters - support tigers well and properly. Frost is created at about zero degree temperature. During the frost season, the non-irrigated dry patches of sugar crops become ideal spots for tigers. The essential soil heat in form of radiation is constantly emitted. It is high in the night and low during the day. The canopy of frond is too heavy and continuous; it does not let the heat escape, which facilitates the creation of a green house like effect. During the sharp bouts of frost towards January tigers live here, (as prior to harvesting irrigation is discontinued) and these develop into warm spots.

The expanse of tall crops does help the tiger to inhabit areas in numbers that is not possible in the jungle and would not have been possible earlier when the area was a jungle.

And finally, like other cats, tigers are quick learners. Through observations they exhibit defense and caution against wandering bands of people that share their range. They show distrust towards humans and rely more on their keen vision to preserve themselves from dangerous proximity of human enemies. Thus they thrive better in the country where the lives of people and wildlife are intertwined with mutual respect and tolerance. (These traits are indeed select for fitness to survive in a given environment. Survival of the fittest is often misinterpreted to mean survival of the most aggressive. Fitness is a much broader term.)

Even in the dry period, when the fields are an empty waste of charred and smoldering desolation, tiger's presence in them had been proved. For example in the summers of 1979, the officially documented fifteen attacks on humans were mostly from these tigers. The partially-eaten human bodies, which were recovered from Mohamdi and Mailani area of Kheri in the months of March, April, May and June, proved the presence of a micro population of sugar tigers ranging up to four animals. The latest attack in this series had come in July when a youth from Ayodhya village in Mohamdi was attacked about eight miles away from the forest area.

Repeated surveys have revealed one more key factor for this presence of tigers. Human interference and cattle grazing have degraded many outskirts of reserved forests in the Tarai. Herdsmen with their hundreds of cattle cross the threshold of forest, going three to four miles inside in search of fodder. As a result peripheral tiger population prefers to move out of jungle into sugarcane plantations, using it as a daytime lair, to lie down and snooze than to face constant disturbance in the jungle.

In this case, even the presence of huge buffer prey population entering the jungle is not an inducement enough to hold them inside and not to transgress the imposed barrier of their natural home, where they are presumably safer.

It is argued that sugarcane plantation is not a pleasant habitat. The edges of saccharum have silica deposits (silicon-dioxide, used in production of glass) which makes full-blown sugar leaves unpalatable. In some varieties of cane, leaves tend to become crudely rough and knife-edged and worry the cat by disrupting its movements. Yet, as tigers take to this habitat, it is possible that the gradual physiological adaptation to undulating fronds of sugar cane creates conditions which make a tiger's tactile adjustments with plant communities almost effortless.

Wildlife in Sugar Farms - A Prevue

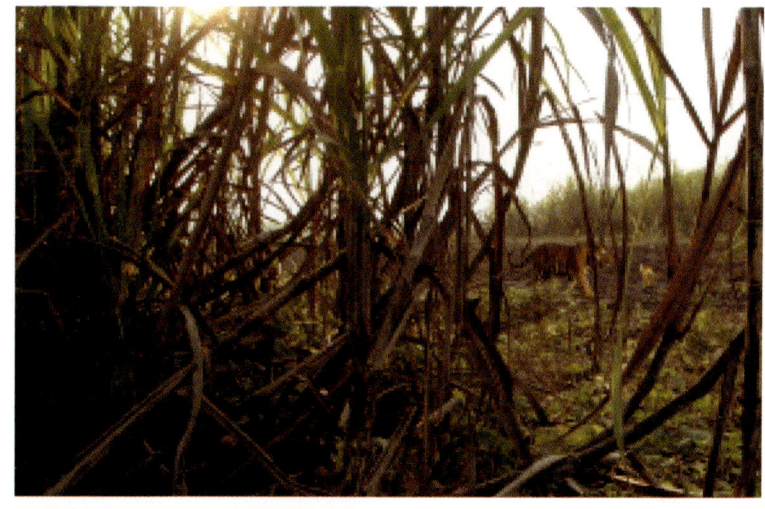

Wild animals are eminently adaptable to changing environs and even tigers are no exception to this rule.

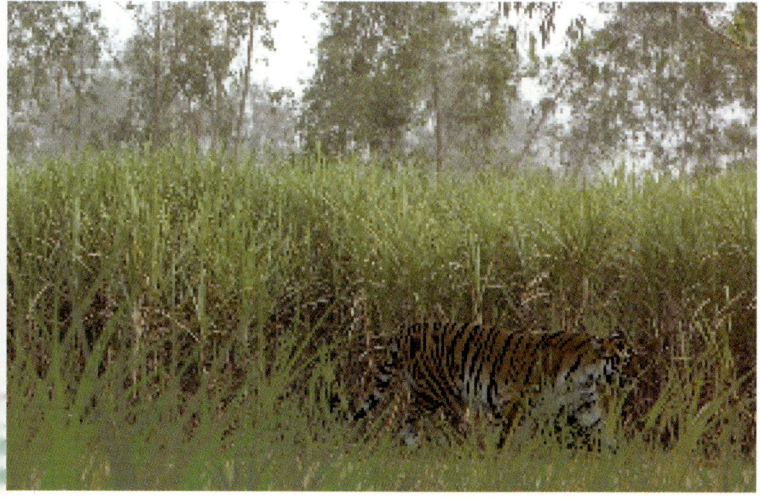

When the man manged sugar-grass is at its bloom, it is particularly a good predator habitat, no way inferior to jungle grasslands that work for the advantage of tigers.

The tracks deeply rutted by *Lehru*, and often ankle deep in dust, are frequented by tigers from dusk to dawn.

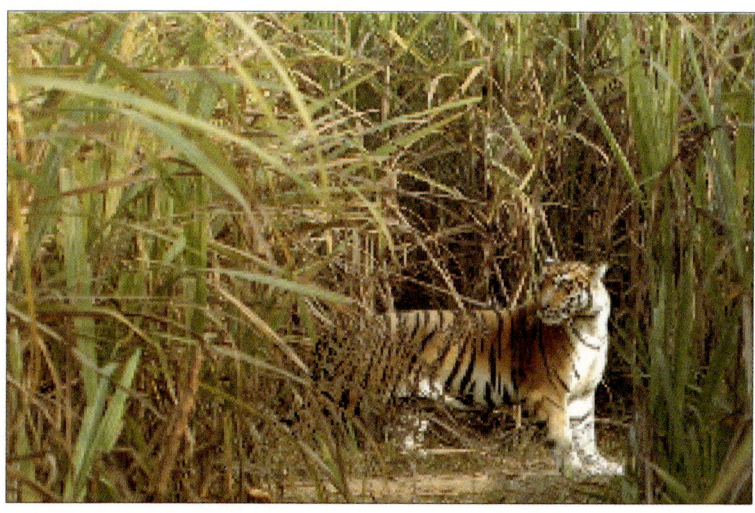

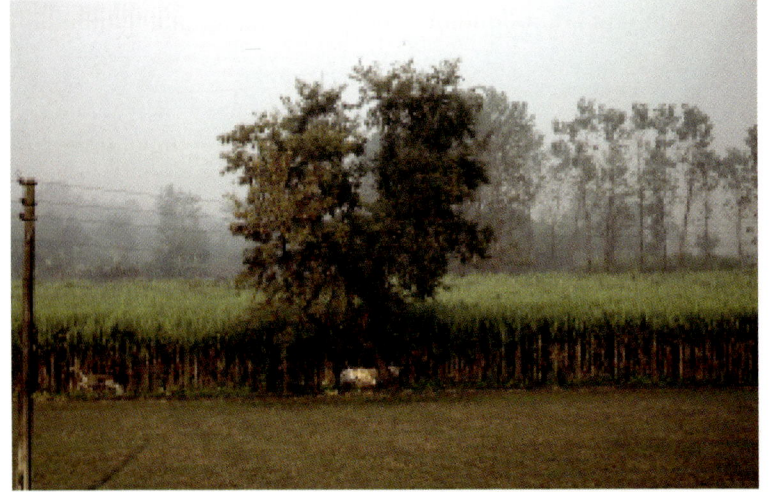

The croplands carry all the specific elements of wildlness such as water, cover, shade, sunlight and food.

When the pressures of farming, animal husbandry, forest product collection and huge developmental projects, degrade the physical quality of tiger habitats, sugar plantations provide quality concealment to farmland wildlife.

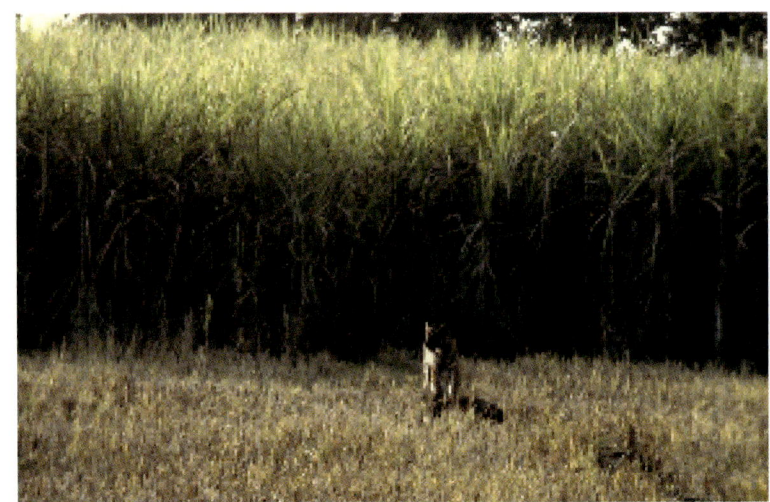

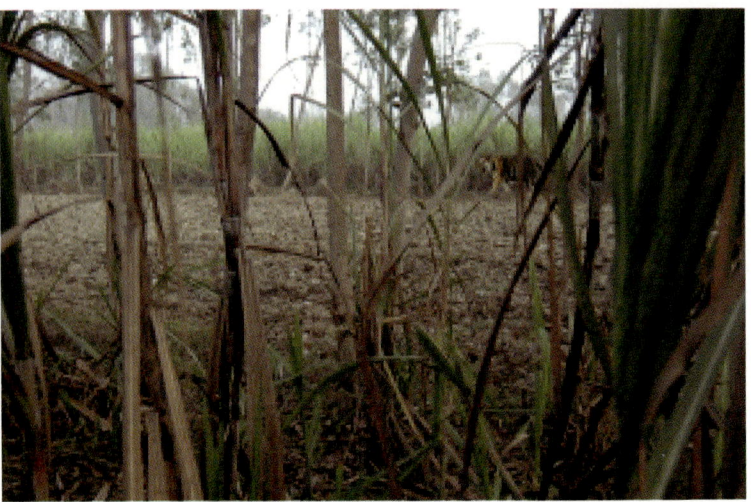

Breeding activity is closely linked with extended movements of large predators as well as with their 'ecologically surplus ability': when the activity level exceeds a location-specific threshold, it is probable to see tigers coming out in selected farmlands.

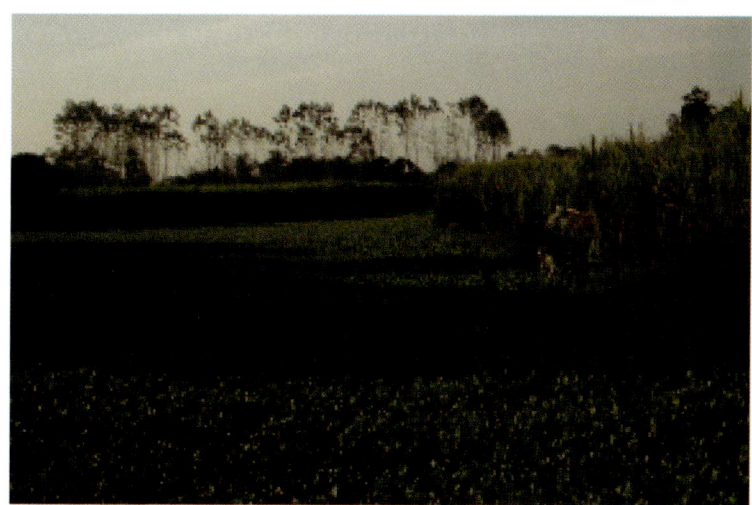

During monsoons, sugarcane crops develop knife-edged leaves that gradually wane off in strength after rains becoming droopy *patawar*. Tigers appear adjusted to this cycle and don't easily leave sugar farms.

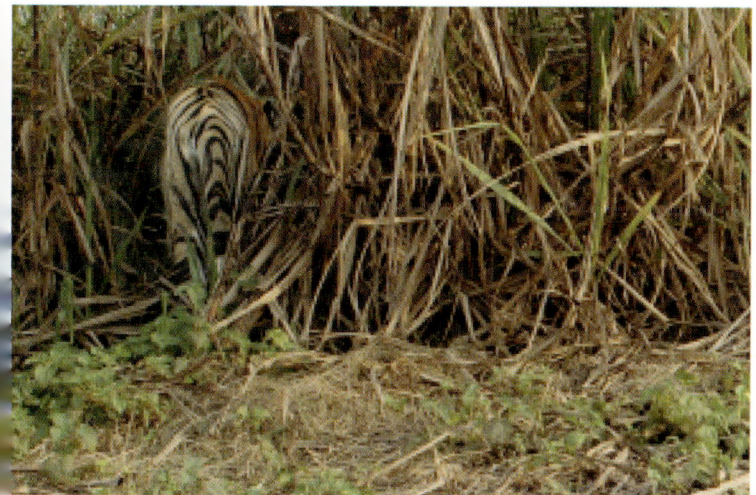

Some people consider tigers in sugarcane as nature's danger signal set as a warning, while others take it as nature's friendly signal and accept it as a reality.

There are no proper management strategies to protect wildlife outside the forests and the foresters, in their ecological ignorance continue to show the signs of confusion about the status of these tigers, which continue to live quite comfortably amidst human activity.

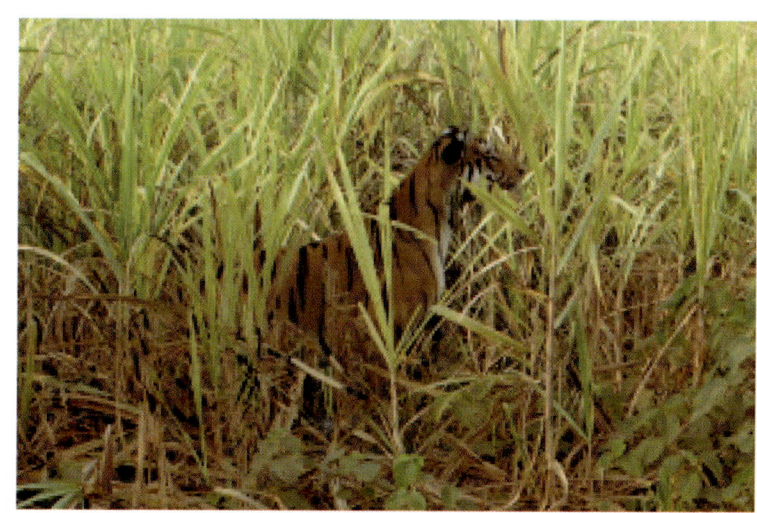

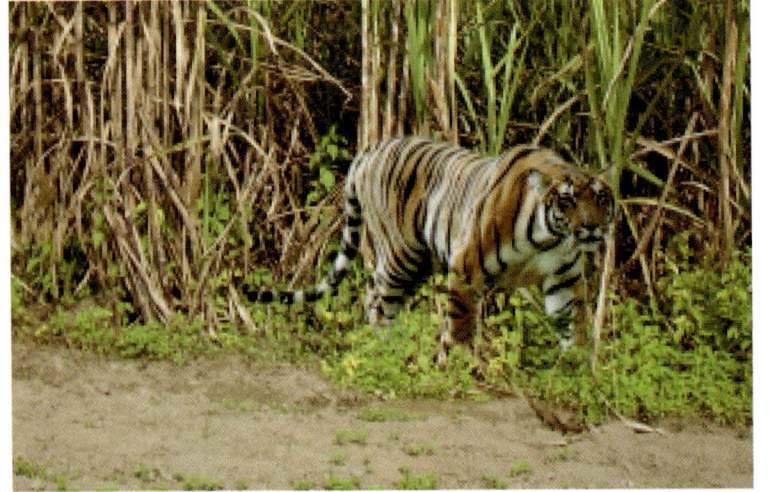

It is definitely surprising that big cats can hold on, on their own in a rural landscape that are often hemmed between thickly populated townships, and even people, not disturbing the quiet of their lives, are glad to pass on unmolested.

A tigress naturally searches for a dense cover to make nursery that should have well concealed interiors. The spot should also be located in a position from where it can be readily defended. These preconditions are instinctively sought by tigress, for her cubs are born blind and helpless.

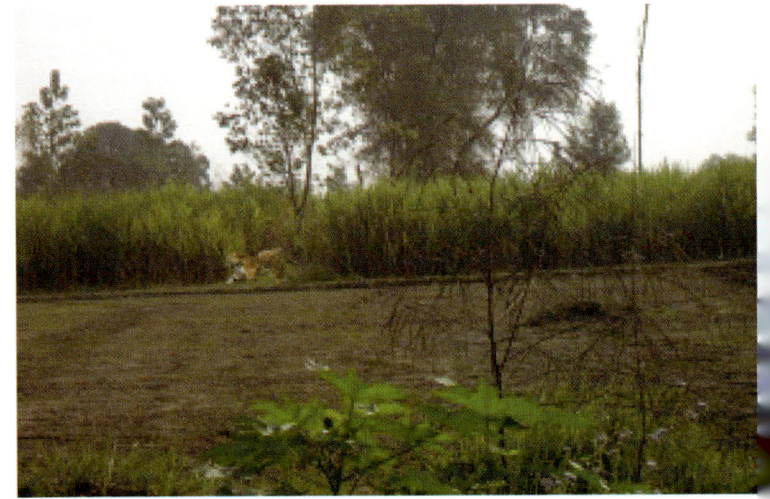

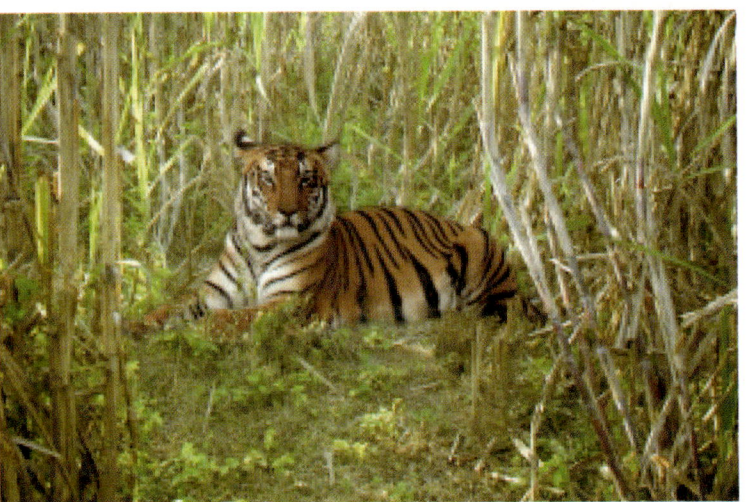

Anthropogenic pressure is a bigger controlling factor of tiger movements in farms than the movement of their prey and tigers do this with a decision of safety issue that under the circumstances would necessitate extraordinary restraint or caution.

Regardless of the scarcity of natural prey in some areas of Tarai, livestock losses to predators are never high and almost everywhere in the Tarai farmlands, unwanted feral cattle top the list of natural prey for tigers.

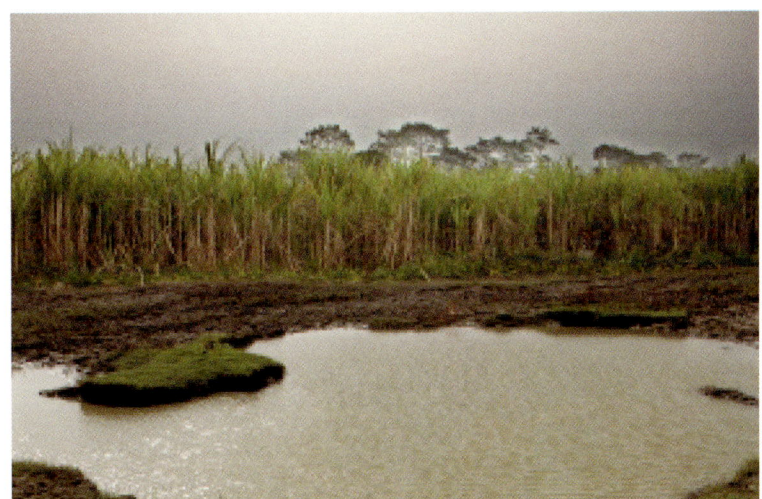

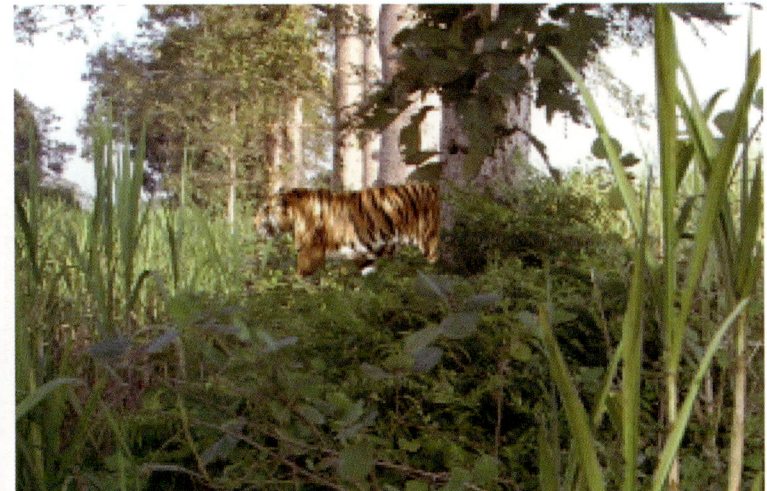

Tigers in farmlands are the compelling evidence of their former continuity- perhaps the progenies of positive 'eco-types' - whose gamble to change their habitat proved to be of advantage to them.

GPS points clearly indicate that these tigers live in farmlands 24x7.

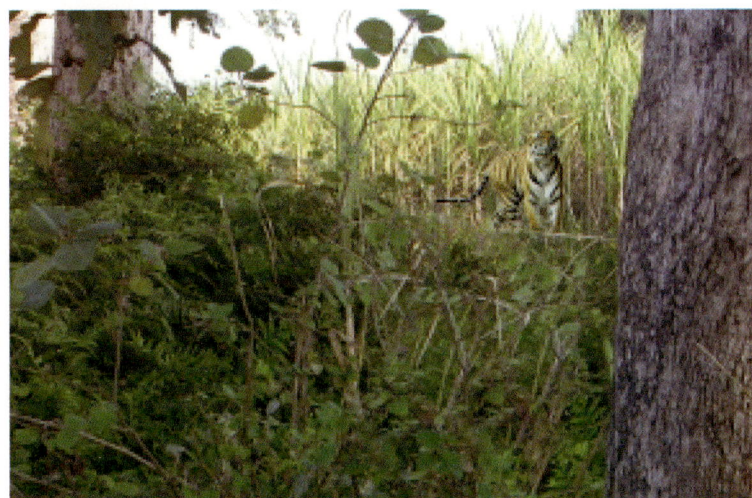

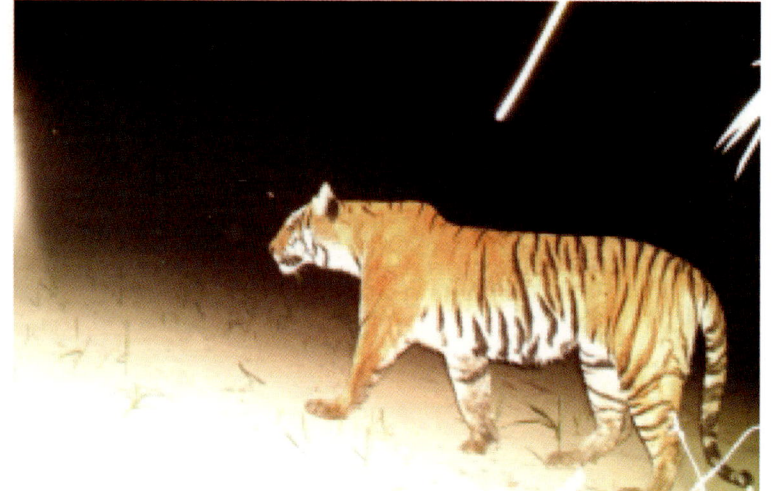

At some farmlands tiger is really trustful of man.

Tiger is no competitor of man but the killing of livestock spirals the man-predator conflict.

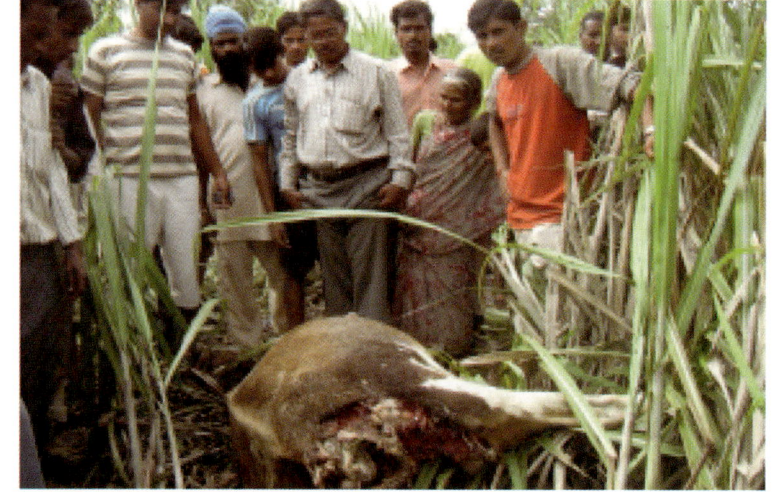

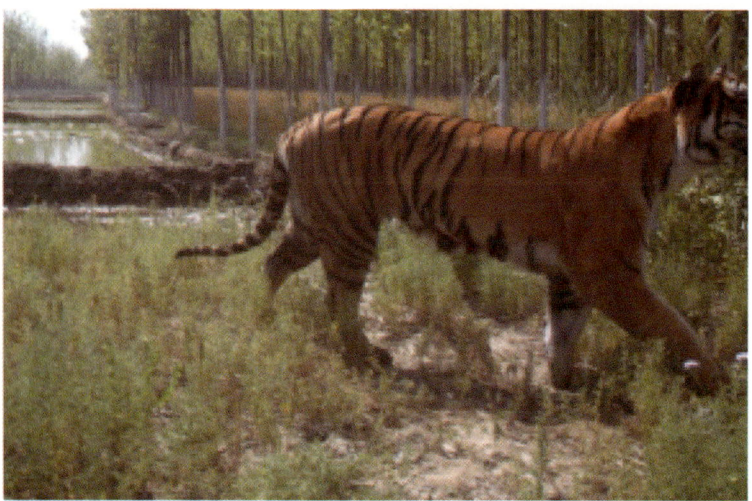

Tigers presence in sugar farms breaks through the scientific dogma that tigers belong only to the jungles. The established prejudice is a total nonsense or better to say a scientific passivity.

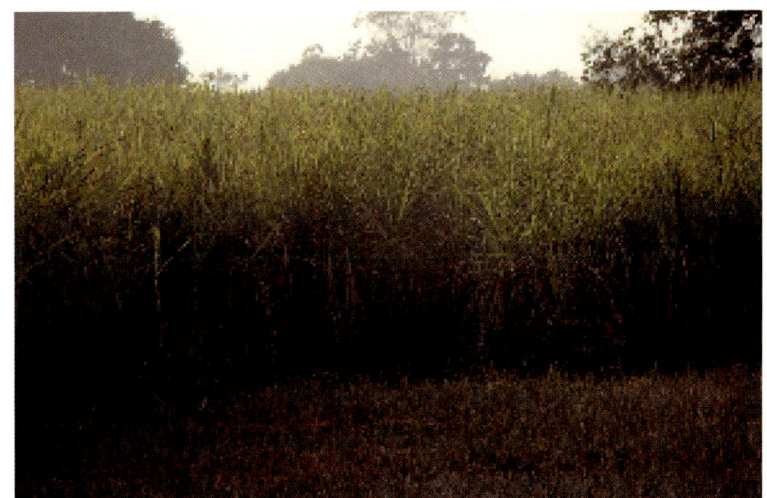

A young tiger cub does not have to proclaim its tigri-tude.

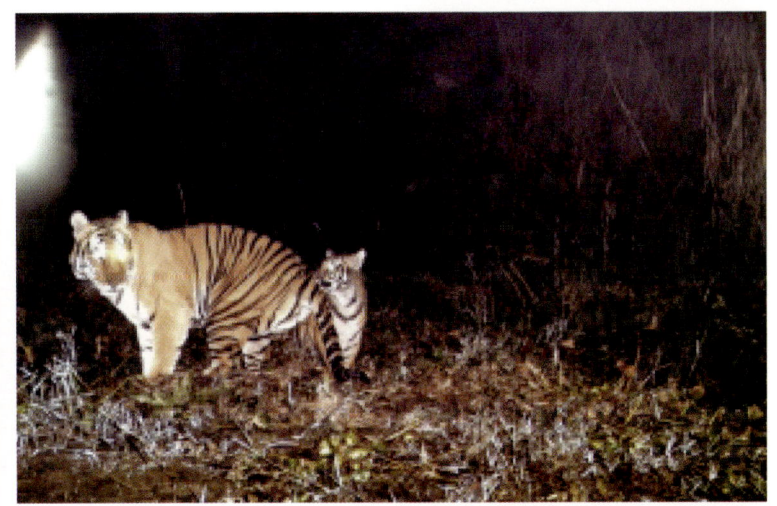

Because of the loose sandy texture of the soil, tracking was easy when we found this tigress with her cub.

Everything was in tigress's favour in this growth.

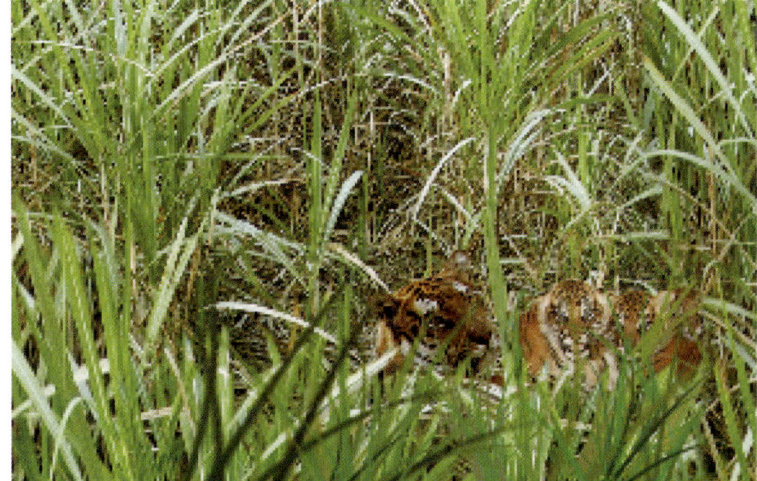

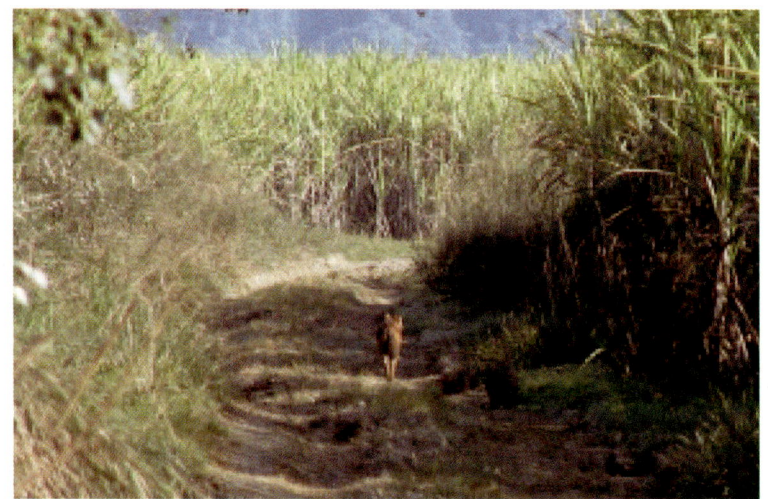

Jackals abound in sugarcane and relish its stems.

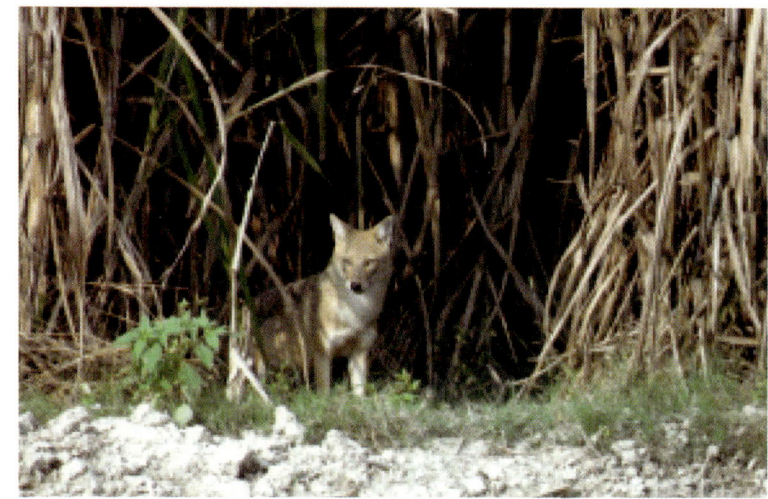

The sound of Tarai landscape is not the rumble of a tiger or the trumpet of elephants. It is the voice of the jackal that gropes through the coy virgin darkness, seemingly coming from nowhere yet everywhere.

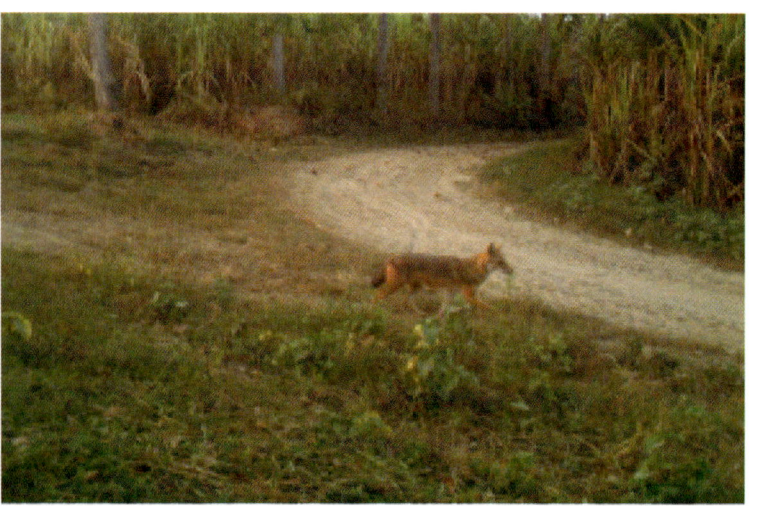

Like the croaking of frogs in South American Pantanal, the laughter of Hyena in Africa, the yowl of Cayoti in Prairie and howl Wolf in Taiga, the jackals caterwaul is indeed the apex spirit of the Tarai.

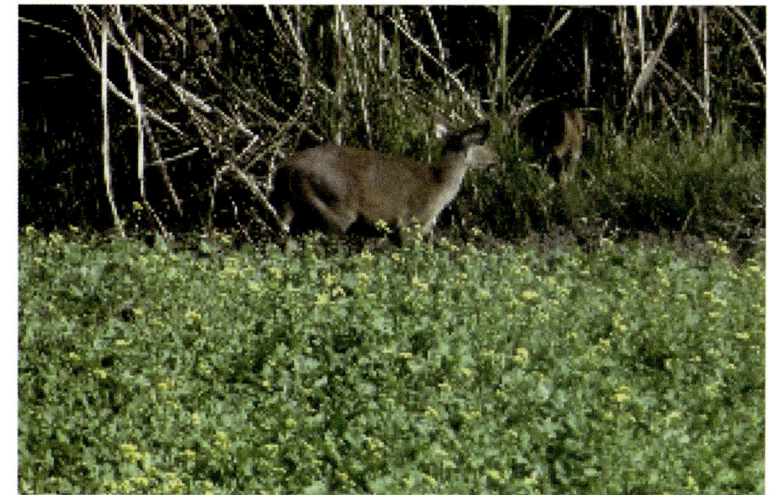

A hog deer finds refuge in sugarcane.

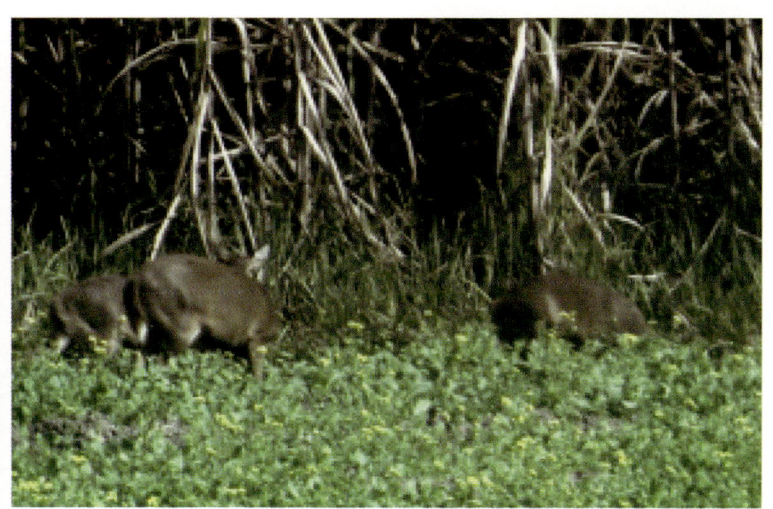

Hog deer, essentially a grassland animal considers sugarcane as an extension of grassland habitat.

These deers also serve as staple food for tigers in sugarcane.

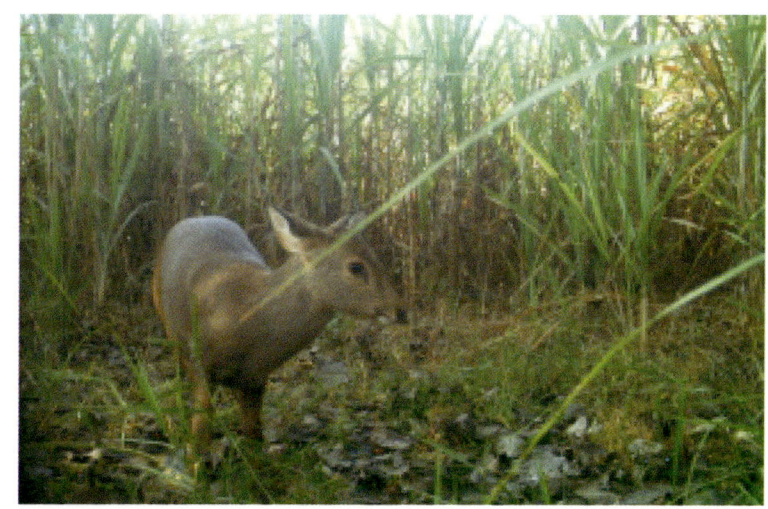

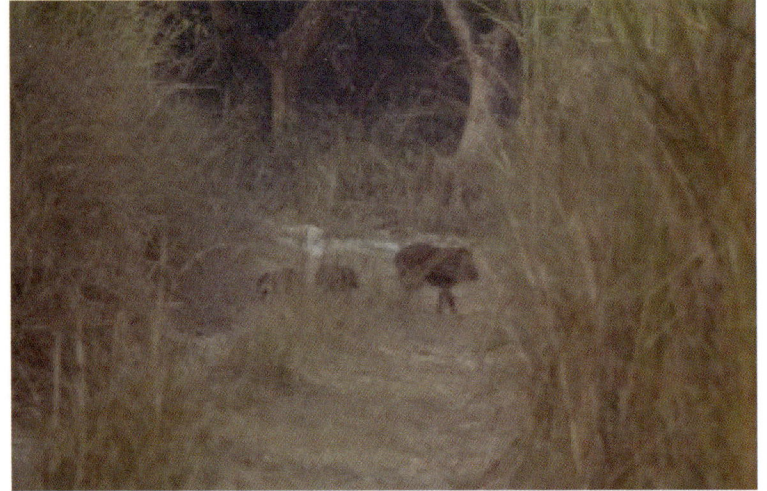

Wild boars delight in sugarcane.

A sow may deliver 15-20 piglets in one pregnancy.

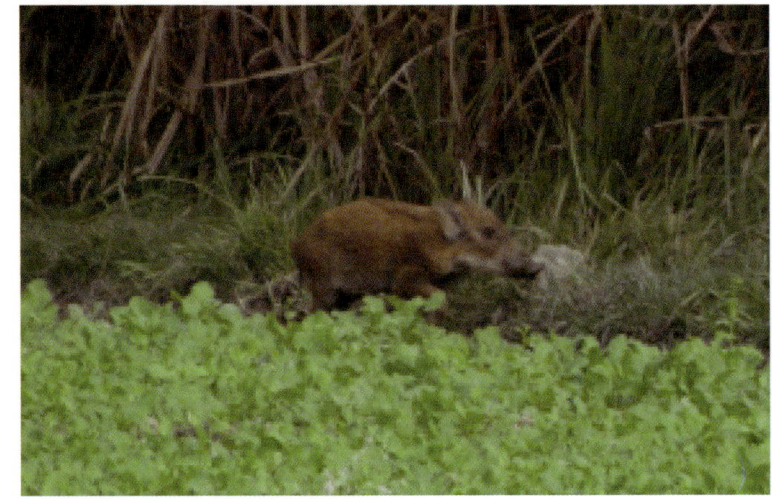

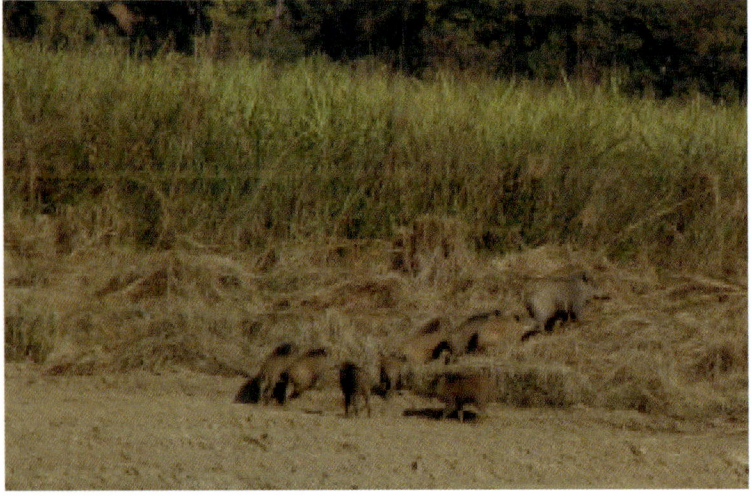

A wild boar sounder making way to a sugar plot through a ploughed field.

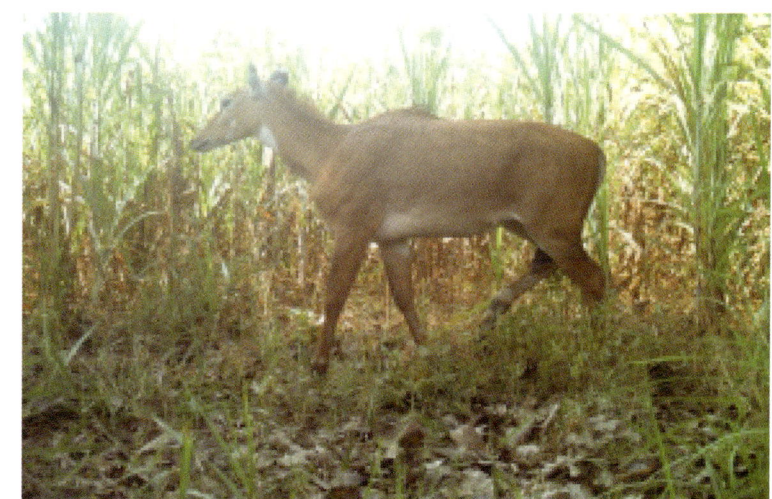

Nilgai is India's largest antelope.

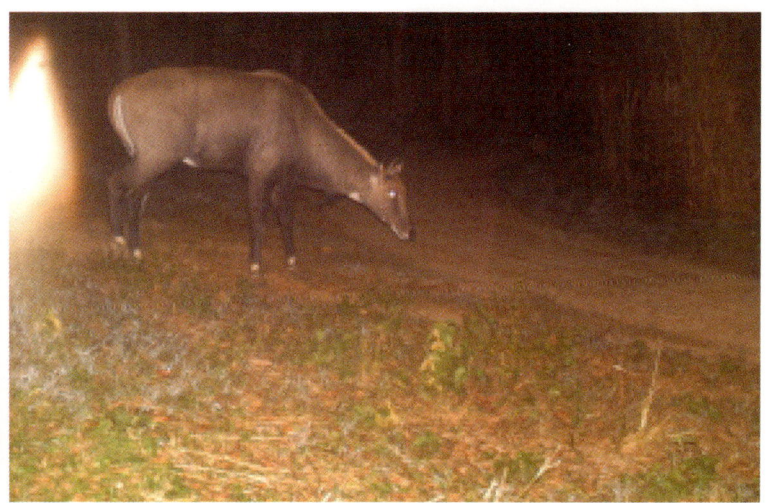

The burly, slate grey bull with its sloping withers, contrast sharply against sugarcane with their white stockings.

Black buck antelopes now extremely depleted in numbers still frequent remote Tarai farmlands.

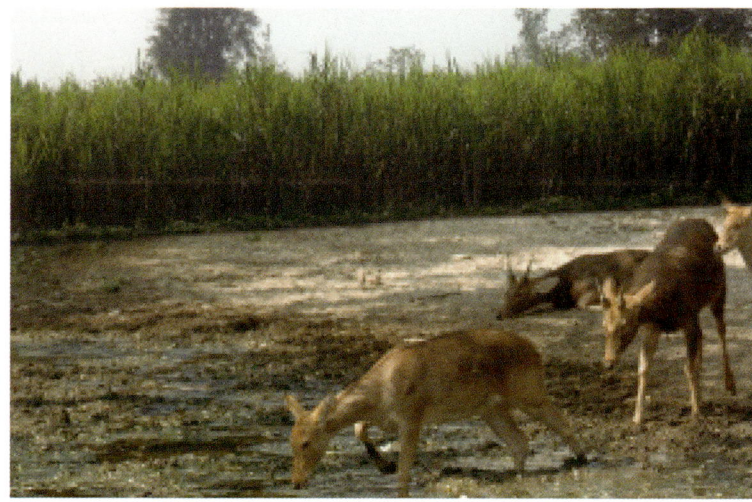

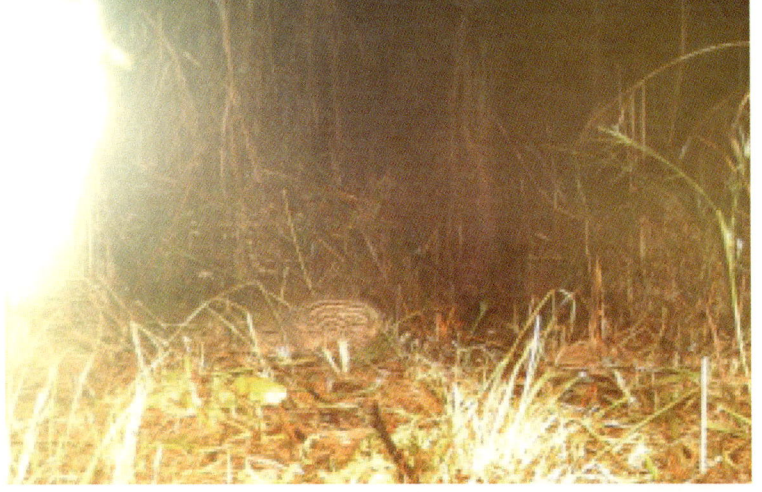

Small jungle civet in sugar farms near Palia.

A jungle cat in the sugar farms of Bela.

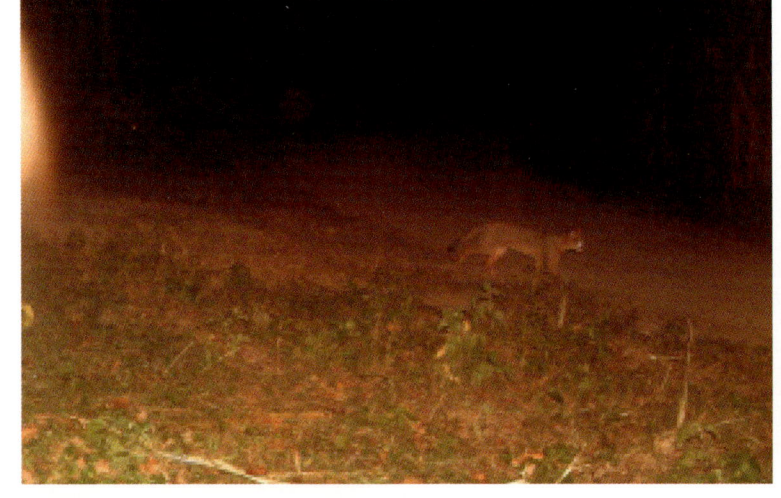

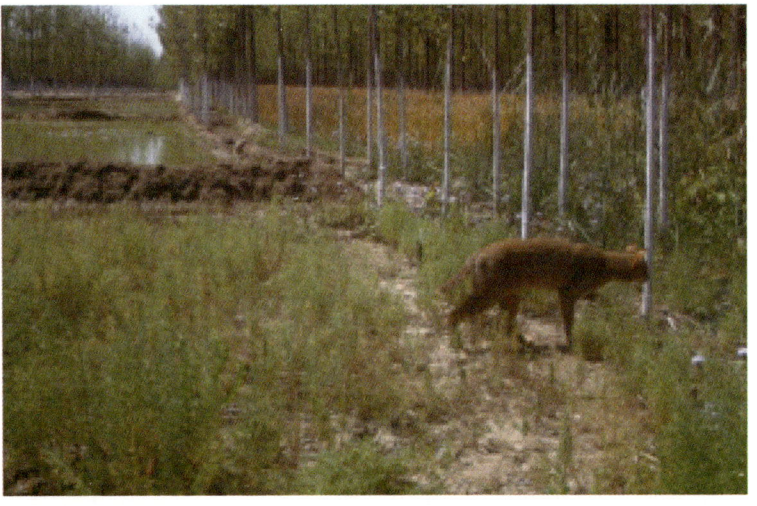

A fishing cat near Santgarh farm, Kishanpur.

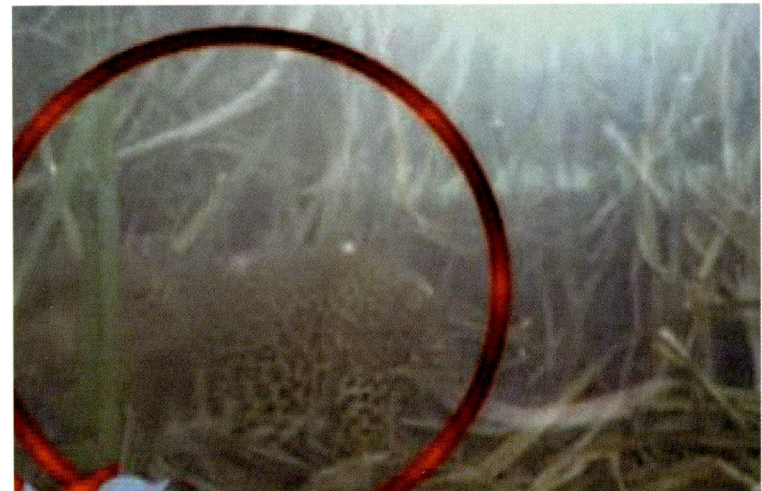

Leopard in sugarcane - census camera shot.

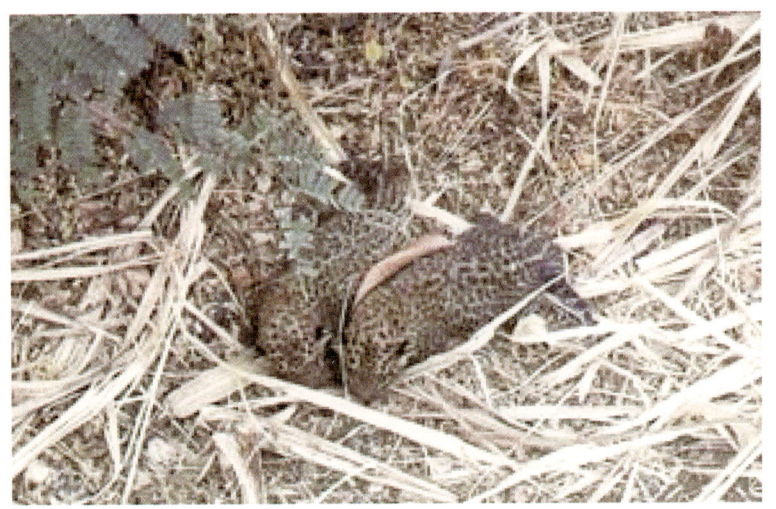

Leopard cubs are often found in sugar fields during harvesting.

A leopard caught inside a village house.

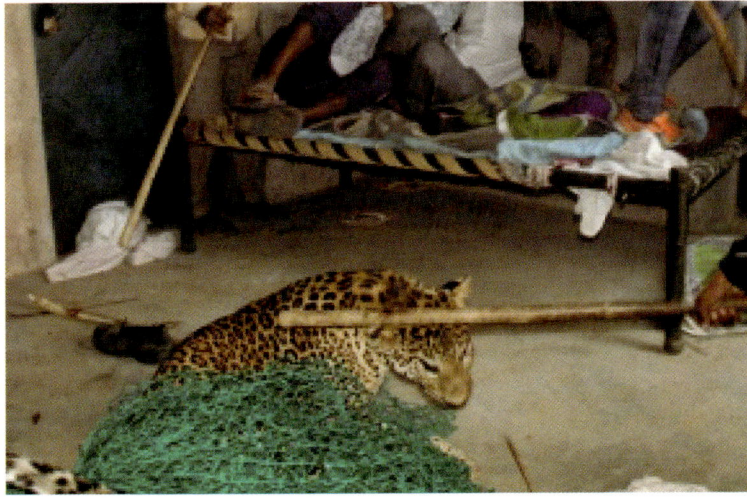

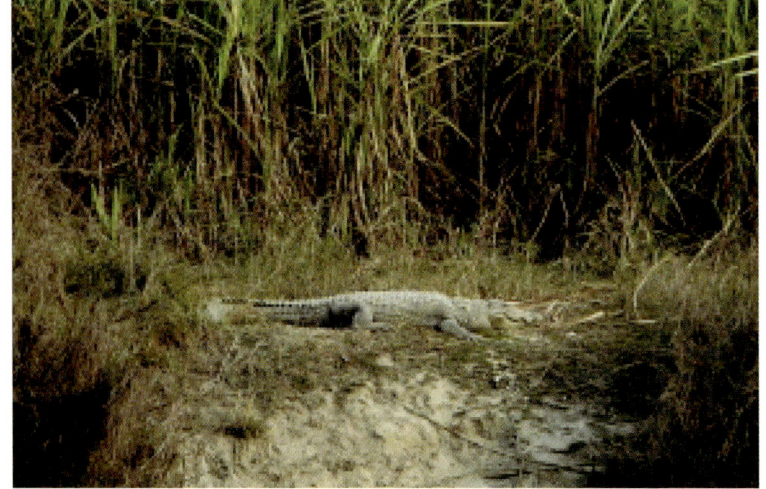

A crocodile basking in the sun near Katna sugar farms.

Tarai farmlands, once the favorite grounds of partridge shooters still harbor their remnants.

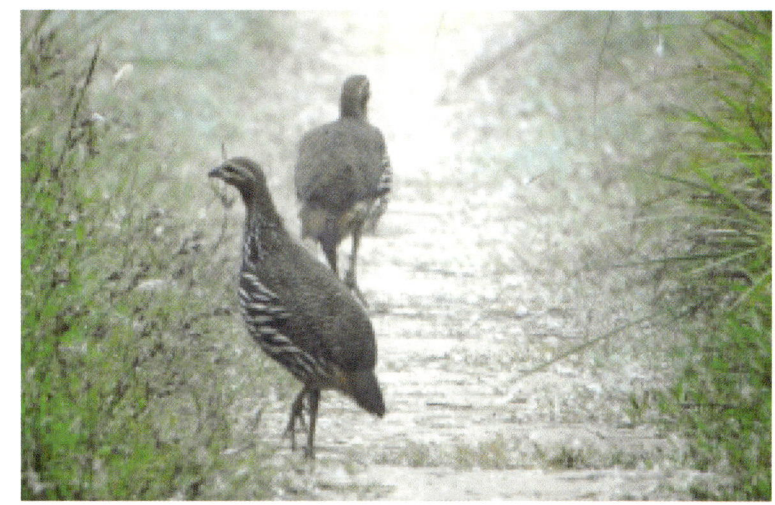

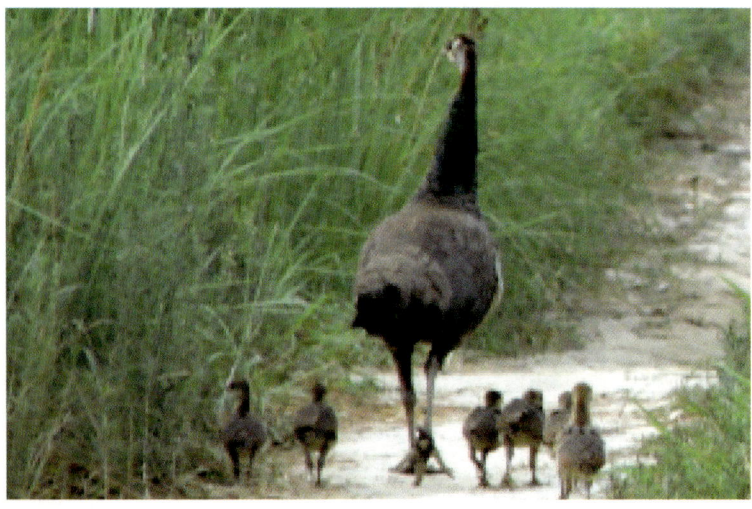

A peahen with her youngsters in sugar crops.

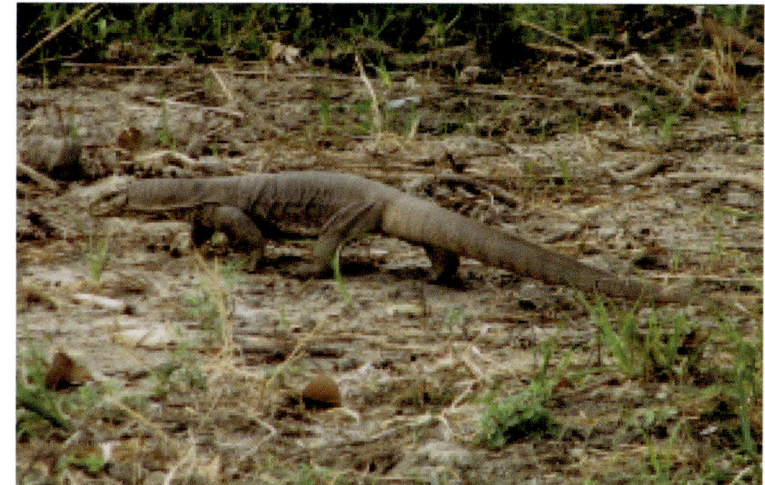

Iguana lizards are common residents of farmland areas.

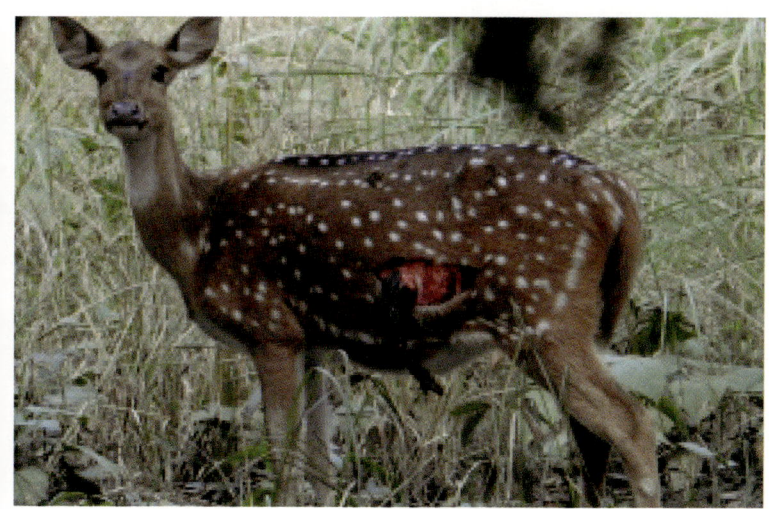

A pregnant chital doe injured by some predator.

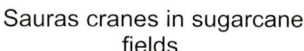

Sauras cranes in sugarcane fields.

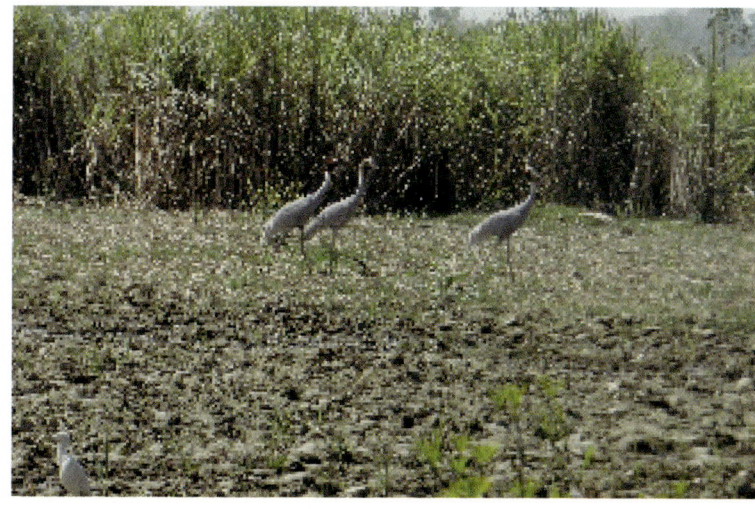

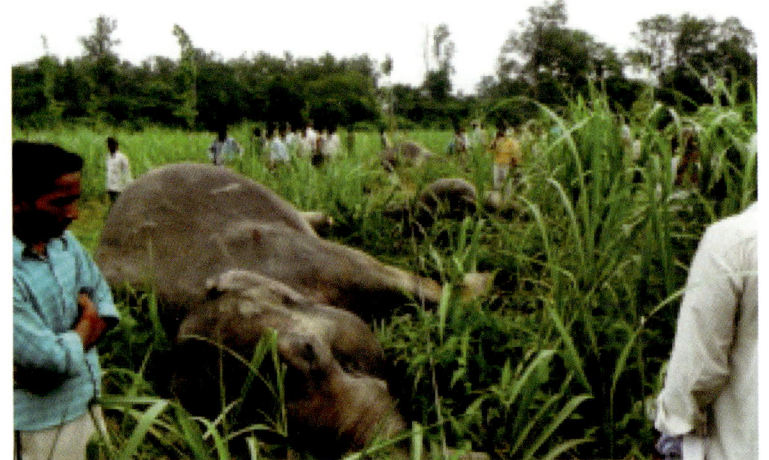

Wild elephant electrocuted by live electric wires.

Elephants also drink sugarcane wine and sleep for hours.

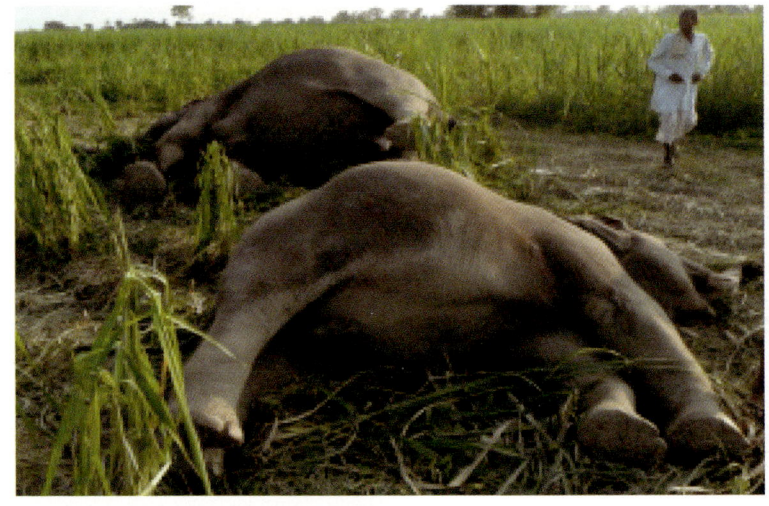

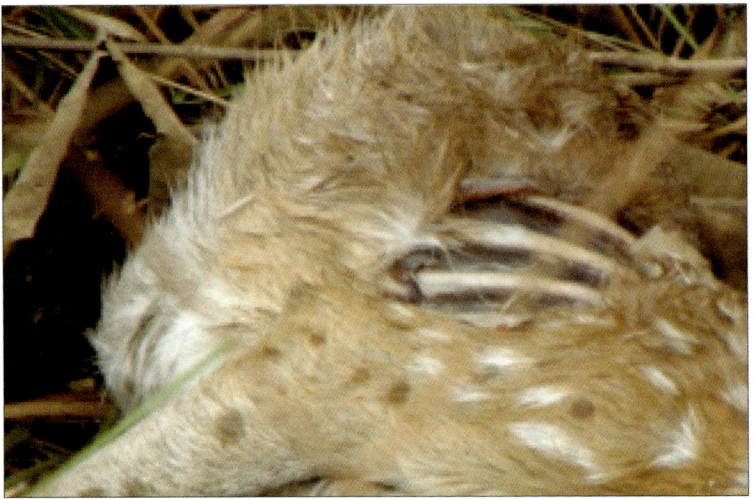

A chital killed by Jackal in sugarcane.

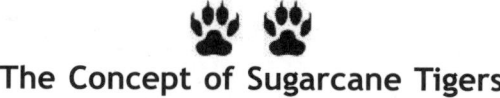

The Concept of Sugarcane Tigers

On man, on Nature, and on Human life, Musing in solitude..
- William Wordsworth

The more I watched these tigers, the more I realized that there are those stay-at-homes experts, who save tigers on computers, know nothing about the facts and conditions appertaining Tarai farmlands. These were tantalizing glimpses into the secret world of sugarcane tigers offering trains of thought for the future where I could put on my thinking cap on great logistical lines. As I contemplated their population increase in the farmlands this process became comprehensible on Malthus' analysis. Now it was becoming integral to my understanding of evolutionary mechanism of biologizing this ecological phenomenon in which the preponderance of animals was cut down by nature's own safety valve that is also called the nature's selective scythe.

Sugarcane plantations are an important land use in the Tarai and are a food resource for many omnivores. But this landscape is of low conservation value, for it does not fit into the way ecosystems are valued and governed. Moreover in agricultural landscapes no conservation strategies can be applied to protect the habitat loss for the wildlife that takes place at harvesting. Dangers for these animals include exposure to roads and vehicles and exposure to poisons such as pesticides. But a modicum of protection given to waste land patches and expanses of local unprotected forests, where various animal groups migrate during desiccated periods, is sufficient to make micro populations of cane tiger survive. These forests outside the protected area network fall under the legal jurisdiction of *gram sabhas* and play a critical role in conservation of farmland wildlife by providing important additional habitat for animal and plant species.

With the discrete surveillance of a researcher, these were the aces up my sleeve, the subtle stepping stones on which I hoped to get across to solid solutions. The pursuit of tiger, conducted on such lines, will afford ample scope for breaking new ground regarding their supplementary habits and the character in sugarcane fields, where they lived on a completely different scale from jungle tigers as if to suggest that they were quite at home.

As was always with me, it was a slow motion leap and I had to break through a scientific dogma that tigers belong only to the jungles. The established prejudice was a total nonsense or in better words a scientific passivity. I wondered as I always did, as how such a simple thing, so strikingly obvious, had not been obvious to wildlife managers in the past? Obviously one needs to be more attentive than natural to notice such facts. We needed to speculate this development under the process of natural selection, hence it was no extraordinary and odious instinct of tigers to search for cover anywhere, even inside human altered landscape.

The only obstacle in the growth of this tiger was the tremendous anthropogenic pressure they endured. The involvement of this factor in petite percentage might serve as a component, adding to the improvement of ecology and generating managed-wilderness of sugarcanes. But the increasing percentage essentially creates a diametrically opposite effect and perpetrates crisis. This absurd and self-contradictory juggernaut interestingly happens to be a key factor in determining the etiology of a tiger's adaptation to the farmlands. Tigers living here are forced to live in an area surrounded by humans because the sugar-crops are an entirely man-made environ; planted, watered and harvested by none else than the human agency yet paving the way for tigers to walk in. Thus human agency is a mandatory component of this feature, which maintains essential ecological processes and life support systems, to ensure the sustainable utilization of species and ecosystem.

It is my gut feeling that when the habitats, supporting larger breeding populations have already shrunk to a minuscule of about 1 per cent of their former range and are also biotically messed up, then in order to survive the species have to harden against anthropogenic pressures or eventually lose the battle. Thus many a tiger seemed most responsive to change that determines the qualifications of fortitude at much stronger levels than the jungle tigers because behavioral adaptation is a top quality trait which can happen far more quickly. The more intelligent the animal, the faster it can learn to make behavioral changes in order to survive.

The species with useful adaptations to the environment are more likely to survive and produce progeny than are those with less useful adaptations, thereby increasing the frequency with which useful adaptations occur over the generations *in situ*. Along this line of reasoning, sugar tigers are definitely more equipped to absorb multiple pressures. These tigers are reconciled to the crop and land use pattern and as the pattern exists unabated tigers also continue to exist in farmlands. The concept should not be confused with rhetorical tautology of survival of those who are better equipped for surviving; but it also contains an independent criterion of fitness for a segment of species to turn into a putative creed.

There were not many experts to contend like Billy but there were people in formidable authority to contend with, viz, the Director of Project Tiger, the Chief Wildlife Warden and many stay-at-home armchair conservationists. These individuals were emotionally loaded to save tiger in their strategies that were mutually exclusive and diametrically opposite to each other, that generated more heat than action and lead to policy paralysis regarding conservation of farmland tigers. They would bemoan the death of tigers in sugarcane but not alter their views.

The 'Ferocious Boundary Keeper of Dudhwa' Billy negated the cane tiger theory for sheer pseudo-scientific and obstructionist reasons asking me, "What a tiger will eat in sugarcane?" I reminded him that he had himself answered this question

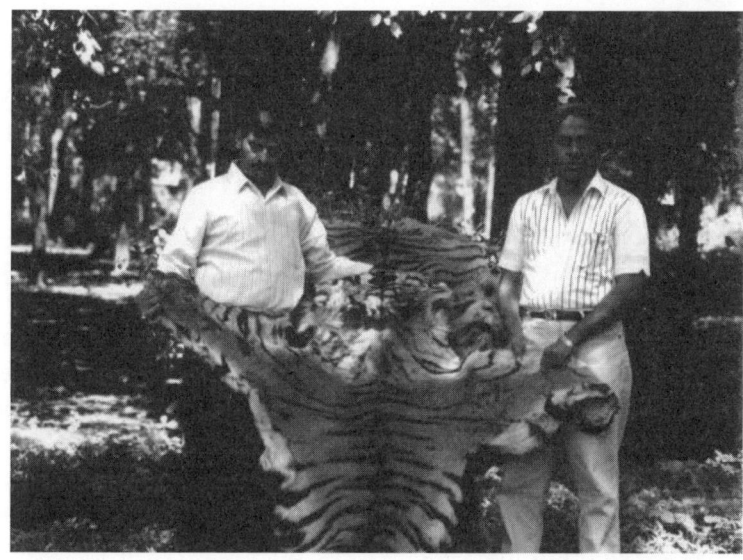

Author with two big tiger skins, he recovered from Banjara poachers in 1997. Standing with him is Yogesh Kumar IAS, then Commissioner & Secretory Revenue to the State Govt. (*Photo credit : J.V. Sharma, IFS)*

in his book *Tiger! Tiger!* as to what tigers eat in farmlands. He writes on page 52: "One reason for the respite was that although much of the virgin land had been cultivated, the tall grass had been replaced by an alternative form of cover almost equally well suited to tigers – sugarcane, which grows to the height of ten to twelve feet, and offers dense quiet shelter through the winter months. Tigers which spilled over out of the forest, when populations there became too high, lived and bred in sugarcane and marshes, and lived on wild pig and deer, which themselves subsisted on farm crops."

I told Billy that sugar farms harbor a complex biota of prey life and I had just added the names of few more species, like *nilgai*, feral cattle, pea fowl, *langoor* monkey, monitor lizards and pangolin into this prey list of tigers that were perfectly naturalized in farmlands, while their youngsters prey on species with which the bigger ones do not naturally meddle –dogs, goats and even chickens. And all these are normally available to tigers in human zone. Considering the preponderance of large mammals in a predator's diet, as they are evolved killers of big herbivore species, *nilgai* is the only large mammal whose viable population is not confined to the country's network of wildlife reserves. They are open terrain and farmland animals which are plentiful in Tarai.

Moreover there were also authentic reports of non-selective intake of small prey by tigers from many farm areas where ostensibly no leopards were reported. In fact in the farmlands the pyramid of life is bottom heavy with feral prey with no top predator to feed on them. Jungles may stand denuded of prey but farmlands are never devoid of ungulate prey base hence it is an extended buffet table for a tiger for its protein requirements.

Billy writes that tigers don't like eating beef while Brander gives a similar statement but in the context of hardcore man-eaters: "Confirmed man-eaters usually decline to kill buffalo or bullock but will often kill a pig or a pony, if these are tied up as baits, I have known other tigers, not man-eaters, to have a similar preference, but the disinclination of man-eaters to eat beef indicates that their palate has undergone some definite change."

I don't know for what reasons Billy twisted this statement for general disliking of tigers for beef and repudiated even George Schaller's findings that "Livestock had assumed an important role in providing the cat with prey in many areas." Is there any scientist worth his salt who would deny an iota of this truth in the fanciful claims that Billy made about tigers not liking beef? There are many researchers in the ranks of tiger studies, including Ullas Karanth who support this finding, yet Billy denied them with steadfast certainties and thus also my findings that feral cattle provide a great biomass to sugarcane tigers for their sustained living in the canes.

However Billy, living by the very floor of the unremitting phenomenon, continued to view it and kept his head buried in the sand on this point - while in theory, he continued to differ with me at any rate. His erroneously wide off the mark statement that tigers don't have much liking for cattle flesh was his oft-repeated wisdom. Though once held responsible for degrading habitat and potentially out-competing wild prey, the cattle have now been arbitrarily elevated to the status of buffer prey by scientists in recent reports. This punctures the bubble Billy lived in.

It is a fact that breeding females, rearing three or four cubs need more prey than a single tiger and scrutinizing all these points they carefully chose sugarcane farms as their nursery. Then how it can be expected to result in lowered carrying capacity of prey animals? Clearly, lowered prey densities would substantially depress the rates of survival of the cubs from the first day because in absence of proper food even mother's milk goes dry. Even juveniles are nutritionally dependent on their mother to a considerable extent. Hence my reasoning was that the tigresses knew better what suits them than the experts knew.

On reflection, I find Billy's arguments generated more heat than light and had many drawbacks. He spent more energy in criticism of my work than in understanding the phenomenon. Like half-mummified professors with an authoritarian style of functioning, he was ultra-conservative about cane tigers, whereas empirical appeal of my observations only served as a bombshell to boost my 'bad-boy' image - schooled in every sin and was prepared to invent a few more to preposterous extremes. However it took him years to evolve from being reactive to become protective of these tigers but as it happens, much biologically tragic loss had already occurred by then.

Science explains a phenomenon in logical framework experimenting with methods and outcome. However, in keeping with the biology of the species my synopsis steadily evolved. After years of critical scrutiny I was finally able to classify these tigers into three basic categories; A- the ones that come and go or cross the terrain, B- those that stay here by personal predilection, and C- those that have lived in canes for more than a generation. Experts believe that cats nurture complex behavior; some are predisposed to learn through human interactions (Prepared) and some are predisposed not to learn at all (Contra prepared). Keeping this in mind, I further classified these tigers into two more categories; the oriented and the disoriented ones.

The oriented ones used their energy with tranquility and thus knew the basic knack of survival in this landscape. Habitat reclamation for human use seemed to have no permanent impact upon them. Such tigers born in sugarcane do keep coming back to sugar farms as they reshape and mature. I am sure it is genetic memory that generates familiarity with the landscape, with the air and everything and they feel at home, like salmon or sea turtles going back home to their birthplace. They know the ways of sustenance in human altered landscape and hence they are *in situ*. They prefer hunting feral prey rather than frequenting the prey deficient jungles. Once this new prey composition is stabilized the offspring of these farm dwellers viz, transformed predators, easily naturalize with these dietary changes. R.L. Singh, who had first conducted the census of these tigers in farmland finally called it conclusive.

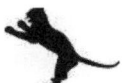

The Model of Behavioral Adaptation

Tiger is a creature of remarkably open modes of life and wherever they are living they are at their best for their presence by definition is the indicator of the strength of the environment.
— Author in a meeting of WWF, New Delhi

The fact that the tigers were living in the canes for years could be a tentative demonstration of the hypothesis that could help me arrive at a comfortable conclusion. The more I browsed my field notes, the more convinced I became of the challenge to discover such beasts and establish their identity. In the struggle for life, the chosen are those with some adaptive edge, some physical or mental advantage, which means they survive to leave offspring; they were being naturally selected. These are beasts that are capable of absorbing utmost pressures generated by humans like animal husbandry, developmental projects, poaching and habitat loss at the same time.

It is not a misery for wild animals forever multiplying and struggling for food. If so, then their death rate will be unimaginable. Cut-throat competition from over-population, caused by animal sex drive worked by thrusting out weaker ones, is a mysterious law, the central point of matter governing the extinction of species - the nub that Darwin hereafter called his theory 'The Natural Selection.'

It was vague but man is a creature of reason. To my mind, the problem lay with the behavioral adaptation of some animals, their ancestral blood ties with their homeland, where they were born and which repeatedly made their progeny return to the same environment and place.

Even this theory had to ultimately rest upon deep history and what is truly *terra incognita*. An ideal example of this can be found in sea turtles. Of the five species of marine turtles in this region, four nest on Indian beaches. Their nesting extravaganza takes place in Tamil Nadu and Orissa where over 200,000 Olive Ridley turtles come to nest for a week between February and March. Humans, dogs, birds, jackals and monitor lizards know when the laying season starts and where the eggs will be laid. Despite the colossal destruction of eggs and their hunting, turtles always return to the same beaches. In the way they pass by several uninhabited islands, which might serve as safe havens for egg laying and also keep the turtles protected, yet they travel to a disturbed zone. This clears a ground for a bigger debate as we rush towards understanding this practice because the source of their problem lies is their behavioral adaptation for the place and they can't get rid of it.

Another example comes from leopards in the western state of Maharashtra where, as per estimates, around 600 leopards are reported in sugarcane farms alone. They live there as they find ample food in them. These farms serve them as a good hiding place and if these leopards are displaced by wildlife managers and sent back to the forest, a region foreign to them, they panic and try to return to the place where they belong.

The repeated return of leopards from 60-70 km distance of a release site not only signifies their penchant for the sugar habitat but is also the problem of behavioral adaptation which the foresters well understand. In this case the leopards' home is not jungle, but sugarcane plantation where the common stock is living, their kin, cubs and mates and of course their prey.

However leopards are not at all a slandered model on which tigers living in sugarcane can be gauged because both the animals differ in body size and operate differently but behavoriul adaptation to land terrain is definitely a solid model. Similarly when the mother tigress brings up her cubs in sugarcane nurseries and as they mature they get to know their home and its laws under the tutelage of their parents, triggering their steady establishment in the land. So the question was – whether indeed just a miniscule part of this population could be acclaimed as a compulsive creed of sugarcane tiger; the hard-core dweller of this habitat with farmland life-history characteristics that lives here by propensity and improvement. Because when the cubs are almost fully grown and the tigress leaves them to

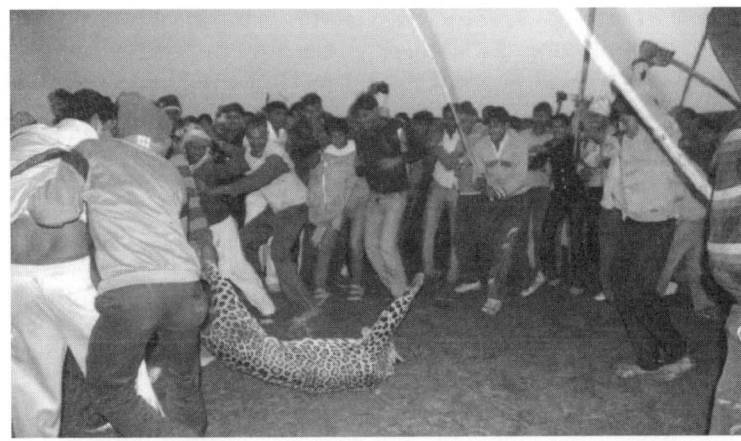

A scene of man -leopard
conflict in Maharashtra
(*Photo credit : Vidya
Atraya*)

prepare for independence, some individuals are presumably more familiar with the
habitat where they are raised and where they feel naturalized, and thus are better
able to take on.

Naturalization is a process in which an organism becomes the citizen of a different
environment other than that its birth and the naturalized citizen always renounces
allegiance to its native land and slowly but directly becomes committed to allegiance
to his adopted environment. Now I had a concept, I coined a new term to encapsulate
it, calling these the sugar-cane tigers. This mint fresh nomenclature first appeared
in my book *Killing Grounds* in 1993.

Disregarding this hard practical fact gained from innumerable hours of fieldwork,
Billy questioned me as on what biological basis this classification was determined
whereas Kailash Sankhala, the pioneering Director of Project Tiger, was delighted
to call it a "remarkable discoverer achievement." He had bought a copy of my book
from the market. He even said to me at his home in Jaipur: "For me a tiger is tiger
whether living in the jungle or farmland, a zoo or a circus, but strain counts. It is
basically the strain which divided tiger families into eight sub-species, from Siberia
to China and from India to Bali. Moreover, a zoo or a circus tiger doesn't represent
a wild strain. These are out-of-the-wild tigers. They can't cope with the hard living
of true wilderness. If they are left in the wild, they will die. After reading your book
I feel sure that generational cane tigers might be representing an eco-type strain
and they are equally at high risk of extinction from poaching… Poachers must be
playing havoc with any putative strain which might be evolving in these tigers…
You need to generate a considerable media attention to support funds for this
cause."

Scientists believe that over the years, neuron conditionings of some animals
evolve, predisposing them to interact with their environment in a certain way and
this lot transforms into eco-type animals, and therefore these predators have now

come to be called as sugarcane tiger. This nomenclature may be disagreeable to many experts but the neologism is not. Similarly animals may be less in numbers and may not be noticed much till their number multiplies, but I believed that cane tigers were least known to the tiger scientists of the world. I wanted the scientific community to undertake such research and carefully review their matrix. For it could possibly be a behavioral code of putative strain if not biological. This is what qualitative researchers call filtering science through logic.

Although survival and fecundity rates for tigers in moderately healthy populations were known to foresters but changes to these rates due to poaching and prey depletion were poorly understood. Moreover cane tigers were no body's chattel or even worse an ignored lot, though equally endangered, rare and valuable lot like jungle tigers. Therefore no demographic modeling could be used in recording their decline, the cause of which seemingly did not rest on the prey depletion but more on anthropogenic forces. The mortalities of tigers (both adults and juveniles) resulted from systematic poaching through poisoning, electrocution, netting, trapping and of course illegitimate sport shooting. And all these deaths, called poaching-mortality, would ostensibly have more destabilizing effect on any possible development of a putative strain if there was one in building. Poachers were least concerned with these biological intricacies as to which strain they were eliminating. Tigers were just money for them.

Death by poaching is entirely different form the background mortalities of tigers that are attributed to disease, dispersal into inhospitable habitat, inter-species violence and poor survival rate of litters due to starvation, which is a significant effect of prey depletion.

Reports affirmed that cane field tigers are generally known to local people but are often not known to foresters and therefore these never find a place in national statistics.

Arguably when we can't restore their lost wilderness and the goal of tiger conservation is to save each tiger, then each native individual in tiger-operated farmlands is the key to farmland wildlife preservation for we lack a wildlife set-up authorized with exclusive assignment of controlling hunting in farmlands.

Years of focused study had helped me establish benchmarks for tigers' presence in farmlands. But I had also observed that foresters hardly knew about selective occupations of tigers in rural areas though the natives knew. Natives were the first and last agents that ever guided me to these tigers for it was they who had suffered from the problem animal and tolerated the death of their cattle. And in face of worst conflict they became allied to anti-wildlife conservationists, and clandestinely helped poachers, smugglers and trophy hunters. It was their resentment against conservation that the tigers were poisoned in reprisal and it was by their will that the super-predator could live on their land or diminish away. It was principally through natives that I learnt about these tigers.

To my mind the natives are the unproclaimed stewards, not captors, not owners but keepers and unwilling custodians of these tigers. Their assembled know-how often represented an impressive chunk of tiger craft. Yet, the situation is highly anomalous for they don't know that the existence of flag-ship species is greatly threatened; it is getting ready to disappear from their world. Throughout Tarai when a tiger dies its cadaver is essentially discovered by some native. A grazer who takes his cattle far off in glitches to feed or a honey collector who scales swamps or a grass cutter is usually the first neutral informer of such deaths. Long before the media and officials reach the site, the natives are already there, standing, surrounding the dead god.

Like a honeybird which has inexhaustible knowledge of the whereabouts of beehives, the native remains first and primary in my research with their inexhaustible bank of information about local tigers, adding new shades and colours to my spectrum of understanding. Ordained by destiny I was determinedly set on generating a new fund of knowledge on farmland wildlife, which then in the 1980s and 90s, was something, unprecedented in the history of Indian wildlife conservation.

Post publication of my book *Killing Grounds* I worked like one possessed, writing letters to Forest Department, Project Tiger and many other international wildlife organizations to take conservation initiatives for the cane field tigers or at least send their envoys to gather a firsthand appraisal of phenomenon. Though the response of individuals as well as of organizations was that of acceptance towards my findings and sympathetic to the cause but it was least proactive. I was a non-official player, and assisting recovery of tiger population in farmlands was an idea that sought sanction of official players whose official response was always unclear. The importance of animal rights was sidelined by the supremacy of human rights. Reputed national magazines like *Outlook* and *India Today* cared to publish grand photographic features on the subject. But the plight of the wildlife in the farmlands remained unheard and no conservation organization came forward to help me in preservation of this microcosm.

The idea of 'tigers in sugarcane,' and 'sugarcane tigers,' 'hardcore dwellers of sugarcane,' slowly gained traction in wildlife circles. Though these remarks were only in the nature of hypothetical theories but one fact was firmly established that tigers were there, living in the sugarcane farms and perhaps some of these had already developed eco-type tendencies. There was no denial of this phenomenon by any agency. This debate had transformed a non-subject into a significant issue, becoming a pain in the neck for forest officials, who looked at these tigers as an additional burden foisted on them. The only problem with experts was that whether these were 'tigers in sugarcane' or the eco-type 'sugarcane tigers' as I called them. These were real wild tigers in farmlands whose genes were inextricably mingled with those of other tigers in the park and whose descendents might well continue to tenant farmlands for generations to come if not poached. For better or for worse—and I was convinced that it was for better, they needed protection seriously on similar scales as jungle tigers deserved.

Experts also had no answer to my question whether these tigers were a result of conservation success or conservation failure. They rather liked to content themselves with the responsibilities about health of their jungles and constantly blamed the Central Government for the paucity of funds and for the lack of technical and financial expertise in wildlife issues. The lack of funds for salary of field staff and filling of the posts that had fallen vacant due to the retirement or death of the guards seemed to have deterred them from fulfilling their constitutional responsibility to protect wildlife outside reserves.

Regarding lack of staff, this is no off-track information that in Uttar Pradesh State, no regular selection of Forest Rangers and Assistant Conservators of Forests (ACFs) has taken place since 1988-89. This is 2016 and a piled up volume of vacancies in State Forest Department is yet not advertised while real field staff is reduced to more than half of its strength.

The Secretary of Environment Ministry dismissed this idea, pointing out that the salary component was very marginal compared to the amount given by the Centre for Project Tiger. In addition there were strict guidelines to protect landscapes around wildlife reserves. Lands falling within 10-km boundaries of national parks and sanctuaries were yet not notified as eco-fragile zones. Foresters still did not understand as to which factors drove the tiger population dynamics in sugar farms, or what made them leave the forest cover and reside in this artificial landscape. Their only answer was that the forests are fragmenting but had no plan as what could be done to de-fragment them. While all this wrangling was going on, I was continuing my work, disconsolate and alone worrying for my overreaching goal of protecting farm tigers.

Appendix to Chapter 4

My studies had taken off on a steep tajectoy and villagers were willing to repose their trust in my insufficient efforts to protect these tigers despite the turbulence and enormous difficulties caused by sporadic incidents of man-tiger conflict

- Author in a WWF Symposium, Lucknow

A simplified analogy for paradigm is a habit of reasoning on old lines inside the box that is analogous with normal science. The box encompasses the thinking of standard science and thus the box is analogous with paradigm. And on these lines there cannot be any sugarcane tigers because tigers don't live outside jungles. But I was thinking "outside the box", this is what science historian Thomas Kuhn calls revolutionary science. It is usually unsuccessful, and only rarely leads to new paradigms but whenever it is successful it leads to large scale changes in the scientific worldview.

The classification of sugarcane tiger though presented some difficulty and varied according to the views of individuals. But as regards their protection my contention was that all the tigers wherever they are found, are essentially the same beast though they vary considerably in types according to the environment in which they live. Thus the tigers taking to farmlands must also be included in tiger conservation schemes outside the protected areas.

Immediately after the publication of my book *Killing Grounds*, I applied for a fresh project with WWF and Project Tiger in 1998, asking for some monetary help. My idea of farmland wildlife was rejected by both the bodies (incidentally now both bodies acknowledge this issue as important in their agenda that needs to be handled with all seriousness.) The self-proclaimed experts were just unable to believe that there is a plethora of wildlife in rural areas, which can support a tiger's living. I was perhaps portraying an erroneous picture - something so odd like existence of a strange man-eating elephant or something similar, whereas the animal in question is supposed to be strictly herbivorous. I felt lost for some time as there were no takers for my initiative. It even created a crisis of confidence as what the hell I was doing, but if I abandoned the cause I could never live with myself.

I reminded the Forest Department official in 1986 when 14 tigers were found poisoned in sugarcane fields around Dudhwa. It showed that harassed people really did not feel compensated with the money and had attempted their own clandestine resolutions to the conflict by poisoning livestock kills made by tigers. It was a biologically tragic loss, as most of the dead were healthy breeding females and the situation warranted a warning signal to guard against future ecological disasters. But a wildlife department official was arguing on logical lines: "With all noise and activity in farmlands it seems beyond reason that any wild animal would risk its life in such surroundings."

"You need not look surprised at these curious facts. They show that my investigation is not only taking the right direction, but it is something to reckon with as extraordinary," I told the doubting man, with much irritation within myself. "Project money is nothing to me in this case. I can burn it if it can be of any use in enlightening you to the truth. Tigers are living there. These tigers are a unique resource for scientific research, and you must understand that. Any way if government is not interested in their conservation I cannot force them to be," was what I could say.

The heavy clouds wrapping the top mandarins' brains seemed immovable. My emotional speech was for him some kind of fiction conjured up over years, while within me there was a realization that what the hell was happening. In light of such fundamental differences, I was fighting with my own government to protect this eco-type tiger. Henceforward it was a battle that could only end in defeat. The problem is that our great grinding bureaucracy doesn't take advice - it only gives advice, pressurized as it is by the attitude of politicians.

It was tragic for me and even more tragic for tigers. The official had grown to associate size, stealth, strength and carnivorousness of a tiger only to wilderness and his gratuitous statement was: "no super predator can inhabit the farmlands." The eccentric argument easily sounded convincing when rendered in an air-conditioned office in Delhi but in Tarai fields it was disconnected from reality where presence of tiger in sugarcane was actually re-colonization of an animal back into their homeland. "If it goes everybody will be a loser, including you, me and finally the tiger," I said as I finally accepted the homage of his irrationality to my reason and left the room.

I must confess that I applied for no less than six projects but none of them materialized. The possibilities of my project were always shattered because I was no zoologist by education and I was not expected to work out things with a scientific temper. Moreover since it was a matter dealing with the Tarai's turf then Billy's expert opinion was ritually sought on the subject and it is needless to say he too was no scientist. Billy never missed an opportunity to launch entirely unprovoked attacks on my projects, even overemphasizing the untoward consequences likely to follow if it was approved by mistake, though at the same time underemphasizing the impact of man-tiger conflict in sugarcane zone with rigid attitude.

Somehow on my part, I felt that these developments were unlikely to radically change the thrust of my research and I had yet a long way to go. I thought of the loneliness through the years that I had gone through while on this venture, I had worked alone and was accused of being highly subjective in my performance though I was just slamming the hopelessly distorted views about tigers, portrayed by conventional pundits and the professional coterie of biologists - mostly zoo-keepers and wildlife academics, that were invariably absorbed in learning the biology of tiger inside reserves without any understanding of its behavior outside the sanctuaries. My objection was at the lax empiricism of contemporary conservationists and their facile tendency to treat all ailments with same prescription. They felt I was relying too much on haphazard uncoordinated individual experience of natives about tigers that could not generate any intelligible record of results.

There I was - without funds, but money or no money, like a warrior, I felt committed to save these tigers, and at the same time, if possible prevent further human casualties. It was a key challenge to farmland tiger conservation, a magnificent enterprise and I had to take a positive step to bear this formidable responsibility. Conservation of farmland wildlife was not an opinion to be held but it was

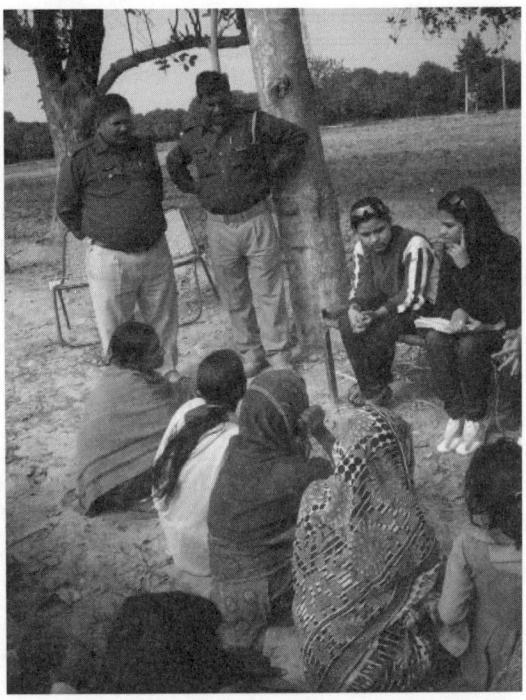

Shrivridhi and Samridhi counseling villagers.

work to be done. Least I knew that by offering sugarcane tiger theory I was laboring hard to lay the foundations of a new chapter, where nobody's attention had yet gone; the importance of farmland wildlife, making their survey and marking out fort hem their proper and distinctive fields.

I had learned from long experience that when one follows a separate chain of thoughts one finds some point of intersection which should approximate to the truth so the foresters were needed to be educated on this line of reasoning. To start now they had to understand that there was a commendable cycle between sugar plantations, tigers and farm animals that kept both the prey and the predator energized. In some cases where the fields were far off from the regular forests, such as the area of Barotha tigers that opportunistically eat jackals, as the excessive increase in the population of meso-predators had created problem in the area. It was an absolutely independent growth with almost no co-relation with the jungle scene that left me believing that small to medium size carnivores are definitely a benefitted lot in absence of large carnivores and their population often rise to excessive numbers that might upset the ecosystem functions.

The phenomenon also demonstrated that nature in its infinite wisdom ensures its balance with the survival strategy of the predators as they by their territorial demands have to depend only on the prey that is easily obtainable.

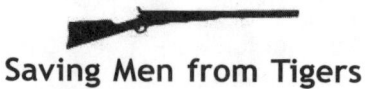

Saving Men from Tigers

The conservation community went passed out in 2004 when scientists discovered that Sariska Tiger Reserve contained no tigers, even when government records maintained that there were 20 tigers. Foot print, scats and scrap surveys, camera traps and other indicators showed that tigers were long gone and ironically I was trying to save tigers in Tarai farmlands where they were far more vulnerable to poachers than any Reserve.

- Author in Wildlife Symposium of U.P Forest Department. 2013,

Dr Karanth and Rajesh Gopal's studies prove that "given the pattern of human population densities across India and the highly clumped distribution of tiger populations, the extent of conflict is relatively small. Such conflict zones perhaps cover less than 1% of India's geographical area, and involve an even smaller fraction of tiger population. Therefore in micro ecological sense, human-tiger conflict is relatively localized management problem. However by its very nature, the conflict poses a serious dilemma for conservationists trying to promote human-tiger coexistence."

However, besides Sunderbans the Tarai, seemed to qualify for over half of that 1% of India's geographical area that the scholars mention as prone to conflict. Man-eating may be called the "last ditch activity of a big predator rather than its standard behavior," but unfortunately it is the ultimate expression of a max-out that triggers an extreme hatred for tigers. And, despite the animal being fully protected species, it generates a natural reaction – a call for revenge on the part of natives. This was going on not only in Dudhwa area but almost in entire nine districts of Tarai which are contiguous to principal jungles and where sugarcane crops were preferentially planted and where tigers had overcome their natural fear or repugnance of man.

McDougal's worrying prediction that "as the existing habitat outside parks and reserves, where tigers are multiplying, becomes progressively fragmented and degraded owing to ever greater human encroachment, we may expect increased incidence of problem tigers," seems to have come true here. As incidents grew from killing of livestock to accidental killing of humans and even occasional predation on humans by tigers, it led to their retaliatory killing by natives. However, none of these tigers were mainstream killers; as most of the villagers who had been bumped off were squatting or bending over to cut grass for fodder. A squatting man is half the size of a standing man. He offers twice the spread of back with folded knees flanking his sides. This shape resembles a medium size deer that makes him vulnerable to predation. Among these, many of the tigers had never shown their inclination to kill humans. There was no evidence of their stalking the victim or returning to look for the body, yet these tigers were eliminated on the suspicion of

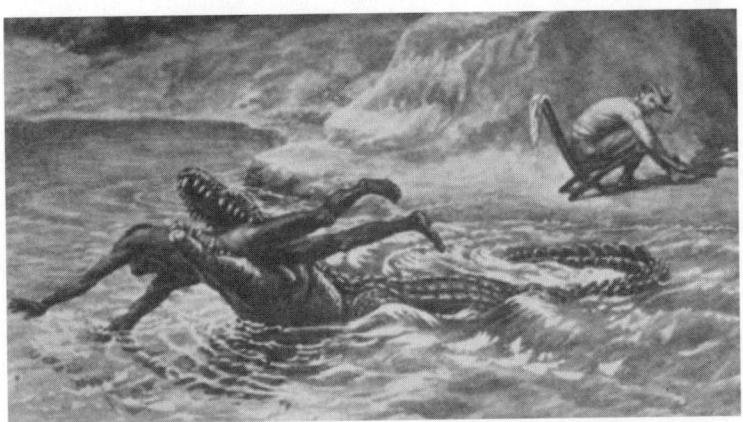

Crocodiles are also deadly killers. A conservative estimate approximates one human being a month is essentially dragged off by Crocs in Tarai. The figure may be higher because successful Croc attacks leave no trace of the victim.

being man-eaters. This unfortunate development had put paid to my efforts to conserve farmland tigers. It had rather become counter-productive.

Villagers live in direct competition with wildlife and often resentment grows amongst them when cattle are killed and they don't get adequate compensation or it is belatedly granted with a substantial cut. Then the involvement of local population stems from this resentment which often grows into monster of commercial poaching and visiting poachers often act as cover for their illegal activities, where locals get benefit of doubt. Back in 1984, I learnt of a case of poaching of a young tigress in Bangawa area. Her presence in human landscape was within my knowledge for a couple of years and as a noted cane-dweller she was in my list of prospective studies but involved with important datelines I could not visit the area and then by an accidental chance I had to investigate the case of this tigress after her death.

Kanjars and *Banjara* tribals are most destructive people in Tarai. Their potential as game killers is still not known to the government and the conservationist world. The damage done by them though not so dramatic as is of natives is certainly a serious problem. They do it silently and quickly move away from the district using trains.

The *Banjaras* tracked the tigress and concealed an iron jaw-trap in her path. The trap weighing over 40 kg was secured to the ground by chains and pegs and with a juicy hump of flesh placed in its centre, into which the tigress ventured and was caught. Sometime in the night, the villagers heard the peacocks screech as mighty predator's roar after roar, agonized and tormented, rent the primordial darkness. Towards midnight some villagers trooped along to see the catch. The tigress rushed at them but the trap had been pegged down so firmly that it only came to the length of the chain. However the ground was sandy not giving too stable a hold on to the peg. The headman noticed that the mighty predator would be able to pull the trap adrift without much impediment so he drove the natives back home. Sometime afterwards she made a desperate plunge and the powerful wrench eventually but deceivingly freed her.

Next morning the *Banjaras* came and found that the moorings had been broken and the tigress had walked away tenaciously with the ugly trap held to her right front leg. She had gone into a dry drain, from where the hollow clang of metal was echoing out as the chains rattled. As the nomads approached her, the furious animal reared up on hind legs waving 90 pound trap in the air, clambering out with a violent effort. Even with their magic and ancient sorcery, the *Banjaras* felt afraid of her desperation and vanished from the scene.

That very evening, they returned with some natives and found the tigress had moved off further. They followed the trail and found the beast stuck-up at a place where the trap had got entangled in a tough creeper. She was lying down growling and snarling. Nature may be "red in tooth and claw" but there is ruthlessness in human inventiveness which seems to shock her, nevertheless.

The poor beast had broken its ankle bone in her struggle to get free; its paw was still attached to the trap by sinews and she lay motionless as if quite inanimate. The *Banjaras* threw a rope round its neck and strangulated it. They were conscious that no spear holes should mar the skin. Tigers needed to be a perfect trophy-flattened in death, to rest glass eyed, on polished parquet floors.

It was a historical time of man-tiger conflict and as such the worst of the time. Post the Bangawa tigress investigation and to get an idea of what was happening around, I surveyed 22 villages in Kheri and 16 villages in Bahraich district where tigers had gone on a killing spree increasing their human toll inexorably higher. The situation was chaotic, communications were chaotic, and the press was apparently offensive as there also seemed to have emerged a segment of opportunistic man-eaters. Everywhere I went people reported confrontations with tigers and wanted me to shoot them. It was clear if I had to save tigers and at the same time forestall human deaths I had to take a positive action. This motivated me to counsel villagers and start up a programme of "Saving Men from Tigers" to serve the cause of nature.

I might not have attained government funding but I had august friends namely Yogesh Kumar, N. Ravi Shanker, Prabhas Kumar Jha, all IAS officers of Uttar Pradesh cadre, and IPS officers Balraj Bhalla and Vijay Kumar in state bureaucracy, who regularly went on official tours to Tarai districts. I accompanied them periodically and took them into tiger affected areas. Their presence with government paraphernalia created a great difference. Presently I observe a newly emerging trend that conservationists of my generation are now calling celebrities like Amitabh Bachchan, Akshaye Khanna, cricketer Sachin Tendulkar, M.S. Dhoni and Hollywood actor Harrison Ford of Indiana Jones fame on their side to voice the plight of tiger on television networks and generate awareness about its importance all over the world.I don't shy away in telling that my friends' co-operation proved critical in my venture. They were no TV icons but their visits in remote rural lands with me, with assisting Deputy Superintendents of Police and Sub-divisional Magistrates including

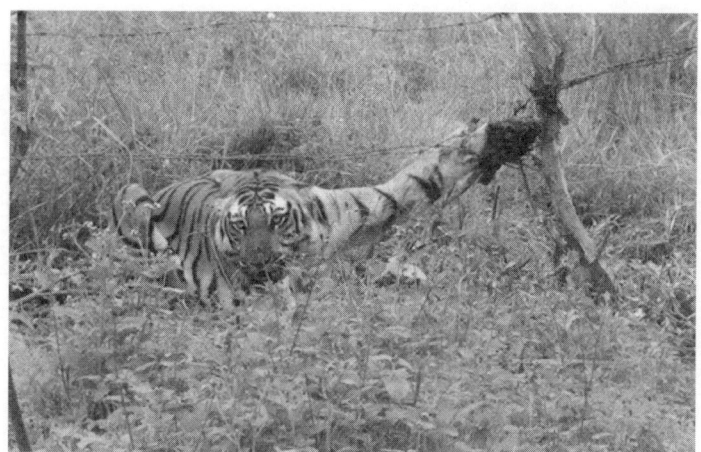

The suffering of a trapped tiger; notice its left foreleg is all torn to shreds in its efforts to break free from the barbed wires. *(Photo credit Karnataka Forest Department)*

Rangers and Foresters, were taken as no less than a film shooting affair and they as great celebrities. Their potential of vehicle cavalcades, beckon lights and presence of police, attracted grassroots and helped me immensely in addressing masses in implementing my non-profit public service announcements of 'Saving men from Tigers'.

Years later, my daughters Shrivridhi and Samriddhi also stepped in this venture. By fortuitous chance, I had to deal with a problem tigress at a village named Maurhawa-Burkharya in Bahraich district in which they accompanied me. On March 16 1997, N. Ravi Shanker, then Secretary (Home) in the Uttar Pradesh Government, facilitated me with adequate police force and skilled labor for the job as I drove the tigress back into the jungle some eight miles away. But after a month she returned on the same village fields, starting her nefarious activities again. Then onwards she frequented the area for good three years and finally in June 2000 was brought down by a large excited mob of 500 people, netted and beaten to death mercilessly. This proved that the same ecological factors including landscape linkages and topography that induce a problem animal to primarily seek living near human settlements force it to continue in the area unabatedly and even if driven away they return again and again.

The lack of expertise and control over the situation on part of officials had lead to the treacherous killing of the tigress for when she had already been captured in the net then she could easily have been sedated and saved. The last thing I wanted to overlook was the unnecessary killing of farm tigers before my eyes, when in my small way; I had already put in two decades of hard work to restore their relict population. On one hand sugarcane fields were uniquely important laboratory for the study of Tarai tigers, and on the other equally extraordinary in terms of gaining insight into the tigers' political dilemma.

However, this death moved my daughters deeply and they voluntarily engaged themselves as social scientists to study public opinion and their approval for the

The problem had surfaced because the relationship between man and tiger had changed. Shrivridhi later acquired her Masters Degree in Social Work from Tata Institute of Social Sciences, Mumbai and contributed new points to my old blackboard with the measures that addressed man-tiger conflict in a scientific way. For two years 2009 to 2011, before proceeding to U.S., she served as a full time co-researcher with me and having recorded over 100 personal tales of native encounters with big cats, she deliberates that public involvement in carnivore policy can have extremely positive results and proper counseling can change human behavior. She structured a questionnaire, which helped me understand current trends of public behavior and find practical ways to protect the cats within the human landscape.

For preventing and mitigating human-carnivore conflict, she carefully crafted a questionnaire for villagers, which was approved by Chief Secretary of Uttar Pradesh, N.C. Bajpayee, presently chairman of Planning Commission, U.P. to be used for research purposes in Tarai villages by Forest Department to determine the intensity of man-animal conflict and find the ways for people that live within the confines of tiger domains. It was also endorsed by the State's Wildlife Advisory Board of which I had been a member. The questionnaire ran thus:

1. Number of Years you have lived in this area:
2. Were the tigers always there?
3. Since when the problem was first registered?
4. Give a reason for the problem?
5. Since when the problem increased?
6. Has recovery of carnivore population escalated the conflict?
7. Are land use practices exemplified by re-growth of sugarcane?
8. Why do tigers live in the sugarcane?
9. Frequency of the sighting of the animal.
10. What do you think is the main food of a tiger?
11. How do you react when you see a tiger?
12. What is your opinion about the tigress that lay cubs in sugar field?
13. Do you let the tiger eat the cattle or drive him away?
14 Whether the compensation for a cattle kill is sufficient?
15. Do the tigers often threaten your cattle?
16. Details of the last attack:
17. Measures taken for protection after the attack:
18. Do people around kill wildlife for the pot?
19. How do you perceive a tiger; valueless or important?
20. You still want tigers to live in the sugar fields?
21. Whether threat from this animal is molecule as compared to death from car accidents, snake and dog bites or fever like dengue and malaria?

The analysis of various answers, based on scientific data both biological and social, gave us the opportunity to address the most challenging question of motivating the people living around large carnivores to support their conservation and acknowledge the fact that the threat from this animal was really miniscule in comparison to the deaths that take more toll of human life in their neighborhood.

The answers also gave us a good understanding of carnivores' behavioral ecology based on empirical knowledge of people's experience. Some people considered it as nature's danger signal set as a warning to its victims while others took it as nature's friendly signal to accept it as it is, a reality. The later contention, in seemingly acceptable and morally agreeable ways became a valuable booster in the initiation of my campaign 'Saving men from Tigers.' It encouraged communities to participate unreservedly in the process of proactive conservation and also earned me the good will of local population besides reducing the human cases of carnivore mortality.

The responsibility of a social scientist is to study the public problem carefully, find out situation specific solutions, co-ordinate between public and policy makers and see that locally feasible options are implemented for the apparent welfare of wildlife and possible co-existence of humans with carnivores in human-dominated environment without much lethal options.

Herdsmen are more concerned with their livelihood than with understanding what biotic or a-biotic factors motivate a tiger to live in their farms. The wildlife sanctuary does not seem to provide them any tangible material profit. They are not proud that their land harbors one of the last great sanctuaries of the Tarai land where they also enjoy the sight of tigers and hear their roars echoing across the agrarian landscape. They are more concerned with the grim realities that impose restrictions on them such as forage for their cattle and their cattle's future and where predation imbalances along with variegated interpersonal dynamics makes for problematic feelings. All the study finally focuses on one and only fact that affected natives will have to accept tigers and leave poaching at first because the animals tigers eat are also irresistible to human predators. And when the principal prey base is slaughtered en masse, its effect is equally devastating where any normal tiger will easily land in competition with man or turn into problem tiger.

Shrivridhi's assertions that despite so many odds cattle killers do not confront humans easily and run away at their intrusion were largely gleaned from fact-based accounts of natives. A perceptive theory, mooted by Stephen Mills, a British naturalist and film-maker, who studied tigers for more than 20 years in Tarai, postulates that unless tigers become man-eaters they do not normally attack humans for they visualize a standing person as being larger and taller than them. Citing his own example Mills declares that to a tiger his own height of two meters would appear formidably five meter tall to a tiger, which is a convincing deterrent to attack. Though the question may be raised that a full-grown *sambhar* or swamp deer with large horns, when their necks are fairly straight, often stand more than two meters in height, yet these remain the preferred prey of a tiger. Mills' statement is no doubt magnified but the hypothesis seems partway logical when applied upon two-legged animal that stands erect.

However, the existence of many Tharu settlements inside protected areas that harbor larger number of tigers does not generate much conflict, despite presence of their livestock as much trouble is generated in farmlands where there are much less tigers.

My campaign is now 32 years old and its gradual evolution laying emphasis on the change of human behavior in some important pockets of Tarai involving non-lethal solution for a problem carnivore is significant. Predators are ordained by nature to prey or perish. The key to co-exist with master predator is not to compete with it, so its natural prey must remain inviolate. The need to reassure public on this line would determine the fate of these tigers and the people around them.

The only fault of farm tigers is that they are viewed as a threat to the livelihood of communities and not as a heritage resource to be conserved. Shrivridhi's targeted solutions, based on hard-worked data have helped change people's hostile attitude towards carnivores and promote their rational conservation actions in some areas like Kaanp-Tanda and Ghola sugar fields. Here tigers are reported to occupy crops in every winter and location specific scientific understanding of tiger biology and preserving the prey base has drastically reduced the conflict. At the time of writing this book on 20 April 2016 a tigress had killed and eaten a farm worker Anjani Kumar at Beharipurva village in the north Kheri yet his family doesn't want the tigress to be killed.

Book 3

IN THE WILDERNESS OF SUGARCANE

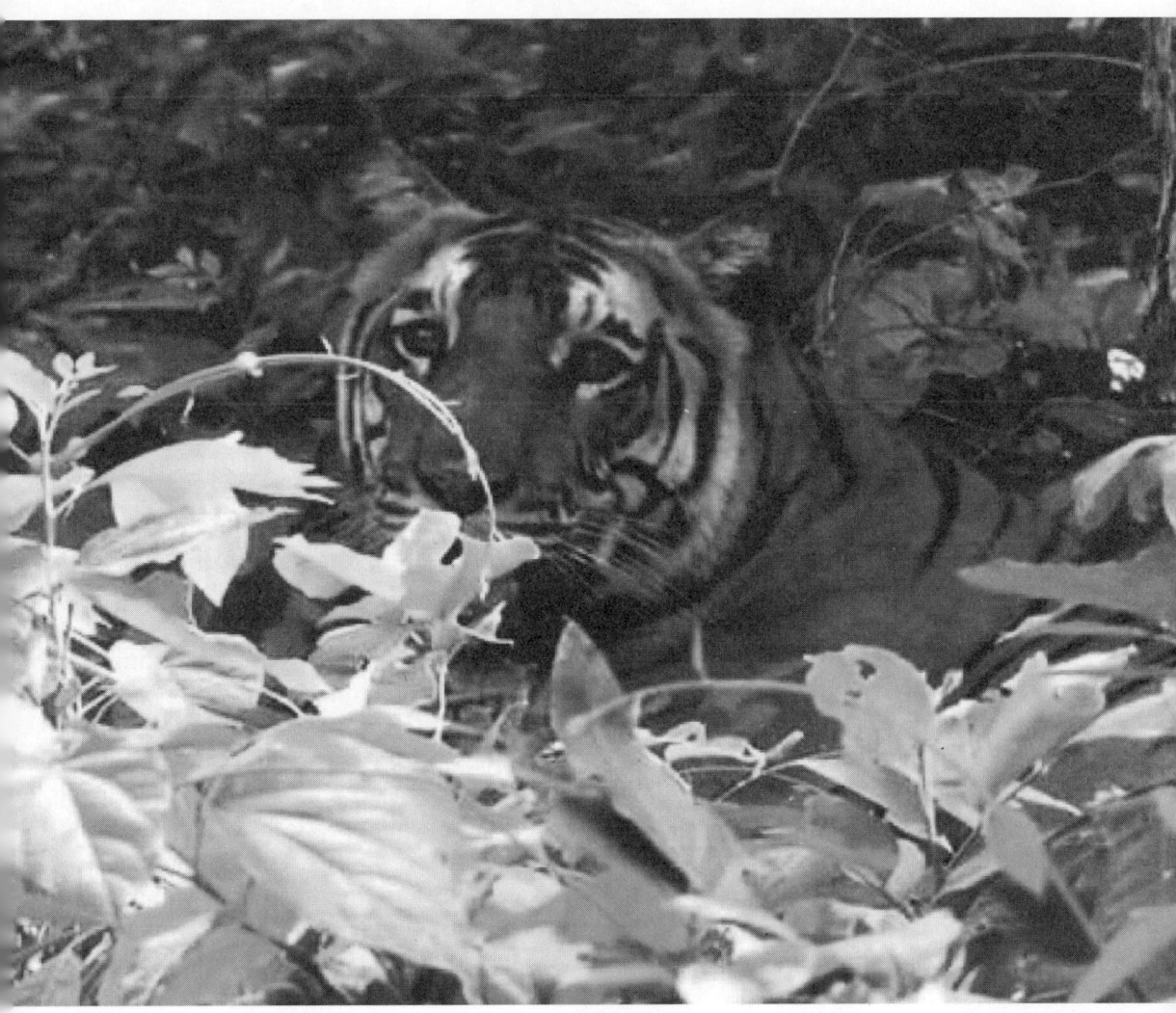

CHAPTER 5
THE PUZZLE OF BIG TOMS

Chapter 5

The Puzzle of Big Toms

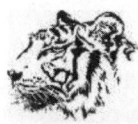

Do you have any idea what it means to follow tiger tracks? A tiger is not a sable who would walk a few miles and·is done. This tiger could be fifty miles away by now. It could be a hundred and fifty miles away."

— Valdimir Shibnev, a hunting inspector in Taiga

RESEARCHERS HAVE THEIR OWN UNIQUE WAY OF SETTLING THEIR questions. They never lose any opportunity of data generation. They decide their questions independently, formulate hypothesis, develop methodologies best suited for their work so that statistically viable samples are generated. While a terrible man-tiger max-out was going on in sugar fields of Tarai, a queer question was flashing in my mind – how many years of life a tiger might spend in farmlands? Do some of these spend their full life cycle in farmlands? Do others, bigger in size, having increased perambulations and their inherited instinct for the jungle having grown stronger, naturally move into deep recess of woods and adapt them as their ultimate home? And finally but not the least, what is the average age and size of these animals that give priority to cane as their habitat over jungles?

The average measurement of farmland tigers was an important factor in my study as these could help me determine their biological age. The most important question was whether all of these were young carnivores in the first flush of youth, a doomed surplus that dies before reaching the reproductive age. It is this category of tiger that creates trouble with the human neighbors for it rejoices in hunting and only needs hunger imperative to grow into a troublesome predator. And if it is so, then all the cane tigers could not be accounted into a matured lot. They must fall under three years of age with a size not exceeding more than seven and a half or maximum to eight feet, and if some are bigger than this, then they are definitely mature and over five years of age. This shows that the matrix of tigers in farms was no different from that inside the jungle and perhaps there was an interdependent singularity. It held all the age groups from grandparents to great grand children in both the zones. In fact the intermixing of such intricate biology and ecology between sugar farmlands and tiger range jungles regarded as environmental crisis from human angle was an entirely natural phenomenon produced by inherent capacity of sugarcanes to provide food and cover as grassland ecosystems to tigers and their prey.

Normally bigger tigers are found inside principal jungles but here was the contrast that some big specimens were also roaming in the farmlands as their saucer-pan and dinner-plate like pugmarks showed this truth. In case even if we accept that sugarcane tigers were peripheral tigers of jungle, that are displaced from their home ground by the bigger ones, then which were these bigger ones in the farmlands? How did they leave the safety of their remote jungle homes and come here? Did they hold this area within their hunting territory or they had arrived here chasing the juniors for the heck of it? Or had deliberately come here to court with females? All these conjectures were possible but one possibility was even stronger that the big ones on farmlands were perhaps so called provisional transients. They were making use of cane cover to cross over from one jungle to another regardless of the separating distance between them.

This seemed a right answer to my question and when analyzed in this way it also held the answer that these tigers were covering the cane zone too because their large territory extended up to 500 sq km. In the light of this fact, that there were many cub-nurturing females inhabiting farmlands with which they mated, while crossing over to other forests.

October 2002, in Tulsipur sugar fields of Pilibhit district I once watched the association of a large tiger with his female and two cubs. It was more an exhibition of greed and selfishness on the part of a freeloader male than of any matured fatherly role. Seated high up on a tree with a pair of powerful 7x50 Zeiss binoculars, I watched the tigress pull down a hog deer. The male adapting the bullying tactics, immediately fell upon the carcass and begun devouring it, tearing to pieces. Though a little apprehensive of grand male's aggression, due to his greater size the female also joined the feast sheepishly but when her half-grown cubs, somewhat less than an year old, and already emaciated, tried to participate in the meal, the male or possible father did not approve the idea and instantly chased them away.

Being too far away to hear anything other than loud growls of the admonishing male, I could imagine those cubs giving pathetic wails for their share in the carcass. They sat some ten to twelve yards away which is considered a safe distance but soon their patience gave way and they begun to walk in a wide circle while the parents remained busy in gorging their kill. The cubs tried to close in once again when the freeloader growled at them threateningly staging a violent exhibition of disapproval. It was curious to note that how his ferocity seemed to be stirred by eating or possibly the impulse of defending what he considered belonged to him. He jerked his tail up and down in protest; these made the female jump away quickly and sit at a distance from him.

It was a rewarding observation about defined table-manners and protocols among tigers. The way the younger tigers wait without complaint while their parents feed is remarkable. I feel no hungry human child would behave in half so tolerant a fashion. But here the situation was different. The cubs were jumpy and nervous.

They sensed danger in their father's behavior and finally lay down under a shady tree, evidently hungrier than their parents. They watched their father in frustration who feverishly finished the entire carcass, stripping it to bone. Then the big one walked towards the shady *pipal* tree; the cubs immediately vacated the place for him and he sat grooming himself and licking his paws.

The cubs then took the possession of remains but practically there was nothing left, even for the vultures to pick anything edible but for a few bones, innards and offal. The look of disappointment and complete defeat was largely written on their face when their mother came at the remains. She symbolically licked the leftovers, demonstrating that she intended to feed them. Like a good conscious provider she prompted them to share the spoils and then in order to satisfy their demands she perhaps regurgitated some meat for them. I say this because I could not see properly but I could well understand the desperation as those two starving cubs gulped down something, perhaps the meshed meat, as their confused mother continued to threaten the treed watcher for whom those hours of discomfort had been infinitely worthwhile.

Even if in an irate mood, the males don't practice infanticide on their own progeny to bring cub rearing female into heat. As far as he is concerned as father, their genetic value is high in his eyes. It is the new male taking over the range from the old male that tries to kill any cubs he finds. Moreover for pairing tigers, it is highly probable that in the impenetrable, closed environment of sugarcane, prolonged proximity of a male or an exposure to his strongly overpowering sexual hormone called androus pheromone makes an attached female impulsively inclined to go in for mating, thereby solving the male's problem of having copulation. The male in such condition do not need to kill her progeny as the female is already inclined to mate; the killing of the cubs is only done to bring female into estrus.

However, the father tiger's sheer presence with female sometimes spells trouble for the cubs. Males appropriate all the kills and make cubs totally handicapped, not allowing them to approach until they have had their fill. In such rigid conditions as I had witnessed, how long the cubs would survive the fatigue and hunger is anybody's guess. Their emaciated condition was a testimony that they had not been getting proper food for many weeks, perhaps since their father had joined their mother. I felt convinced that until the mother hunts again to satisfy their requirements or luck turns the dice in their favour they would soon fall prey to starvation created by the big tom's tyranny and lack of sympathy towards them.

In Barotha farmlands, I had observed a male performing their family duty with surprising connubial-paternal attentiveness. He was in the habit of issuing loud hollers after securing his kill to let his females know that the meal was ready for them. But here the behavior of the male in question was different yet there seemed no reason to me to suppose that this could be an isolated case of tiger depravity. Undoubtedly many such tragedies are enacted in the Tarai jungles and farmlands

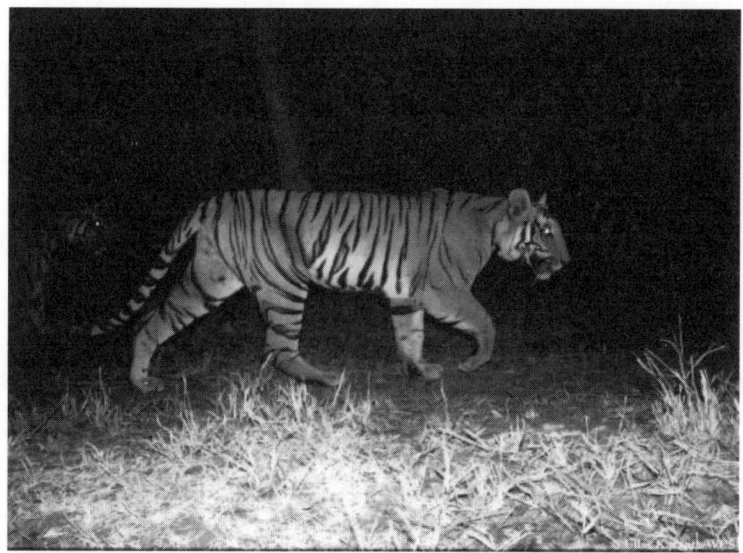

Territories are temporary parade grounds and a source for permanent food supply for the nuclear tiger families. The extensive estate is also shared by related members of the clan. *(Camera trap shot; Credit Karnataka Forest Department)*

that escape human observation and go unrecorded. I have listened to several stories of similar nature from the natives. Indeed they consider it quite a normal practice and none of them takes it as unusual.

This might also be one of the reasons of cub mortality in the species that the big toms don't let them secure their proper meal. Any disregard for the rule very often ends fatally for the young ones. The verdict almost in every case is starvation and even death for the weaker. But this is the way the tigers have flourished for millions of years and the fact that the species still survives in the wilds is a proof that it works as nature's law.

The presence of such a large male in the human-dominated landscape clearly indicated that it had arrived here from the jungle; or to say from the scientifically managed reserve, into the high density of human population area. It was definitely not the component of sugarcane tigers - as I called this segment - that was comfortable in the sugarcane farmlands and that considered the vista their ecological niche through ecological succession. This male was different with a different name that I called 'tigers in sugarcane'. But at the same time, he was no strayer in the strict sense of the word; he was in his prime mating years from 6 to 11 years of age, and sugarcane farms in fact formed a part of his territory, where all the females were included in his harem. The landscape though offered somewhat ecologically disturbed niche, a dangerous land for such a large passerby, but crossing this terrain was mandatory for him to touch the other points, far-off inside jungles trails, that fell yonder but undoubtedly within his territory.

Since mega sugar farms hold the basic requirements of a tigerine life, a segment of females, with cover, water and food as well, it is indeed a biological corridor for jungle tigers; a corridor that marries two far-off ranges, across the immensity of space, this also demonstrates the falsehood of belief that no tiger which has lived truly wild would intentionally prefer to navigate through farmlands. The habitats of jungle and farmlands, though are ecologically distinctive but the Tarai tigers on the eternal and evolutionary standards are used to this "justifiable legality of crossing". They have merged with this variegated nature of habitat over generations; because on balance tigers are closer to true cats in biology and disposition than lions with enormous potential of adaptability.

This conjecture was like a conjurer's rabbit to many foresters. They thought that I was drawing on my fertile imagination with no foundation in fact. For example north and south Kheri divisions are two separate forest trails that run in liner horizontal beat from each other with great rural landscape of thirty to forty kilometers stretching in between them. Their simple question was how can a real jungle dweller go from here to there crossing such vast a zone of farmlands? And what is the need of this exercise? Yet many curious foresters found this possibility fascinating because it was formative while some others who partially believed it, found it worrying and destabilizing, perhaps more perplexing than my belief of sugarcane tigers. However, I had still not developed my knowledge base to test this speculation of mine, so obtaining measurements of matured animals' appeared a significant dimension for further studies.

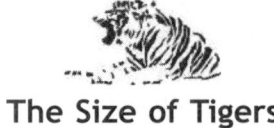

The Size of Tigers

To say that a tiger is an 'outside animal' is an understatement that is best appreciated when a tiger is inside.

— John Valliant

I was wondering that any tiger, whether sugarcane tiger or for that matter a tiger in sugarcane, can compete with the lengths of the biggest tigers shot and recorded by big game hunters in deep jungles. For example, Shakespeare shot a tiger of 10 ft. 8 in., Maharaja Bikaner exactly of 11 ft. (7 ft 8 in. body and 3ft. 4 in. tail). Simpson obtained two of 10 ft. 4 in. Colonel Geoffrey Nightingale mentions of a man-eater "with head like a tub" he shot in Deccan. "The tiger was old, nearly white, and his teeth were stumps. His skin was 12 ft. 1 in. long and 5 ft. broad and he was 2 ft. 8 inches round the neck, and such a forearm." Two generations - four brothers and their father - of Shillingford family, the indigo planters of Bengal, killed 170 tigers between 1865 and 1878. These were registered by J.L. Shillingford as one being of 11ft. 5 in and four of 11 feet in length. It is also recorded that the father C. Shillingford had claimed a tiger earlier in 1849 in Purneah district measuring as he fell 12ft. 4 in. across the zygomatic arches.

These measurements are open to objection, unless we acknowledge that the pituitary gland of some tigers plays havoc with them increasing their size and volume by extra secretion, one cannot accept or reject them instantly but reaching an age, where the body size is more than 9 feet, enriches the chances of a tiger's survival against natural calamities and competitive existence amongst its tribe. It is these large tigers that win females and rear their genes. However, on saner side Nightingale's second largest tiger was of 10 ft. 2 in., just 3 inches short to Corbett's Bachelor of Powelgarh that was of 10 ft. 5 in.

There was no way to determine the body size of tigers in farmlands but to measure their length and weight through paws but this could easily become a vague approach in absence of knowledgeable *shikaris* like Chhotey and Kararia Kanjar who, by carefully observing each footprint could give precise measurements of the animal, were no longer there. It is worth mentionable that these men were no less competent than that duo of Corbett's trackers that had predicted the exact size of the Bachelor of Powelgarh by its footprints, as maximum up to 10.7 much before the tiger's death and it was found 10.5 after being shot. The other option was disconcerting but practical - to keep an alert about tiger death news and measure its body that would slowly generate a record. In that phase of years, tiger cadavers were occasionally being found in sugar fields, killed by accident, poached or even poisoned by people.

I don't have earlier records of tigers found dead in agricultural fields but for one big tom that was found poisoned in 1984 near Paraspur fields. It was since 1986 when 14 mature specimens were discovered poisoned in sugarcane fields of north Kheri that I started to keep their measurement records properly. It was a biologically tragic decimation of predators as 11 carcasses were of young females. However, I myself measured some of these full-grown dead tigers and later also collected the data of the measurements of other tigers where I could not reach physically. I found that a full grown prime breeding female is invariably one to one and-a-half feet shorter to a prime breeding tiger.

Brander says that "classification of what is a mature animal presents some difficulties… out of 39 tigresses selected as mature; the smallest was 7 ft. 10 in. and the largest 9 ft. 1 in. The average is 8 ft. 4 in…. the shortest tiger classified as mature was 8 ft. 9 in. and the longest 10 ft. 3 in. The average works out to 9 ft. 3 in".

I was surprised that their average length of matured male specimens (found dead in cane zones) came down to 9 ft. and females to eight feet. These were not over curves, where one gets opportunity to increase the length because much depends on how much the tape is pressed, these were just straight line measurements from the tip of nose to the tip of tail, thus fairly accurate readings. However, the tail played a great part in increasing the size of any animal. The shortest length of tail I measured was 30 in. and the longest was of 41 in. and the vertebrae in the tail has been recorded as varying between 29 in. to 40 in. I don't know if the length of the tail has to do something with the flight reflex of a tiger but a jungle axiom maintains that long tailed tigers, like leopards, (whose tail is proportionately longer if compared with a tiger), are expert tree climbers. They are extremely accurate in pulling down hunters from trees if injured.

These are conservation times and in jungles there is a comparative immunity from serious hunting or poaching. This gives every tiger an opportunity to survive against human odds and grow to the fullest size. Hence one abnormally large tiger that was found dead near Paraspur fields and who had survived a 450/500 bullet in his upper thigh, only to die of bomb-biting was measured about 7 ft 4 in. in body with a 3 ft. 5 in. long python size tail. The mind boggling carcass even exceeded by 4 in to Sir John Hewett's record of 10 ft. 5 and a half inch tiger, the longest he ever shot in the Tarai.

The more improbable the event the stronger the evidence demanded in order to establish the same. Jerdon in his *Mammals of India* (1874) does not acknowledge even an 11 ft. tiger while he must have come across men who claimed to have shot such hell of an over-length animal. Had Jerdon been there at Paraspur, he would have revived his opinion that phenomenal supercats haven't seized to materialize, they still do exist in Tarai.

Scientists believe that when trophy hunting and poaching removes the largest and bigger ones, the population of species may increase with new induction of modest genes but size and the weight of the progenies often gets badly affected. Such animals no longer seem to grow as large as they once grew. A parallel example of this can be sighted from Moose that inhabits the forests of America from Maine northwards, and from Alaska to Nova Scotia.

The mega bull herbivore, weighing in neighborhood of 1500 pounds with well-developed symmetrical and broadly palmated antlers afforded a grand sight. Its trophy hunting slowly reduced its body as well as antler size that the scientists call as "Trophy engineering". During post - Second World War phase, sport hunters competed for best moose trophy and the biggest animals were methodically removed from the gene pool while the smaller animals, with small antlers were spared to pass on their moderate gene for the survival of the species. This happened year after year as the large antlers gradually disappeared from the vista but the moose population rebounded to a sustainable level. The present moose and even taiga tigers are regarded as lesser beasts than what their ancestors were in pre - Second World War years.

Debates among large mammal scientists have developed on the effect of sport hunting on wildlife populations. One side argues that hunted mammals adjust to hunting pressure and therefore thrive better than those in non-hunting areas while the other side believes the opposite is true.

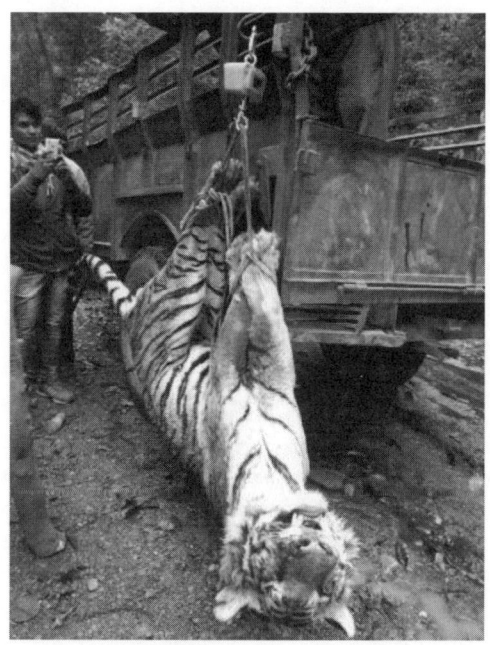

A10 footer tiger found dead in NanitalTarai,
December 2016

Russian scientists have speculated the reduction of size of Amur tigers on the same lines of the moose, which they claim that after massive hunting of large specimens, is presently no longer as big as its earlier size. In fact it is now similar to the old records of large Indian tigers described by early hunters as Royal Bengal (a fanciful nomenclature not recognized by zoologists) though the population of Amur tigers is continuing to be sustainable.

The Paraspur tiger was never weighed before public eye, nor was its autopsy report published in any paper or tabled for debate where everything including length is recorded. But many old-timers believed it to be a five-hundred pounder. In the words of Heera Kanjar, a hardened poacher of tigers, "*Aiso sher, arre baap-re-baap, kabahu nahin dekhyo, aah-ah*" (Such tiger, oh my father, we have never seen in life.) Locals believe it was a huge cat by any period's measure.

However, presently with a total moratorium on trophy hunting, no such records of tiger specimens are meticulously kept. It is rather considered a humbug. Under Wildlife Protection Act consumption of wildlife products is prohibited and tiger skins are classified as top contrabands. The State Government forms an official committee that looks after periodical disposal of contrabands by consigning them to fire. In the capacity of Honorary Wildlife Warden of Dudhwa I have been the member of two such committees but at that time I was nothing special. I remember having requested the authorities to preserve the big tom pelt for research purposes but the officials, who had burned dozens of pelts to keep them off the black market, didn't hear me at all and the specimen was reduced to ashes.

I may add that Hewett was probably the only person who possessed the most extensive records of Tarai tiger measurements, covering some 241 animals which he has seen shot during his active hunting career. Brander tells that out of 241 animals, Hewett measured only nine tigers who were 10 feet or over and ten tigress were 9 feet or over.

Tarai tigers are generally amongst the largest in India and in some areas these beasts spanning sugar farms are known to have shown constantly nasty track records. This may be due to the fact that villagers constantly harass them and provoke them off their wild kills for meat, and therefore their patience slowly becomes short-tempered with the man and makes them aberrant. A short-tempered attacker or a cattle killer easily qualifies to be poisoned sooner than later.

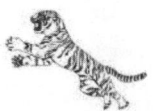

Territorialism of Big Tigers

The gauntlet of trials and initiations a male tiger must endure is long arduous and deadly, and the survivors are truly formidable specimens.

— John Valliant

Big toms operate on a larger scale with more resources and superior profile. Their periodical shunting through sugarcanes worried me and I spent a great deal of time in understanding the morphology of the tiger's paw. It was this phase when I travelled with no less than ten plaster casts of great tiger paws in my bag, trying to understand if male tigers took such a long journey of 40 to 60 miles, much part of which is covered moving through cane corridors to reach distant jungles, precisely shifting between north and south Kheri jungles or even further into Nepalese trails.

Ecological monitoring of such tigers was needed at several spatial scales. At human dominated landscape level we needed to understand sugarcane corridor connectivity and crop pattern where tigers emerge from jungles, from a selective occupancy and far from human presence, cross the human landscape through it. At the point of individual tiger, it was essential to understand its behavior in order to meet his physiological needs; keeping cool and conserving energy. At tiger population levels we needed to examine whether these were stable, increasing or decreasing in sugarcane fields. On life history parameters, the survival and dispersal of their populations, living cheek by jowl with human invader, where no expansion of space was possible needed to be empathized with much critical thought and lastly the impact of baleful human activities on tigers, their changed prey composition in farmlands and their silent adjustment with it through the period they crossed it. Were these jungle tigers were also partly farmland tigers, the multigenerational beings and the voice of their forefathers that had frequented the farmlands with same frequency?

From today's standards it was a poor quality data for it relied only on pugmarks but I had no scientific tools with me to apply and address these issues. And as expected in all the cases I had to look at forest department who too only relied on pugmarks.

I presented the measurements of tigers found dead in farmlands in a conference of Forest Department. The average length of mature male tigers' coming to 9 feet

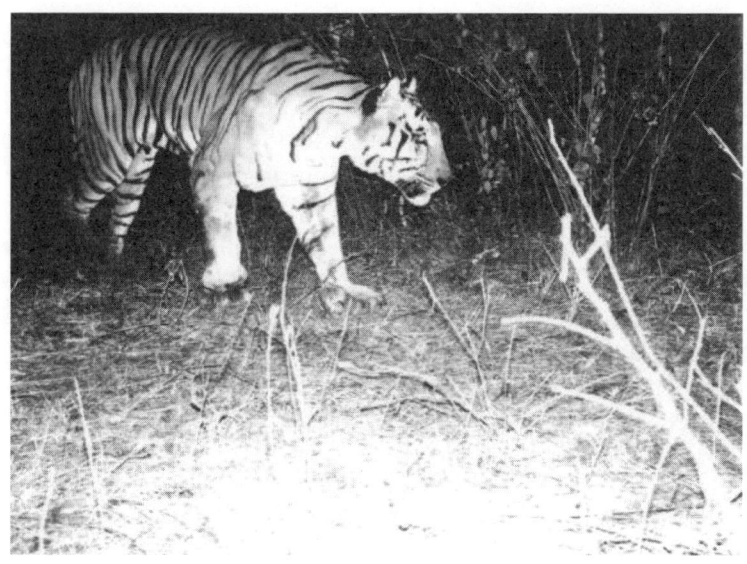

For young males the hole and corner existence often lasts for years. They hide and scavenge successfully without anyone knowing about their living including resident tigers. *(Camera Trap Shot; photo credit, WTS)*

raised the question of their status in the sugarcane farms; whether these were regular farm dwellers or it was a different kind of giant lot that was coming here from jungles to maximize their breeding opportunities with farm dwelling females besides using sugar farms as corridor to cross the human dominated landscape safely and reach other to extend their influence and claim more breeding rights for themselves. Furthermore big cats are big wanderers and all this is inbuilt in their biological mechanism, because the distribution of new genes is dependent upon the successful dispersal of strong males.

During winters the big toms were certainly not crossing the dangerous land in a marathon tread but crossing in unhurried installments, taking their own time, making short perambulations in cane fields, killing blue bulls and feral cattle and resting at halting stations at leisure, when some of them like Paraspur tiger lackadaisically fall to vengeful design of humans. I wondered if these jungle tigers were disoriented to live in human dominated landscape, and while staying longer in cane fields, they showed the lack of adaptive edge for their lives which were a bigger competitive battleground of wits, than their natural jungles. They rather behaved shy in the farmlands, trying to escape unwanted attentions of human aliens, yet aliens behaved belligerently with them, and like a fugitive in the land of their birth, they paid with their life for no misdemeanor of theirs'.

In Tarai farmlands there is no love lost between animals and poachers. Poachers still set gin traps, wire snares and nets to catch the game for meat and in the night when they are safe in their homes the trapped animal stands wearing a necklace of wire, pulled tightly around its chest or throat. The catch is often collected by poachers much late as it is first preyed upon by scavengers like jackals that tear the helpless animal in hunting packs and eat it as an easy meal. I have seen a hog deer disfigured by jackals and a snared ratal completely eaten by a leopard. Traditional techniques are inconspicuous and less in coast. Endlessly useable, snares kill and mutilate wildlife unselectively; it can be anything from a wild boar to a blue bull, a jackal, a tiger, a stray livestock and sometimes even an unwary human.

Human race may be called civilized but is not free from the fear of great predators and there are men who have little respect for any creature that they fear. Their terror inclines them to battle. Valdimir Troinin endorses the fact, "That is the way we are; our interactions with tiger are a problem for us."

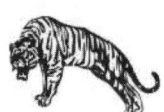

Wildwives of Sugarcane Savannah

My mind is presently a concoction of scientific and historical cocktails - those three days on the tiger trail and I am left with half a lifetime of mental chewing to do...
- Author in the State Wildlife Board's meeting

Young powerful tiger males are in a habit of forming large ranges despite the fact that enough food is available in their local area. For these mercurial animals the hunting ranges are not exactly the same where they search for food but are more of a conjugal nature, where they fraternize and assume possession of females, and mating with unguarded tigress they meet. These may be called mating ranges of somewhat extraordinarily powerful testosterone-rich males.

Breeding is a class of behavior concerned with maintaining integrity of species. No matter how much there is to eat, a great deal of energy consumed must go into the activity designed to maintain the species, or the food is wasted. On the other hand, howsoever prolific a species may be, but it will snuff itself out if there is not enough energy to feed it. Long ranges of males are a nature's way of transmitting healthy genes so that the progeny population should contain a considerable portion of standard material, simply by the laws of chance. In such conditions a genetic line will not be at much risk, for it will not easily lose the struggle against an unfriendly environment at any stage in an animal's life.

The restlessness created by male sexual hormone testosterone inspires large tigers to create large breeding or mating ranges, more by nature's command to counter the adverse effects of inbreeding in small isolated populations. As sugarcane plantations provide plenty of room to such tigers to maintain their genetic strength, as they take to such long journeys.

Apart from the influence of nature and environment the male of all species, including humans, do indeed seem to have propensity for aggression. It is through aggression they extend their dominance and this again comes down to fact that it is because of the overload of testosterone. Some scientists call this male sex hormone as 'warmone' that triggers aggression, competiveness and overabundance of guts. Females are not devoid of this '*chemical-locha*' it is just that their levels of testosterone are far lower than those in males. Moreover as a potential mother, they are programmed to naturally love and take care of the other rather than indulge in excessive mating and establishing ranges.

To many in first instance this seemed like a sweeping statement but perhaps there was more than a grain of truth than imagined. These were long-term resident tigers that maintained great ranges and needed investigation from qualified naturalists.

Clearing of mental cobwebs is a prerequisite for honest thought. I felt that by mooting this analogy in the essence of scientific temper, as this fact needed to be thought over and examined from scientific point of view, I had struck both the world of farmlands and jungle tigers for an advantageous brainstorming, where a complete new horizon would emerge for wildlife experts, helping them to come out of the cave of their own. But in the meeting of State Wildlife Advisory Board my revelation was ridiculed by none else than Billy Arjan Singh as 'utopian dream', and 'kindergarten-hotchpotch.' Such strong-worded condemnation, more of political nature than scientific, coming at an official meeting from people too senior to you in age, may not earn them a nonprintable abuse or a slap, but does make your civilized sense rebel.

I was continuing to be the Honorary Warden of Kishanpur-Dudhwa. A year after this meeting, during summers when all the crops had been harvested and the fields lay barren, resulting in scarcity of food as well as of cover; I reached Paraspur to meet my old companions Mintoo Mama and his sons, Ombeer and Shyamu. The pinch period had set in- it is an ecologically depressing phase the consequences of which result in poor nutrition for the carnivore, increased intra-specific competition on kills and decreased attention towards cubs. Ombeer and I came across a fresh trail of tiger on the fine sands of Sharda banks. Naturally curious, we measured the spoor properly; recording pad length, total length and total width of the front and back spoor, as well as the stride and straddle distances. At places the great pads of cartilage had expanded with tigers shifted weight until these had grown bigger than a dinner plate. When I placed my foot in one impression of big paw it made my booted foot look small. By far these were the biggest tiger pugs I had ever seen, or for that matter have ever subsequently seen. In awe and admiration I exclaimed "*Grand Master*" in a pertinent gesture of salute for the great cat.

"Seems strange that he has moved into scorched fields leaving behind this cool shade," wondered Ombeer. The spoors looked absolutely fresh and we decided immediately to follow them. After a quick bite and packing our lunch boxes, we started from Paraspur on a Jeep. With a pack of five dogs and following the favoured path of this Grand Master we travelled through barren lands hoping to come across the trail-maker any moment, resting somewhere in a grass patch. Wherever we found a high density cove of trees we halted the vehicle, the dogs jumped out wagging their tails, barked and bolted ahead and then came back, giving us a feeling that they sensed the tiger but it was not to be seen.

The animal had evidently crossed the terrain in the darkness of night and walked the whole distance without any break moving at a moderate pace. He had briefly halted at some points just to mark some trees with claw and urine. By the end of the day it was clear that the tiger was keeping high pace, as if feeling vulnerable without some cover to mask his presence and there was no scope of meeting him.

The summer was at its peak. The day temperature was already over 40 degrees Celsius or more in the shade, the hot ground-level air currents (called *loo*) and brief dust storms swept in from the north-west and spiraled in the fields, raising whitecaps over sinking water ponds. The size of an individual's spoor is substrate specific, hence we had to stop recurrently and the measurement exercise was repeated at many places where it was possible on various surfaces – fine sand, soft earth, ploughed field and of course on ashes of the burnt crops that lay here and there to fertilize the soil sand etc. It took us some eight hours to cover over 15 kilometers under the scorching sun and finally tired of the day's exercise we dropped the trail halfway and returned home.

Next day we picked up the trail from the same point we had left. The tracking ended ten kilometers further as around midday a dust storm intensified, making the sky turn hazy with powdered dust. As light diffused, once again we had to leave the trail midway. On the third day, of course we had taken more time on our part in traveling the terrain than the tiger, and finally the affair was resolved when we noticed the footprints entering the jungles of Mala. I followed them for over 300 meters inside the forest up to a point where banyan and flame of the forest trees were shedding their leaves in thousands and strong gusts of wind scattered them in showers, sending them to every nook and corner of the forest. There was a brief audible sigh as the sun lowered itself quiet gently and sank and we returned home feeling amazed at this gargantuan feet of a big tom through barren farmlands.

I returned to Dudhwa headquarters and reported the case to Wung Longwa, the Deputy Director of the Park. The tiger had covered that distance of over 30 kilometers in just one go under the concealment of stygian darkness and we had followed it for three days to confirm his crossing. Incidentally it was *amavasya* (no moon night). Perhaps the tiger had some intuitive calendar in his mind that kept track of the moon's progress, much on similar pattern of Sunderbans tigers that keep track of genuine high tides through moon's movement and use them to vacate the island and seek refuge on high grounds.

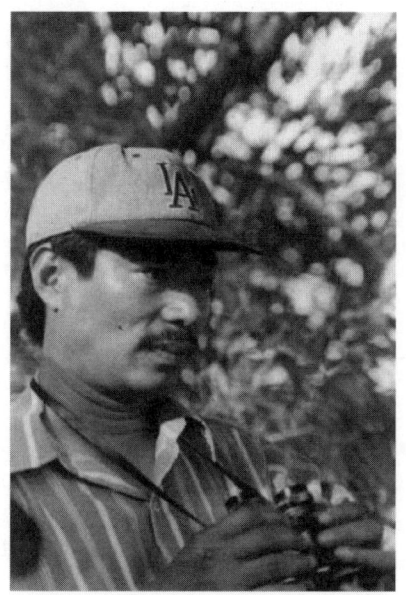

WungLongwa IFS, Chief Conservator of Forests Uttara-Khand, a man of daring and physical hardihood; we have covered many miles after tigers together.

It may be added that physical characteristics of Sunderbans are dynamic. It is a contiguous network of islands, creeks and estuaries of swampy mangrove forests which straddle Bangladesh and India along the shoreline of the Bay of Bengal. The great patch of over 10,000 sq km changes daily with changing tide, where landmarks emerge and submerge constantly; hence tigers have leant to use the lunar calendar for survival in this ever-changing coastal environment.

Next morning, not losing any time, Longwa sent a full-scale expedition of his rangers to investigate the trail. After three days, their team confirmed that they were finally able to match my plaster cast sets picked from the accurate tracing of a big tiger paw recorded at starting point of Paraspur, with the soft earth impression-pads made at Mala forest range in Pilibhit district.

Vishnu Narain Singh, later Honorary Wildlife Warden of Katarnia Ghat, and a strong hand of Billy's anti-poaching projects had assisted the rangers' team, and he also confirmed the findings. He even found a banyan tree, where the tiger, standing full length at the height of 12 feet, with his hands stretched up, had almost locked his razor sharp claws into the trunk and then scratched it down half-inch deep. The deep lacerations showed the strength of claws that once fully engaged in a prey's flesh, they enable the tiger to literally ride its victim into the ground. It was terrific the way the big tom, young and yet a veteran publicized his presence to communicate with con-specifics through markings in the sugar fields while journeying hurriedly.

It requires several years of dangerous existence before an amateur male tiger acquires enough skill as well as the will to create and defend a territory of his own and become a Grand Master. But as powerful as he may be and even if he wins the battle for the territory, it can leave him grievously injured because these animals are so lethally designed that any real conflict between them is equivalent to a hand grenade contest that inflicts serious damage to all. And the ones that survive are truly awe-inspiring specimens.

Ranges are lifelines to tigers, providing a year-round supply of prey species as well as females to court. Though each territory is fluid in its extent, varying according to seasonal changes in prey availability but there are some permanent ranges that are not limited to arbitrary points on a map. It made me assume that in winters, tigers crossed the terrain at leisure, knowing all the possible variations of their prey's paths, and they stayed and hunted in cover of canes. In summers, since there was little or no cover, they undertook the same journey but in just one go. Indeed they knew the terrain well and thus took the straight route that would take them to their destination in one night. In 1998 again at an official meeting of Wildlife Advisory Board, I presented the new data, authenticated by forest rangers, breaking the news that a 'Grand Master' from Jhadital was covering two great jungles of Kishanpur and Mala in his single beat.

This was a remarkable discovery, leaving no reasons to doubt the rendition of the story as this time the Deputy Director of Dudhwa was also officially involved, providing sufficient scientific evidence. But Billy was again furious. He said, "Tarai tigers are more or less local beasts with great attachment to their ranges, which they don't easily leave. Taking this into consideration, it is impossible to say that they will cover such a distance. Only man-eaters create such large ranges, as is evident in the cases of Thak and Talladesh man-eaters (shot by Corbett that enjoyed a one thousand plus sq.km range). I think Dr Shukla should not waste the Board's, his own and our time in this futile discussion."

In his official capacity as Principal Secretary Forest (UP Government), P.L. Punia was presiding over the meeting. His reaction was quick as he picked my report and said waving it: "Besides major relocations that are caused by natural catastrophes such as floods and fires, tigers can cover large distances in a short period, when they require so. The cane tiger theory is not so brittle so as to crumble down to echoes of few critiques. Their data is immense which is endorsed by foresters. It needs understanding." This apt comment tended to dampen some of the nastier observations on my professional integrity.

In any case, it needs many years of dangerous existence before a male tiger assimilates the craft and determination to move out and create an overreaching territory. Such tigers are rare but they do exist.

A Russian scientist Vladimir Heptner has recorded several instances of tigers following migrating herds of wild boar, over six hundred miles (1000 km) in Taiga area. When northern tigers can cover such gargantuan distances unabated then why Tarai tigers were doubted taking a 50 to 60 mile walk of their old beaten routes, especially when so many wild boars resided in sugar plantations, enough to feed them when they crossed.

Parenthetically on these lines my attitude was that the reason should prevail and we should be able to give as definitive as possible a picture of Tarai tiger, that must appeal to village communities and specialists alike. But Billy's contention was that confusion should triumph and his opinion should be sought on every point. I listed my points of disagreement with Billy and accused him of prejudice for he did not seek my view on the subject or asked for any evidence which I could have given him. He was powerless to impress mandarins as my findings had approval of

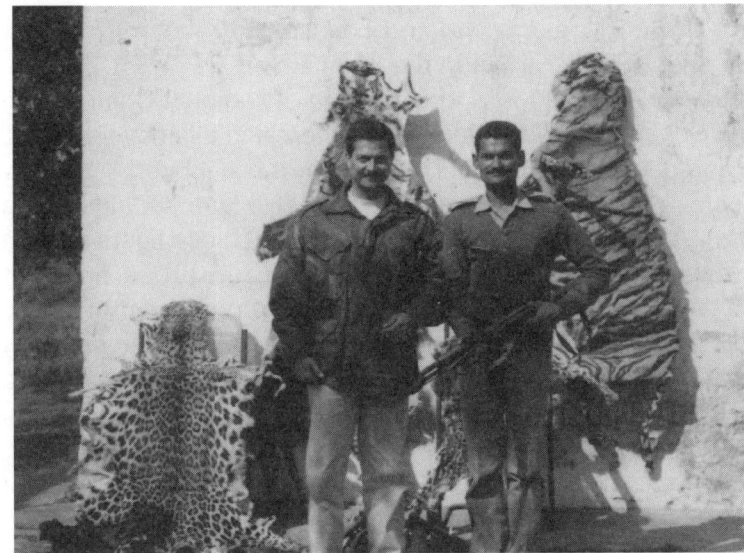

VishnuNarain Singh "Billoo', Hon Wildife Warden of Katarnia-ghat Sanctuary with recovered tiger pelts; a few men have lived life more fraught with peril than him. (Photo credit : Harish Kumar, IPS, STF, Uttar Pradesh

the field staff but he did enough damage to my standing in wildlife circles, perhaps injudiciously, by giving hard statements against my report to the press as "entirely false findings".

A tag line of tiger politics tells that tigers attract big egos and big egos don't work well together. Billy believed that his knowledge about Dudhwa tigers could not be battered by any one hence he often worked as an instrument in blocking the applications and foreign funding's of many a researchers. Finally due to his adverse reaction to my claim, the two issues, the conservation of jungle tigers and farm tigers could never be linked. Farm tigers remained the millstone of natives while the old man on the record maintained the status quo; a process of attrition which could only lead to grinding down of farm tigers.

I may be pardoned for saying that Billy was the 'Honorary tiger' of Dudhwa and one may not see a tiger in Dudhwa, but he was always spotted roaming in the jungle, friendly to tourists. But he did not like researchers and pollsters appearing on his turf that might score a point over him. Going for the throat of such researchers in an instinctive death grip was his tiger nature.

However, a week later Billy filched a dead cow on a tractor trolley from a village called Makanpur and dumped it close to his farm. This was to facilitate the shooting of a BBC film on his residence Tiger Haven. Longwa was quite upset at the news that a pair of tigers had quickly taken to baiting. Only a month ago a tigress with three cubs had been poisoned by natives in Kaloopura village and similarly there was great risk for this pair meeting the same treatment. Longwa and Vishnu Narain raided the spot, fired shots from .315 to drive the tigers away, got the cow thrown off into the jungle, burnt down Billy's *machan* and confiscated much of his gear that was brought for the shooting of the film in the night.

Interestingly, P.L. Punia (till 2016 an MP and Chairman of National Commission for Scheduled Caste and Scheduled Tribes) took keen interest in this development. In the next meeting of foresters, he skimmed the report and declared it as new White Paper on the spectacle of wildlife in Tarai farmlands. He later sent the same to the Project Tiger in Delhi, supporting my endeavors to protect these tigers against poachers. It read: "Between Dudhwa and Katarnia Ghat run broad fields of cultivation devoid of jungles, but this pocket records a heavy movement of tigers. They cross over from Kheri to Bahraich district and vice versa, using more than thirty miles of sugarcane plantations as corridors that have been planted right to the boundary of the forest. Similar travel is also recorded by tigers in Central Tarai Area (CTA) through crowded farmlands between South and North Kheri forests. Dr Rahul Shukla's findings as Honorary Wildlife Warden of the area, for the first time confirm this kind of marathon movement of tigers."

This report was presented at a joint meeting of Environment Ministry and the WWF at Paryavaran Bhavan New Delhi. It came as soothing balm to my anguished self-esteem and silenced many insensitive voices that had long echoed against me.

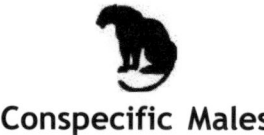

Conspecific Males

Nothing has been done to combat the menace of tigers living in sugar-cane.
— Billy Arjan Singh

In winters tiger ranges increase in size because they tend to become more mobile as the prey spreads. But my own experience led me to believe that these big beasts were shifting regardless of seasons. Taking their natural history and ancestry into consideration, for many hundreds of generations they have inherited this territory. The circle or triangle of travel is habitually completed with monotonous regularity. Occasionally the tour is accelerated or slowed down, subject to success in hunting in farmlands but they make the circle over and over again, perhaps 3 to 4 times in a year or may be more. They regularly cover the outsized terrain that amounts to some 500 or more sq km, containing large sugarcane farms as well as the principal jungles.

In the testosterone-heavy world of tigers, large males are conspecific and intolerant in nature. Their greater sense of territoriality readily objects to intrusion by any outside tiger and especially young males; though the areas well-stocked with prey often allow tigers to coexist peacefully even if overcrowded, but large tigers are better avoided by juniors and sometimes even cub-rearing tigresses. Old data about male tigers found dead in sugar farms is available with UP Government's Forest Department. It mentions that no less than 4 young males, (to my mind, inevitably ones with less regal bloodlines) were killed on the same track falling between Jhadi Tal and Mala block in Pilibhit during 1989 to 1994.

Over the years the resident male had killed all his four rivals in a masterful manner. Perhaps these naive males with no territory of their own were living on the margins. The autopsy reports declared them as killed in outright conspecific aggressions. Incidentally all were over 4 and less than 6 years of age and killed at the same point of their lives when testosterone impact is at its peak.

Tigers, particularly males, are well known for their passionate and reflexive possessiveness when it comes to territory, mates and food. It is a delineating characteristic that wields a powerful influence on their behavior particularly towards males. They become violent boundary keepers and guard their domain as enthusiastically as city gangsters maintain their realm by out-competing other gangs even by heinous eliminations of their fellow beings.

I had every reason to believe that this slaughter of young males, though brutally expensive in biological terms, was done by the grand male, which looped the loop on his long journey through cane fields. For the moment there was no one to challenge him from roaming wherever he pleased. Going by facts that he inhabited two different forest ranges in south and north Kheri respectively with equal ease that are separated by the distance of 30 kilometers of farmlands plunging in between, this human dominated landscape was indeed the heart of his territory. He was the real monarch and lord of this sugarcane range.

His last kill - a a strong tiger - had been messily disemboweled after slaying. One of its thighs was eaten and its appendages had been scattered astride the battle ground. The commencing phase of skirmish was witnessed by Jal Singh, a grazier, and his nephew, who described it thus: "The big one came galloping from behind the junior tiger and landed upon it, seizing its neck in his jaws. His hind legs were still on the ground while his forepaws had clutched the victim from both sides. He appeared to be copulating the rival, thrusting him forward violently from the back with his belly while at the same time puling his neck back with arresting force, which the junior failed to withstand and his neck broke with strain. It was a two minute affair, then the tiger dismounted and begun to disembowel the dead in savage ferocity. We felt so horrified by his anger that we ran back home."

I did not doubt his version at all. For, all tigers evolve, learning to hunt wild game under the tutelage of their mother but some tigers, soon after leaving their mother develop an entirely different killing technique, which is also quite helpful in countering a competitor. Such tigers when hunting a competitor adopt the same method of ambushing from behind. Until the rival tiger becomes alert and counters the attack by turning to face the attacker, this move changes the situation and the battle becomes a boxing round, where much time is occupied in circling, and threatening each other rather than coming to grips. The heavily armed predators do inflicted grievous injuries to each other with much active bleeding taking place. But brawls rarely end in death, for none of the killers then easily get opportunity to effectively seize each other's vulnerable body parts such as neck, jugular or testicles. But if the initial attack is not jeopardized than just one grip of the aggressor on the neck of other tiger is enough. It is this technique of hunting and confidence that makes a Primorye tiger go at the brown bears fairly regularly.

In the same time phase of early 90s, there were no less than four breeding tigresses in this circle, raising his cubs in sugar fields. And all these had possibly come to him through a matriarchal hierarchy, who by association with older females or their mother had acquired the knowledge of best sites for giving birth to cubs and ambushing prey, finding water and shelter as well. Perhaps they were themselves born in these sugar fields and had lived in the area as farmland tigress. Indeed their choice of the place, an old but now a renewed tiger territory was based on their firsthand extensive experience.

Once a tigress creates a range in less competitive habitat, it holds that for good six to eight years, until she has produced 3 to 4 litters and is of about 10 to 12 years of age. Such tigresses often become pregnant by roving males or nomads who are in search of a territory but the off spring of these casual liaisons are essentially killed by dominant males to safeguard his genetic interests, unless the tigress intelligently succeeds in befooling the male that they are his progeny and none else's..

Parenthetically when males of impressive size gain control over larger areas, they maintain their dominance over territories for years. This king tiger seemed galvanized by the urge to protect his territory; never more so than now because there were many breeding females in the farmlands and he didn't want his conspecifcs to intervene with them. This substantiates the belief of Prof Agassiz, a contemporary of Charles Darwin, that homelands are determined by the adaptation of some common stock. In this case the tigresses' home was not jungle but sugarcane plantation where the common stock was living, including their kin, cubs and young mates.

Under present conditions this ignorance on the part of foresters was critical, creating an uneasy vacuum. An investigation was needed to support my hypothesis that was indirectly being confirmed by the death of male tigers in a specified area. But though they maintained that killing of a range intruder is a form of population control among tigers, none of them ever agreed that a real big tom traversing this 30-km long beat of farmland was responsible for these recurring deaths in last three years.

Foresters were unaware that such large ranges are a product of complicated biological processes in tiger systems, the classified process by which tigers control

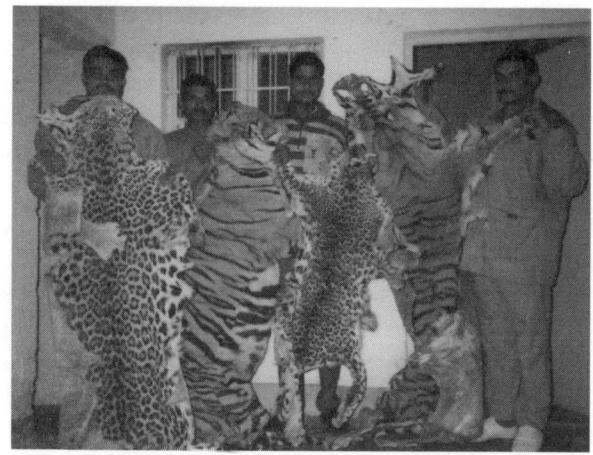

Contrabands caught at KaimaGaurhi and Khajuria near Puranpur border in a joint operation of STF, Author and Vishnu Narain Singh. Left a big leopard, 8'1, shot and skinned at Ghola one and a half kilometers from Billy Arjan Singh's residence Tiger Haven

and maintain their populations (when man is singularly unqualified to deal with its own populations) requiring a considerable knowhow for us as how this works in large ranges. It is in fact an eternal and evolutionary process, which is the eventual touchstone.

At this point I might be accused of talking like a scientist, when exactly I am not. I am just a wildlife conservationist speaking with knowledge, which has allowed me to become too involved with farmland tigers. It has nothing to do with science, it has a lot to do with emotions and commitments as how so many wild animals sustain themselves in a man-made environment that is indeed so difficult a place. My job is to theorize how they do that by allowing myself to get involved with their lives. It naturally opens gates for a bit of science. Yes, I am no scientist but I sound like one when I talk about cane tigers.

Ironically Peter Jackson, the Chairman of the Cat Specialist Group and a gentle Englishman who speaks for much tiger science today, is himself not a scientist. He is a former journalist who got involved with big cats while travelling for wildlife coverage with Reuters. This vocational inappropriateness sometimes afflicts Jackson with disrespect from the very scientist community he apparently represents but he enjoys strong international focus for his personal views about tigers.

It won't be an exaggeration to say that these great perambulations of cats across sugar fields are in fact historical tiger loops, reserved for magnificent and colossal beasts, where their grand forefathers had naturally roamed unabated. Moreover resident males cannot afford to be absent from these places because then other males would seek to establish themselves during his absence and then every female and every selective kill will be keenly contested. It is only at the sudden loss of a prime male, eliminated through traps of any kind, baits tucked with bite-sensitive bombs, or laced with poison that brings about changes in the established order.

Billy Arjan Singh writes in *Tiger! Tiger!* "Just a couple of centuries ago there was ample room for each species to avoid the other. The forests were unlimited and human population was so small that it needed to use only a fraction of the land surface. Between the jungles and the pockets of cultivation were huge buffer areas of scrub and grass. This pattern – idyllic by today's standards – persisted for thousands of years. Then gradually human population expanded, tiger habitat diminished and in past few decades the process has suddenly accelerated with frightening finality. The buffer zones have disappeared; commercial exploitation has reduced the forest to a travesty of its former luxuriance. And humans have returned to live on the edge of the jungle creating vast farmlands."

Keeping this fact in mind it appears that as a result of post-independence deforestation, an extremely complicated pattern of tiger territories made its appearance. It was in fact normal to big resident males because their ancestors had covered these circles as their territories for generations. And now, despite the ecological crisis of newly-emerged farmlands, the animal that had always eschewed humans, had now slowly got adjusted to their presence (though never adopted them as prey species) and their powerful progeny, as mercurial as their forefathers, were still continuing that tradition of occupying great breeding territories, genetically and behaviorally compromised as long the changing conditions allowed them to go on. It is actually urges of generations upon generations of evolutionary selectivity that makes them compete for large breeding ranges.

Every ecosystem, howsoever haphazard a collection of objects and events it may appear to comprise has its own characteristics conducive for wildlife. The basic answer to tigers inhabiting sugarcane plantations is really quite simple. This is an eternal phenomenon that explains as how some tigers take sugarcane on board to aid their survival, making it their home and what is probably the densest but most conducive grass home in all Tarai between September and December. It helps the real big toms to take up patrolling of extraordinary territories as a corollary to the axiom of survival of the fittest.

This is my biological explanation to the complex question of greatly extended tiger territories in the Tarai that exceed from 500 sq km to 700 sq km or more, regardless of the land terrain, whether it comprises big jungles or vast farmlands or jungles partly and farmlands vastly.

Now, some 20 years later, with photographic records of camera trappings becoming viral on electronic screens, these facts are very clear to forest managers. Like the lost piece of a forgotten puzzle this is no hotchpotch but the reality, a first-hand knowledge, a valid data of a fabulous fact, regurgitated by latest quantitative findings of WWF India, that tigers do cover such long distances. But in mid-90s, when my revelation about their journeys was published in *The Times of India* (Lucknow edition) and later made known throughout India, there was nothing revolutionary about it, yet it was taken with skepticism and distrust even by WWF and Project Tiger. The failure to appreciate these facts led to confusion and apparently accounted for many contradictions.

My study of sugarcane tigers was immensely appreciated by the then Governor of Uttar Pradesh Mr Suraj Bhan. During November 1999, he visited Dudhwa National Park wherein I accompanied him. There was a certain amount of worry and burden of responsibility attached to the assignment of showing a tiger to the Governor that we failed to encounter in the DNP but while going to Katarnia Ghat through an immense stretch of farmlands we did come across a large male tiger, sitting on the road behind a scanty bush growing on the central strip of road. It was a handsome animal, licking its paw in the manner of a domestic cat and lazing. We stopped the motorcade and the nonchalant beast kept sitting with his tummy bulging and without changing its posture. Some five minutes later the Special Secretary to the Governor, Har Sharan Das, spotted a tigress emerging 50 yards behind him. She was somewhat smaller and lissome but extravagantly marked. The Governor was overwhelmed at this sight. He whispered to me in surprise, "Such a historic changeover has taken place despite the human pressures that are apparently built up against their existence. To deny your theory needs qualifications."

At a distance, crows were dropping down in flocks, cawing vociferously which was the sign of a kill lying there and the fresh blood smeared on the face of the tigress announced that she had gobbled the leftovers for a long time after the male had finished. Then the sputtering sound of a tractor coming from opposite direction disrupted the scene, the pair first advanced towards us then scowling at the crows went towards them entering the grass forest of sugarcane.

There was no opposition to the tiger's presence in the area, no popular resistance to his ways of existence, for he was known to select only wild game to feed upon, which in itself was a tribute to the non-aggressive reactions of the super predator in a human landscape. On his return to city the Governor took cognizance of my complete work and giving an unfailing moral and material support in defense of the noble animal, was pleased to honor me with an official missive of appreciation. The missive is produced in my previous book *Sugarcane Tiger.*

The glorious history of big toms in the Tarai farmlands has not whittled down at all. In 2016, there are some ten identified big male tigers encumbered with that extra dose of testosterone and they are regularly shunting between different forest ranges. These are recorded by none else than WWF field activist Mudit Gupta and his team stationed at Palia Kalan. Steeped in the wild environment with tiger as his consuming passion, Mudit told me that "Big toms are crossing some 30 to 50 kilometers of rural landscape – as the crow flies – in this hazardous journey. There is no doubt plenty of food but there are dangers too." I increasingly understand that these big toms are exposed to a very odd ecological position when they travel through this terrain, evidently to re-establish themselves but many of these who achieve great age and size have figured out that now with changing times, the safety in this landscape lies in darkness, perhaps also in their good behavior.

The fact is that the climate of opinion and the apparent problems of tiger's presence in sugarcane have changed a great deal since 1994 when these discoveries were first revealed and the idea to protect them in farmlands was first mooted. This is clear that the tigers have survived into an era of better protection both in jungles and farmlands to have the real chance of sustaining themselves. Sugarcane plantations as dense grassed passageways offer sufficient room for them to maintain their genetic strength. And even big jungle toms take up residence in the cane fields during winters, moving gradually to other jungle compartments in bits and installments, not in a swift or clinical sweep as they do in summers.

Capsulated, saving these tigers is a daunting task but still those who moot the idea of essential large scale separation measures, fearing the chances of active man-eating and the melancholy series of deaths, must know that their idea doesn't necessarily apply in this landscape, for simply it cannot be applied with these animals. However, moderately in last five years, rare accidental deaths have been recorded by these tigers, which are no doubt an occupational hazard for humans who work in sugar farms. This corroborates that nature has evolved its own alleviations to steer clear of problems and we need not feel haunted by the memories of malevolent past – that odious phase of Tarai when man-eating had become an epidemic.

There is a principle of contemporary scientific philosophy which declares that great advances in knowledge do not follow exclusively through trial and error but await the occurrences of intuition and the inclination of human mind to accept it. In other words to cite the tagline of television show '*The X Files*', that contends that the 'Truth is Out There'. This is what Mudit Gupta says "It is just a matter of perceiving it with open mind."

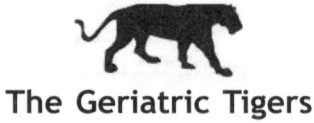

The Geriatric Tigers

There is nothing like staying at home for real comfort.

— Jane Austen

In addition to all this I have also come across three old geriatric tigers, all males in farmlands who spent their last phase of life in farmlands and without becoming a menace to people died a natural death. Just how many tigers die from illness and what kind of diseases afflicts them is not very clear. But fairly large numbers of tigers do attain old age and when they come to this stage they present a tragic feature.

Old age comes to tigers with abrupt conclusiveness as their body colours change with age and health. During youth, the ground colour of a vigorous beast is almost of a brilliant orange with intense black while in an old animal, the black becomes dull and the yellow fades to sandy hue. Their hind quarters become weak, their waist drawn up and their hip bones stick up permanently and somewhat heavy animals quickly reduce in body weight within a few months. Sometimes the effects of malnutrition first takes form of sloughing legs often with ulcers appearing around joints that would not heal but become larger and larger. In such times when the king is menaced and subjected to attack by more vigorous males that are ready to occupy his territory, they better leave the possession of their ranges and shift to peripheral areas of jungles. Not preferring to die in a duel the king is chased out of his territory, such evicted tigers break out into the farmlands and spend their last days, keeping a low profile and hunt only at night when herdsmen are safely confined to their homes.

From 2001 to 2003, a male tiger of old order is recorded to have appeared at Deepnagar farmlands. Perhaps 6 years earlier this area had been an integral part of his extended territory where now, a pale shadow of his former self, he had shifted from jungle to live permanently. He hunted for the possibility of scavenging a meal and the sight of vultures, eagles and crows plummeting to earth always attracted him.

The physiological limits set by ageing, like supply of blood to outsized muscles masses, nutritional problems, loss of agility associated with large body, wear and tear on paws by thorns and other sharp objects including arthritis (all primary cause of man-eating behavior) were all conspicuously apparent. He seemed clearly unable to hunt any large animal but still seemed to attach himself with the abundance of prey.

When towards sunset the herders returned home he felt tempted by the resonant bellowing of cattle and tinkling of cowbells. He often materialized on the scene and followed the cattle from a respectable distance of around 100 meters. Having done this quite a few times, it had probably become his game for he would do this every day yet never attacking them. Once he came nearer up to 50 yards, and when the alarmed herders protested shouting and waving staves in the air the tiger immediately shifted into a muddy waterhole where it sat hidden. Time and again it raised its head to take an appraisal of the situation, but the wind factor was not in his favour, his smell was reaching the cattle, which continued to bellow nervously and the herders shouted.

For a moment the scene was total pandemonium. Finally frustrated the old animal began to growl from his sitting position, constantly raising his enormous head above the pit level to stare at herdsmen. Its half projected head, illuminated by the evening sun and his bellicose roars rolling the terrain advertised his real intentions. At this the cattle ran away and the men also left the place in hurry.

Big cats are catholic in taste but not at all above scavenging and even young healthy game killers take to moderately decomposed carrion quite nicely. Many sick and even pregnant cattle roam far from villages, where they often fall and die and their carcasses are left exposed inviting a volley of scavengers. A chance discovery of abandoned or unconsumed meat is one of major systems that keep wounded and geriatric predators alive when humans are distant or absent. Such carcasses are a magnificent banquet for which they need not so much as lift a paw.

The one and the only time I saw this tiger, he had that gnarled, time-weary look that comes to big cats with advancing age. The impaired animal was awfully thin, his skin was grizzled and I estimated his weight around 100 kg and measuring some 9 ft. 8in. from tip of nose to the tip of tail. He stayed in the area for good 17 months, spending his final months almost incognito. Last time he was seen moving in a gram field, his head lolling from side to side and spittle drooling from his mouth. He was well into his last legs of life. Probably unable to fend for himself properly, he was starving to death. Every so often he used to lay down as if he was too tired to continue in life. He finally died of swathing age.

Here I may make clear that sugar fields do serve as 'homes' for ageing tigers. But scattered populations of old tigers in farmlands are not free from the pressure of roving and nomadic young males, who in a bid to consolidate their claim to the area converge upon them. Nevertheless it is the way of their tribe that forces the weaker to relinquish the tenuous hold from the place.

In such a case, instead of mooching around in the face of inter-species tension and competing predators in a given spatial area, the oldies – like the weaker young ones – prefer to defuse the tension by crossing over to farther lands. The Bangawa male observed throughout 2003 was an example of this. He lived over 10 kilometers away from the main jungle between Bilrayan and Katarnia Ghat sanctuary and sustained himself by scavenging and occasional killing of small animals including frogs. He would sit near the water ponds and stalk the frogs for hours, killing and eating up to 50 in one night. Villagers told me he was seen eating over-ripened bananas and his scats carried guava and *shareefa* (custard apple) seeds. Frank Simpson, the author of *Sport in Eastern Bengal* wrote that he had "once killed a tiger whose paunch was crammed full of grasshoppers or locusts."

Healthy tigers are known to discard innards of prey and eat solid meat from rump and thigh first, gradually shifting to soft bones and viscera. But I have noted in two kills, of course made by aged sugar tigers, one of a feral cow at Salimabad and the other of a *nilgai* bull at Sisaeeya that when prey was ingested, besides rump a bit of intestines were also eaten. In case of geriatric tigers spending the last phase of their life, they feed on everything worth eating. The relevant explanation is that intestines contain lots of nutrients needed for good health and when some young game-killing tigers value such parts then there is no hassle for oldies, whose fangs and cutter teeth have grown brittle or fallen, to go for softer meat.

Tigers can only eat non-grain food crops but I have some times found evidence of *chana* (gram) and pulses in the droppings. It appears that as the pellets of birds of prey often contain seeds from their victim's last meal, similarly, the droppings of tigers that go for innards like intestines do carry such material. Tigers do eat fruits and experienced animals with developing intelligence resort to more diverse diet than naïve unsophisticated youngsters would consider, probably relishing much of non-mainstream food for it helps their survival. However, in this particular case, I have two explanations to offer; the first is that the animal had eaten guava and custard apple, hence seeds were there in the scats or these might have come from scavenging some herbivores' intestines.

Having found some eight scat evidences on this line, I am categorical about it that old tigers do scoff fruits without misgiving as their muscle powers degenerate and nature condemns them to a slow death. I strongly believe that catholicity of their demands with regard to food (not the prey animals) then becomes very wide ranging, besides fallen fruits they even munch mustard, sugarcane flowers and ripe tomatoes, proving that the great predators remain essentially flexible in their resource requirements till the fag-end of their life. Weighted by their physical indisposition and yet ministered by the offerings which are in nature, they linger for a couple of months near human habitations and then wither away into obscurity.

Following the data of geriatric tigers, a carcass was found in the sugarcane fields of Piparya-Bhood village on 4 January 2016 close to Sharda glitches in south Kheri. It offered strikingly fresh evidence of old evictees displaced by youngsters, taking refuge in sugar fields at the fag-end of their life. Found during the harvesting of cane when the field was being cleared, its flesh and skin were completely rotten. The carcass was estimated to be at least three months old. Its skull, bone nails and teeth were intact but the bones of the limbs were dissociated while the condition of its molars and pre molars showed to be a very old tiger.

Catching a free-ranging prey in the jungle is an unpleasant task for an ageing tiger while a small animal is merely a sop to his prodigious appetite. Sanjay Singh, the Field Director of Dudhwa says, "Such animals, half-starved, coming from jungles, shy away from venturing into open but a percentage of them frequents dense sugar cane, eking out their terminal years on scavenging diet of dead cattle, seeking their living on whatever they get in the man-led environment. These are no doubt very hard-pressed animals."

Necrophagy is a powerful tool of survival where most putrescent remains are willingly scavenged by healthy tigers, and were consumed even by early *Homo sapiens* during crisis times spanning the evolutionary chain. Human history records that for millions of years our ancestors empowered by developing brains and evolving technology moved across the great continent of Africa, and survived without lifting a spear to kill. They rather stole their meal from the deadliest hunters, attacking them in groups and driving them away. For in nature, life feeds on death in as much proportion as death feeds on life. Similarly once an old tiger finds the dead bait, practically of anything, it holds him there, and some tigers particularly develop customary feeding habits at the spot where the dead cattle are thrown.

Old tigers with their carnassials and canines broken and their powers waning to overcome normal prey, gradually waste away into obscurity. Though necrophagy does support them for a short time like a bed-ridden patient on oxygen, but soon they fall and their earthly remains rest in the glitches and swamps of Sharda, Girwa, Suheli, Mahona and Ghaghra etc where the dense scrub swallows them in the foliage pattern of vegetation. The same alcove that had once shielded them within its shades now consumes them with its worms, fungi, moulds and microbes and they disappear forever in the recess from where they had once come.

There is no natural history record of an old tiger being pulled down by any one of scavengers in India, while in hard African conditions aging lions are invariably attacked by wild dogs and loathsome scavengers like hyenas who in normal circumstances would flee in terror from the great animal's one grunt of disapproval.

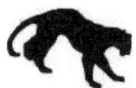

The Blighter Old Chap of Bankeyganj-South Kheri

Old tigers do not automatically take to an alien diet without intense compulsions.
- Billy Arjan Singh

As regards man-eating in geriatric tigers, when their natural prey is driven away by disturbance or they are unable to catch them, they naturally take to hanging around the outskirts of human settlements. Often driven by intense hunger they enter the village and create problems. As this book is being written, in April 2016, a geriatric tiger has been found to inhabit farmlands of Jatpura near Bankeyganj in south Kheri range of Lakhimpur Kheri district. Despite the crops of cane and wheat having been harvested and the fields lying open without cover, he had not gone back to the jungle. As per villagers' information a tigress was known to be raising three cubs inside the jungle and perceiving him as threat to her cubs she had aggressively and permanently driven him out. The old tiger now lived in farmlands; he sometimes entered the jungle, penetrated some two, three hundred yards but due to the fear of tigress, again came out quickly in farmlands.

Hunger, essentially aggravated by decimation of prey species in farmlands, compelled the Blighter Old Chap to seek food around villages and enter human settlements. Consequently he made two human kills that he couldn't eat. On 28 February he killed a shepherd named Rahees Gaddi and on 19 March, a Sikh farmer Tersen Singh was fatally attacked towards the evening. When the victim's companions heard his yells and a vibrant growling, they came out shouting. At their sight the tiger ran away and the man's body was found lying under a bush in a pool of blood about twenty yards away from his toppled chair. The victim had been seized directly inside the premises of his house. This implied that the attack had been deliberate and cold-blooded. After a long gap of activities, in attempting to catch a woman named Kiran on 11 April, he mauled her badly and later killed another named Sunita on 15 April 2016. All these times he was dispossessed of carcass by yelling farm workers who later also burnt down whatever grass cover he could hide in the vicinity.

In the next week, a farmer named Binda Din unearthed several snakes like cobra and krait when he ploughed his field. The reptiles were ostensibly living just below the surface and the harrow disc attached to tractor dug out their shelters and the writhing and sliced bodies of reptiles and rats emerged into the open with freshly broken soil. That very night, the tiger arrived on the plot and enjoyed a hearty meal of sliced reptiles. Furthermore he got a clue to an easy meal in this experience and started frequenting ploughed areas in the cover of night searching for another sliced meal. One morning he was seen hanging about the spot after its nightly meal scowling at jackals, and other carrion feeds which might attempt to pilfer its larder. This determines as how geriatric tigers, although extraordinarily isolated from their own world, efficiently manage their lives.

While tigers are politically unprotected and old tigers are hard-pressed animals, opportunism plays a big role in their poaching. When such crisis occurs and a predatory carnivore starts entering the village; the so-called virtue of not initiating their elimination might mean cows, goats and humans getting killed. Thus, the rationale to not to put down an animal like the wild tiger, is particularly hard to implant among the people most likely to commit the act. The problem is to make the larger and more compelling logic that might drive people to protect the animal than the logic of poachers emphasizing innate savagery of tigers and encouraging people to "get rid of the menace" - a theory which locals, going nuts, easily buy.

Anyway, from the point of view of conservation, death of a non-productive aged granddaddy is non-detrimental to the long-term survival of the flagship species. This in no way endangers the conservation programme, hence there is an immediate clamour for the tiger to be declared a man-eater and shot, which to my mind may enhance the long-term survivability of the species in the area as the female would better be able to rear her cubs and locals sure enough bequeathed unmolested, will not target tigers as enemies.

Old tigers, no longer intrepid hunters, are able to exist as scavengers for a long time. The Bankeyganj tiger seems to be able to manage petty food for his survival otherwise human killings would have been much more frequent. Yet, in the constraining aberration assailed by prolonged hunger and malnutrition, it has started viewing humans as prospective prey species. Consistent and persistent man-eaters, tigers not leopards, are known to go about their ghastly work at any time of the day, picking their victims randomly. On July 8, the decrepit critter struck again near a village called Khareta in broad daylight. Like a characteristic man-eater, having been savaged enough by starvation and injury to attacking man, it

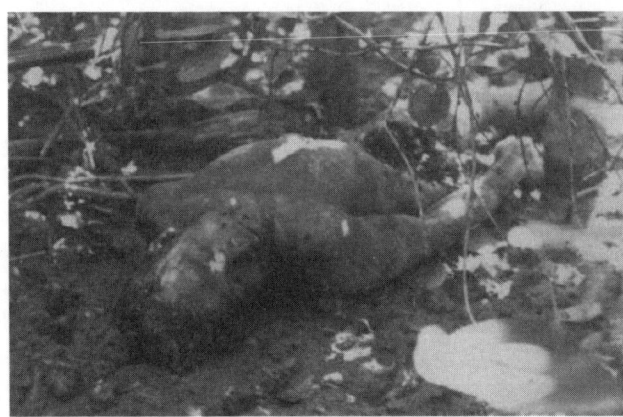

Dead body of Bhogal

killed a labourer named Bhogal. It clutched the poor man between his rotting, broken teeth, and tore the man's thighs and buttocks with his claws, disemboweling and bleeding him to death at no extra charge.

I feared if this trend continued it might soon turn into a master criminal, if not an inveterate man-eater and that would soon qualify him for a bullet but as it happens, the starving cat did not survive for long and by September 2016 finally faded into oblivion. Nobody knows under which leaf mound or undergrowth his mortal remains rest.

Having known exactly half a-dozen such specimens far outside forest boundaries in farmlands and watched a few I can still safely say that old age by itself is not a decisive factor to turn a normal tiger into a man-eater. Essentially adaptable tigers do not automatically take to an alien diet without intense compulsions. Has this not been a fact then we would always have a segment of aged tigers eking out their fag-end years on a diet of human flesh. True that aging tigers with defective teeth cannot readily break up cattle or deer and can easily deal with the bodies of human beings and obtain full nourishment, but the human is not an accepted prey species for a tiger and the punch line is this: Since human progress and population has advanced with high degree of expertise in various fields, the man no longer feels fit or has ceased to have its place into the environment in which tigers seek different forms of life maintenance.

The man's alien habits and his power for vengeance has made him an object of fear for animals that keep a safe distance from him except for those who have learnt by the process of familiarization that human is the easiest and prolific prey species.

The National Tiger Conservation Authority needs to have a thoughtful and caring attitude for the farmland wildlife where, eerie midnight chorus of jackals is not muted and hoof beats of blue bull and loud booming bass of fear-stricken wild boar still resounds at the notice of great marauders. The conservation programme will achieve much more success when this unique glitch of sugarcane plantations as holding and breeding ground of big cats, as well as great corridor is properly understood otherwise sands are fast running out for such mighty territorial colonizers.

IN THE WILDERNESS OF SUGARCANE

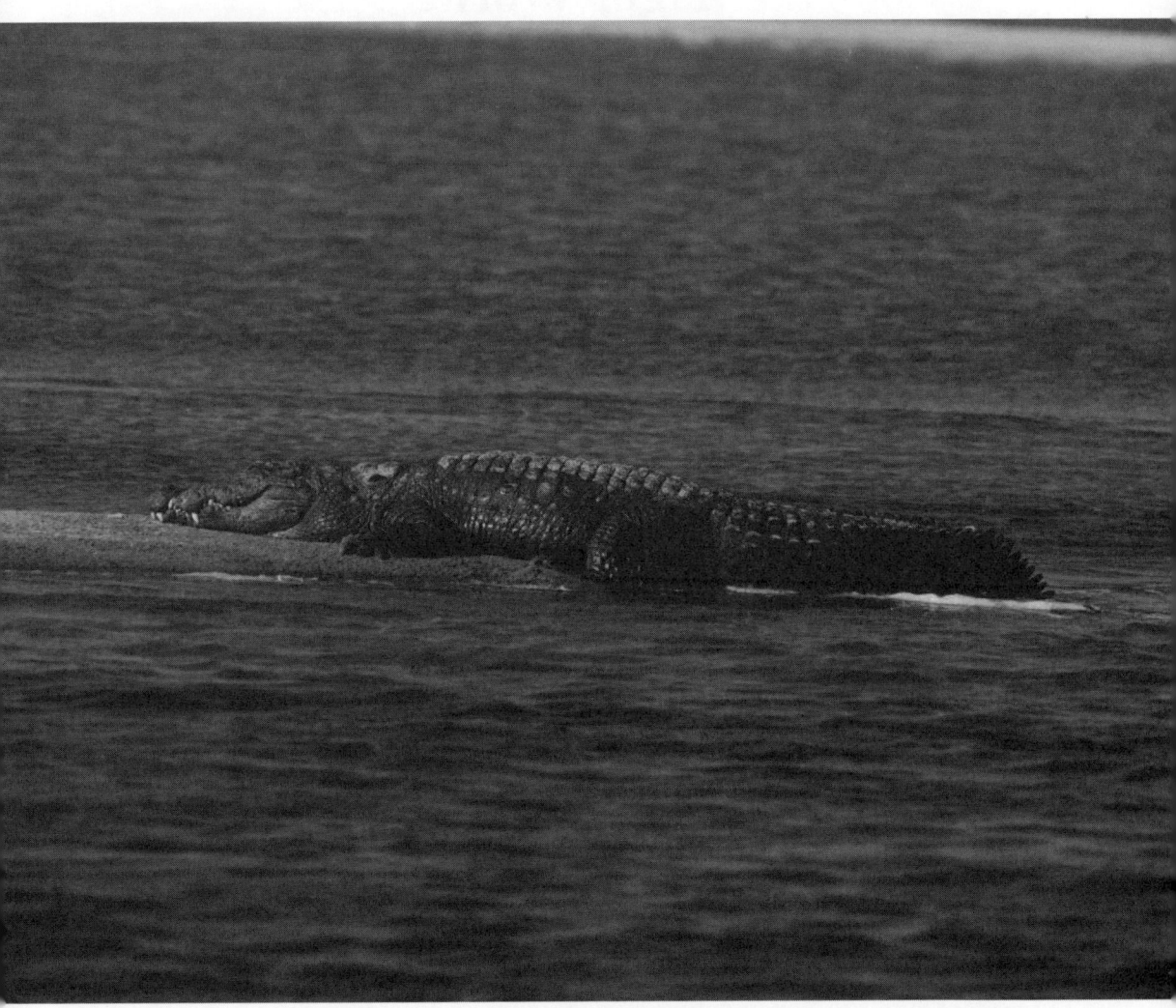

CHAPTER 6
IN THE REMOTE ISLANDS OF GIRWA

Chapter 6

Tiger World-
In the Remote Islands of Girwa

"Our knowledge base of how dangerous animals adapt aggrarian terrain has to be obtained by focusing on how they live without becoming a problem."

- Vidya Athreya

TARAI IS NOT ONLY WILD: IT IS ATTRACTIVE AND MYSTIC IN ITS OWN WAY. It is the Valhalla of bygone hunters and the Utopia of escapists, a photographer's paradise and a sweltering inferno of crime. It is what you think of it and it withstands all interpretations. It is the last vestige of a dead world or the candle light towards a shiny new one. To a lot of people, as to me, it is home. It is all these things with one constant– it is never dull.

The 1980s were a tiger-centric phase and the big cat population in the state of Uttar Pradesh had officially touched the 700-plus mark. This number was sufficient to satisfy even the most pessimistic of genetic prognosticators. I was then spending four months a year in the Tarai on my cane tiger research. During one of my visits, I met a forester named R.D. Batham who told me that not only had tiger population swelled, but the cane tiger phenomena too had increased. The profuse growth of inedible vegetation in jungle had driven the prey out and into agriculture fields. As they searched for food, tigers followed them, exploring new vistas for survival. He told me about a pair of tigers living in a remote island of Girwa river at the border of Kheri and Bahraich district.

"By heavens, they are beautiful tigers Dr Shukla, you would love to study them," the ranger concluded.

This large island of mainland Tarai, comprising three revenue villages named Khariatia, Jasnagar and Makanpur is located between the two bifurcating channels of Girwa river. It is oval in shape, like an enormous egg pushed up out of water. During the 1980s it was largely inaccessible. There was no connecting bridge, dispensary, school or even motorable roads, and only a small network of muddy paths wound into the settlements that were extremely backward. Villagers mostly used ferry to cross the river. The island was 40 per cent covered with the grass and the rest being cultivation. Till the early 1950s, the only inhabitants were a group of Thanaits, a fishing community that once abounded the place like forest dwelling Tharus. Later, families of Sikh immigrants turned up, finding it just right to start sugarcane cultivation.

It was a gorgeous afternoon of February 1983 when I alighted on the island with my old allies Deep Shah, Rajesh Bharti, Chhotey and Phagunia. Sardar Dalbeer Singh, an old friend of Bharti, received us warmly. A leathery and tireless man at fifty, this Sikh gentleman had a certain youthfulness inbred in him – a look of his eyes, tone of his voice – which tells about a vivid and eager curiosity for wildlife and the same passion for the world he lives in.

Our host made arrangements for our stay in his tile-roofed house that stood out in marked contrast to the green verdure. Electricity supply had yet not reached the village. As the dark hours commenced, hurricane lamps were lit and placed at selected places. We could hear islanders beating drums and upturned boats, and whatever else they could find to make a noise. This was to keep the herds of ungulates out of their fields.

It was a pitch black night. There was no moon but the velvet stars twinkled as we all sat under the open sky around a bonfire that cast deep shadows in the fields.. An open fire, whether it is a fireplace inside the house or a bonfire outside does something magical to me, relaxing me to that point where I am completely at ease and conversation comes readily. Peace begins to steal through me as I forget the fretters of civilization and drop off the pressures. It was a moment like this when Sardarji told us about the arrival of tigers.

"Tarai is susceptible to pronounced floods. During 1982, the monsoon had been threateningly heavy and the floods were terrible, resembling the scriptural deluge," he remembered. "The water entering the snake pits drives them out and they take to trees. Only then it is possible to get an idea as how numerous they can be. It was an extraordinary sight to find all the trees in the low-lying area being festooned with a motley collection of creatures like lizards, rats, squirrels, short-winged ground birds and of course hoards of snakes. They were lined up like rolled belts in a cloth shop and any professional snake-catcher could have easily picked them up with bare hands and dropped them one by one in a bag."

❖

As an aftermath of the deluge, low-lying areas, streams, canals and pits continued to hold the tail end of the flood waters. Dozens of dead animals littered the raised embankments of Girwa where vultures gorged on them and the remnants of thatched huts were suspended in the branches of the tamarind trees. One fine morning villagers sighted two tigers sheltering on high rises. Believed to be immigrants from Katarnia Ghat sanctuary and perhaps caught in the fury of floods they had swam across the deluge and reached the highlands.

It is much in the context to tell that Tarai flood have been historically furious. Colonel Keith Warrior (1930) describes one in Katarnia Ghat. "The rivers rose to full spate and flooded the country. Almost all bridges of the area have been breached or washed away including large sections of the metalled road and the entire habitat around sanctuary has been degraded by the water-logging. The water was up to the level of a man's head and at some places only upper portion of trees is sticking up out of it. The barrier of swift flowing water had defied all things that move on legs to cross it."

While a colonial hunter S.B. Simpson (1886) mentions: "At such times tigers used to live for a ten days or a fortnight on trees and... where doings were reported, they used to be shot on branches. These beasts fed apparently on turtles and crocodiles, on fish and animals which came to the mounds for refuge, and on the carcass of drowned creatures which came floating by. Tigers can swim well and I dare say that they used to swim from trees and return to them. I never saw anything of this myself, but I know the country and more than one gentleman who shot tigers on these trees."

The island tigers stayed on small mounds which were a sort of highlands for them. They were regularly seen there for a month, gorging on the stinking cattle carcass. Then gradually as the flood water disappeared, their sightings also reduced but their spoors littered all through the island brashly announced that the random wanderers had finally settled in the area.

Our host's younger brothers Kuldeep Singh and Jamwaar Singh had seen the pair on many occasions, "They are living here for last one year, they are quite okay-types, never interfering with humans", explained Kuldeep.

We talked till late night. After a few more drinks and dinner I reclined in a comfortable chair in front of the fire and fell asleep.

I must have slept for long, for it seemed hours later that I felt my shoulder being shaken and heard an urgent voice: "Bhaiya, wake up, a tiger is reported close by." I got up, wide awake in moments, getting my .375 Holland & Holland rifle and ammunition at the same time.

Whenever I go after tigers, I keep an adequate rifle with me for generalities are a mistake and I have known of several accidents that are exceptions to rules. It is quite impossible to say how any animal will behave under given circumstances, as one may run off and another do the opposite. Therefore it is advisable to keep a rifle handy, which is more needed to drive away the animal than to shoot it, which is a last resort. In that case the bone of contention is that besides offering great stopping power, the gun also ensures better accuracy. When such vital requirements are assured; rest is to the person who handles it.

On way to the river we came across a herd of blue bulls. They were busy in stealing the prosperity of farmers. Their eyes shone in the torch lights, sparkling in a fantastic manner akin to a bizarre kaleidoscope of traffic lights, switching off and on. Hunted animals become very knowledgeable about the methods employed to kill them. As soon the torches roved over the field the herd began to distance itself from us.

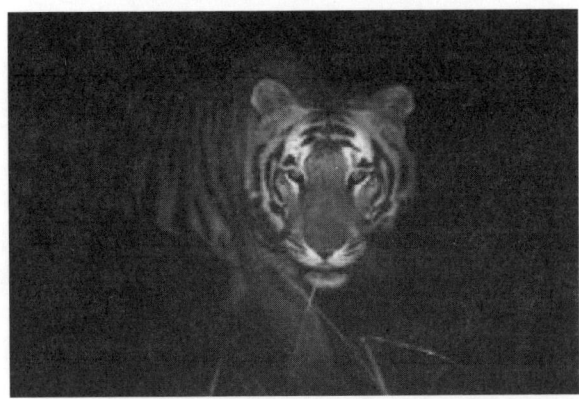

A camera trap shot of tiger in lintel fields
outside PA *(Photo credit NTCA)*

"They recognize light and gunfire so they are moving out of fire range," said the Sikh as the blue bulls quickly got lost in the darkness.

A 20-minute walk finally brought us near a Thanait hamlet. It was on a little rise where nearly a dozen huts were huddled together and canoes were fastened to each hut. The village was silent. We crossed it and descended upon sandy banks of the river. A kilometer away the double headlights of a vehicle emerged on the horizon across Girwa. A duty-bound police patrol was on its nightly rounds and when it was gone we heard a unique hissing sound and next moment our torch lights caught the ghost-like profile of a tiger in the darkness. He was standing half submerged in the water and was hissing unmistakably at the sudden appearance of a crocodile that had pulled a carcass of a cow in the water and was feeding on it.

The splashes in the water confirmed the presence of two saurians (crocodiles are considered saurian by zoological scientists as are the dinosaurs) while the tiger seemed to give vent to its frustrations. He must have stood on the bank watching it for quite long, hissing repeatedly. Rowdily from the river side came the disgusting watery sounds of the crocs feeding on the cow, the tearing of the ripe meat, the muffled clash of teeth, the hollow and heaving gagging sound of swallowing of big bloody lumps of flesh. Then his attention was drawn to the torch beams moving around him. He did not budge and instead of hissing started giving vent to coughing growls that are made to admonish an enemy. He seemed more involved in croc affairs than us but too many torch lights concentrated on him for more than five minutes finally obfuscated him enough and he decided to shift away. Within seconds he was gone, as if having evaporated.

We returned home, smelling the smell of Tarai's bright tingly air in which you breathe greedily amid the lemony aroma of trees; and that distant, out of time retching of the 170-million years old antiquarian crocodiles, our prehistoric friends at such a close quarters, digesting their ghoulish meal. Tarai is always the same, wherever you go. Screeches of the plovers, *did-you-do-it, pitty-to-do-it*, supported by the chorus of scavenging foxes and hyenas in the background with melancholic caterwauling of jackals make the voice of this land. These sounds carry far into the stillness of dark with the music of cicadas, and is a sozzled orchestra sawing through the entire vista.

In these days of moon-landing and mars missions, there is something fascinating, in fact exhilarating in listening to these sounds of Mother Nature. They bring into our imagination a dream and picture of that unknown world immeasurably far in time, fitting with the dawn of creation, that ancient and wise spirit that still exists on this primitive land with the glamour of the nights – ever strong to move humanity and the essential solitude of the spirit.

For next three evenings we constantly ghosted around the spot. Saurians as usual hovered around the banks on sand bars. Their log-like outlines moved at our arrival, slipping into the gunmetal-colored water silently, submerging like a submarine. But there was no sign of tiger. We would see the slow ripples of water, in torch lights, rolling across the calm surface, waving the dark green reeds as the saurian would sail away.

The Real World Lessons

And it seemed impossible that their survival could be so uncertain.

- Billy Arjan Singh

The solitude of the place was challenging. It glowed like burnished silver in the moon-nights with more sharp stars than one can imagine. The sky itself seemed to hang overhead, not unlike a worn canopy of charcoal colored velvet which has sagged and frayed with age and worn into a thousand million pinholes, each releasing a light to form a star.

The island was made of swampy terrain, predominantly cultivated with sugarcane and rice. Towards its northern end lay a big water pond that was bordered by some stretches of alkaline land. Still beyond that, presumably on the marshy soil, grew a moderate block of reeds and bush land, expanding for almost two furlongs with stunted trees. Across it was a great tract of tamarisk grasslands that was waiting reclamation.

The island outers were pitted by tiger spoors and ungulate slots mixed with the sign of human movements. The tigers usually moved separately. Graziers often saw them during dusk or dawn, though hardly for more than two minutes at a time. Even when not in heat the male and female had intermittent contacts and often associated with each other over large kills. This in skeletal form is the social system of tigers which tends to be mutually exclusive. By spacing themselves, both male

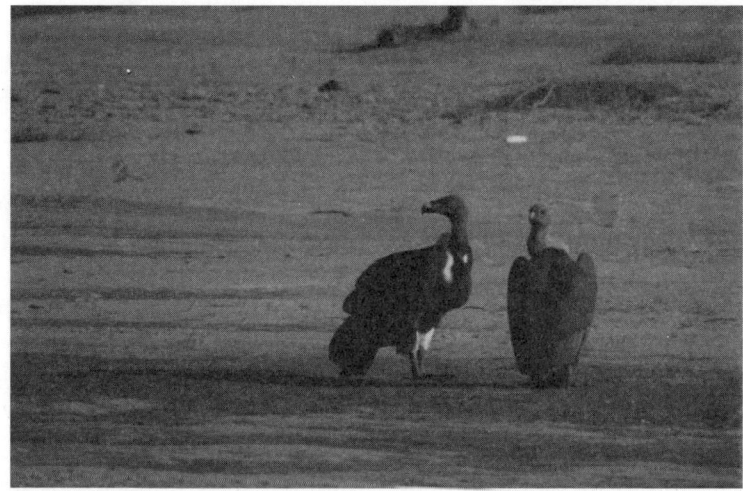

Vultures are useful scavengers. They affect open country, invariably in the neighbourhood of human habitations, picking up offal and human excrement as its diet.

and female are able to maintain separate ranges which contain more food than they need or can utilize.

I announced a five-rupee reward for any news of the tigers, and as the word got around many men agreed to cooperate. On a typical calm morning some graziers arrived to inform that they had just seen the pair sitting on a rise and surveying the country at the edge of Binsaiya marsh. It did not take me much time to reach there and see the tigers from a distance, gamboling like a couple of overgrown kittens but sadly they perceived our arrival and went down the mound hurriedly. It was a neglected area rarely visited by islanders and relatively undisturbed. Accompanied by three islanders I went across the mound.

There were many termite hills bordering the marsh along the mound. We were surprised to find several defunct remains of animals lying there. The place reeked of tigers. There were plenty of bones – as large hard bones of adult animals are not eaten, and peafowl feathers –littered around, indicating that it was their dining point. A strong pungent odor of tiger secretions permeated the area. The bulk of the liquid was tiger urine that includes a whitish discharge from a gland near the anus that provides distinctive odour which is easily discernible by humans.

A flock of vultures sat morosely hunched on a *sheesham* tree, under which lay a severed neck of a blue bull doe and further on, its rear portion. The innards lay discarded with few chunks of flesh here and there, all covered by a sheet of pushing and shoving vultures. There were Egyptian vultures, long-billed, lammergeier and king vultures, all congregated to feed, tearing the carcass through the openings made by tiger. They were flapping, kicking and thrusting each other making raucous voices as they fought amongst themselves for the spoils.

Though the pestilential odour was enough to make one sick, we walked slowly in the direction of the squawking birds. At our approach they stopped quarreling for a moment and looked at us. There were 20 or more repulsive lammergeiers with their snake like necks turned in our direction, their hideous faces smeared with blood. They stared at us briefly then turned to the remains and continued to strip the chunks of flesh. Jackals too were arriving, proving that Tarai is astonishingly efficient in the disposal of protein.

I was told by graziers that tigers did not mind eating animals that have been operated upon by vultures. Having observed this feature several times in farmlands, I consider it a strong variation in behavioural traits between jungle tigers and farm tigers and it is perhaps not irrelevant to compare the two. The jungle tigers seem to dislike the strong pungent odour of ammoniac gases emanated by excreta of vultures and the kills bleached white by them are usually abandoned. But the hard-core farmland tigers do not appear to have such dislikes. Tempered in nature's crucibles, they eat vulture operated kills without a qualm.

Moreover, vultures continue to feed even after sunset, they don't leave the carcass till their stomachs are really full. I have found them tearing and gobbling great pieces of flesh even in the midnight hour. In nature scavenging birds are creatures essential to the operation of the tropical grasslands ecosystem. My conjecture is that the tigers of sugar grasslands – like lions – have to meet the terms of their functioning too. Though tigers also kill vultures and even eat them, this transformation of adjustment with vultures does come in hard farm-dwellers.

Tigers had gone and it was no place to stay. We started for the village through a huge sugarcane plantation, when an old man, who was standing on a knoll about a hundred yards away, shouted that he could see the tigers very much in our way ahead. We had hardy taken notice of his warnings when at some distance ahead the large, handsome animals suddenly emerged before us. The male followed by the female, crossed our path and disappeared inside the flank of mustard cover. We gave them time to move away and then started again. Advancing about hundred paces, we slid past the point from where the tigers had crossed and as I looked left, I caught the glimpse of a crouching low form, as the golden profile of tigress slowly came into view. For a moment she lifted her head over the sprinkled flowers of mustard and glared at me. I stood my ground with my rifle but she did not make any threatening noise.

The speed with which a native can climb a tree in emergencies is incredible. The men behind me were already upon the trees while Chhotey and I were left alone on the ground. I retreated slowly backwards; at this the cunning animal just got up and slid into the matted cover of green, jerking her tail up and down as if in protest. This behavior was slightly puzzling for she had neither growled nor admonished me but had showed no hesitation at all in staying close to the passing humans. She was familiar with human habits and this left me thinking that this kind of adaptation sometimes helps prevent the abrupt nervous reactions leading to non-aggression in farmland tigers. They display the confidence to disregard apparent danger signs – for normally man is not their inveterate enemy.

My consideration is that such tigers make the grade for being a qualified resident of human dominated landscape, for they know the nuances of living in farmlands without creating any trouble.

But tigers are like that. I remember my early phases at Larti when returning home after a day's forays I would make haste to reach home before sunset. At such times jungles could be very inhospitable for a 15-year-old boy. In my rashness I had often passed very close to the spot where a tiger lay hidden. I was totally ignorant of their presence till the fact was confirmed by the evidence of tracks next day.

It gives me a flutter in my bones to learn that tigers had heard me approaching and chosen to stay immobile, expecting me to move away. In two cases, as confirmed later, they had sidestepped into another cover with a complete absence of noise; their protective colouring blending so well with the herbage that I could never see them. Well, they are undeniably first-rate killers of nature but at the same time they are suave and squires as their restraint regarding humans is noble. In many encounters the much focused predators would have nailed me if they desired so, but it is at their generous forgiveness that I relished the freedom of their homelands. So many times I went messing around them and they good naturedly spared my life.

Tigers are rarely found in the same place on two consecutive days unless they have made a large kill. They move an average of six to ten miles per night and male moves ominously further on a day to day basis. Hence my regular trekking for island tigers was a forlorn affair. Any prolonged observation seemed out of question. After this sighting we did not see the tigers for a fortnight. Their movements are largely related to finding and killing prey but they are also intricately linked on the maintenance of rights to an area. They checked most parts of their range every two to three weeks. As tiger scientist and pioneer radio-telemetrist Sunquist explains it as, "Use it or lose it" matrix.

Most of our data was obtained by plotting track records of both individuals. We would discover the points where the tiger had taken a dust bath, rolled on the ground and rested and then leaving the path had descended towards the river banks. The main trail often passed very close to isolated houses and single hutments and went up to Krishna Narain Singh's rice mill near Nishangarha range. It indicated that the beast drifted here in search of dogs as many farmers rising in the morning found nothing but the broken rope with which the dog had been secured. It sounds interesting to say that being of Siberian origin, tigers nurture a deep seated, innate hatred for wolves, and dogs seem to trigger their old wolf killing instincts and they also seem to relish their flesh with vengeful taste.

We recorded their movement on self made topo-sheets and attached that to the Survey of India map, observing that they would enter the jungle for half a mile or so but come back showing their personal predilection from farmlands. The total travel/ range area encompassed by this pair during March, the month of reconnaissance, was about 45 kilometers.

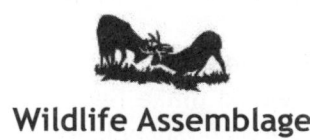

Wildlife Assemblage

"I just sleep better at night knowing they are out there"

— Cory J .Meacham

Many scientists studying highly dangerous animals like elephants, tigers and snakes in India often laud the deep-rooted forbearance of rural Indian communities towards these animals. Drawing on centuries of communal memories, even in the face of conflict, Indian villagers remain largely tolerant to wildlife. It is also because most of these animals are connected with the Hindu pantheon and are considered sacred. Tiger is symbol of power and vehicle of mother goddess. Perhaps this spirit has made tiger flourish on sugarcane farmlands and no free-ranging species has gone extinct in India since independence. The fragile ecological web that binds tigers to other prey creatures of farmlands is yet not ruptured and in many areas natives view wildlife as their old co-sharers rather than a threat to their livelihood.

The sugarcane belt, adjoining forest areas of Tarai is a nine month crop. It is not ersatz as is wrongly understood. It is perennial and a massive habitat for the tiger to smile about. Despite erosion of their primal habitat, sugarcane crops offered an alternative tract that was no less substantial than the previous habitat, rather more improved through human management with less interference. Tracts possessed everything essential – extensive cover, food in shape of wild animals and feral cattle and water. It is natural that such a tract should be the haunt of a large carnivore when his living space is increasingly degrading in tigerine quality requirements.

The Sikhs settled down in the island belong to Amrit Chakha sub-community. They wear long robes with a high turban, carry weapons and follow four don'ts: no wine, no extra marital affairs, no smoking and no meat eating. The last don't is a solid reason why so much of wildlife existed all around.

In the process of tracking tigers we transected the island several times, and this aided us to estimate the status of wildlife at various points. The old sportsmen's belief is that wild animals intuitively know when man's intentions are peaceful or hostile towards them. Eugene Linden, a researcher records that African vervet monkeys issue a different type of alarm call for the people with guns than they do for the unarmed. This proved true with me for here I saw much more animals when I was without a rifle than when I was armed.

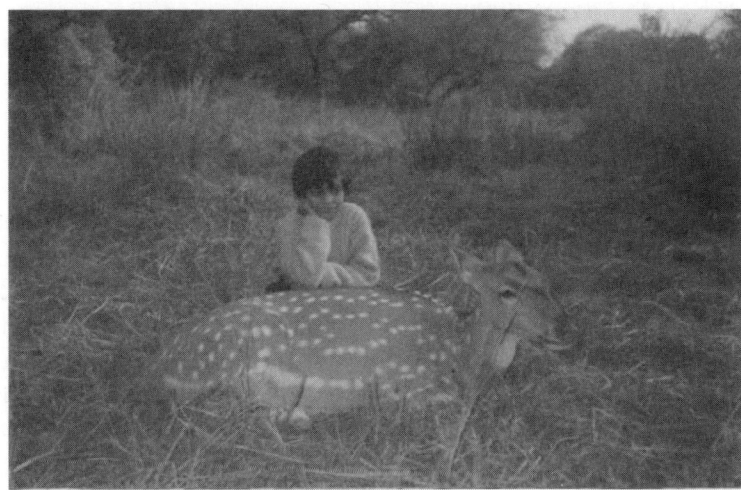

Author's daughter Samriddhi in Bannadavi grasslands of Kahiratia with a pregnant Chital doe which the Nirankari Sikhs had rescued from Pariah dogs

There was a big herd of blue bulls comprising more than 50 antelopes that divided into small groups scattered during the night to graze but reunited during the day under some shady trees. Two old bulls amongst them bore the tiger scars prominently on their half-to-full-inch-thick grey hides. Apparently they had come under the tiger and but not grabbed by neck, and their strength had enabled them to escape the death-struggle and get away. The other attraction of the riverside was a moderate herd of swamp deer, often seen sporting and splashing in the reed beds while their fawns stood in the water up to their necks, feeding and drinking.

We slowly began to recognize all the swamp deer personally. A strong male had a great penchant to stand bolt upright on his hind legs, he was often found in the same position. He stood at the base of a tree sticking his head into the leaves of a low hanging branch, shaking his head back and forth. While attempting to retain his balance, he treaded with his hind legs, churning the soil. Sometimes the whole herd got involved into this practice called preaching but the stags having longer antlers, shooed away the juniors and normally nibbled at first.

There were no rhesus monkeys but *Hanuman langoor* were abundant and so were peacocks, dancing shimmeringly to attract inattentive peahens. Chhotey found the remains of a pangolin killed by tigers. The ant-eater called *ban-rohu* by natives has strong armored plating that is difficult to tackle and when it rolls up into a ball nothing short of a tiger would make it relax and unroll. We also discovered numerous hoof-marks of wild boar and hog deer in the fields.

The grass forest, comprising *narkul*, *phaant*, *ratwa*, reed and tamarisk was a conspicuous component of the island where half a dozen black bucks and swamp deer herds, not exceeding more than 23 animals in all were definitely isolated populations. Needless to say, the small assemblage was well adapted to human pressures.

The area was conducive for *sarus* cranes. Farmers considered these cranes auspicious and tolerating the crop damage by them, allowed them to nest inside their rice-fields. Despite the clash of their breeding and rice-cropping cycle, they kept some portion of fields constantly irrigated so that their chicks might be raised each year.

There were generally green, slime covered sluggish streams in the small forested area, their channels chocked with rotting leaves and decaying vegetation. On withered branches overhanging the stream the abandoned pear-shaped nests of weaver birds could be seen fluttering in the air. It was an eerie spot, yet a haven for a naturalist to sit and probe with a binocular for hours. At times I came here towards dusk to savour the scenery and listen to sounds rising around. One delightful evening, I was at the banks of the river where the trees hung over the water and watching the general scene. A group of dozen *langoor* monkeys sat some fifty meters away, chattering together like so many washermen. Far off a pair of black buck cropped short grass and a flock of dark ibis lazed noiselessly upon a silt mound, scrutinizing the river, where Gangetic dolphins had just gamboled mid-stream.

In extreme silence of sunset I suddenly heard a movement close by and saw several indistinct shadowy small shapes break out of a grass clump. Somewhat surprised, I immediately recognized them as a herd of a rare antelope called *chausingha*. The little four-horned creatures, numbering about half a dozen, stood on a tiny path down to the water. These are very shy animals and I remembered that in early 70s, while camping with Mamman Khan at Nishangarha range, an American hunter, Bum Garner and I had spent a long stint in trying to dig up one or two, seriously cutting the time of hunting other game but could not get a glimpse of these rare animals. They looked round nervously, flicking their tails and quivering nostrils and stood in a line stretching out their front legs and sipped the stream water. Then they happened to see me and within no time all of them bolted back into the same undergrowth.

On the opposite bank treacherous looking crocodiles basked in the declining sun, lying on the sandbars as close packed as sardines in a box. They ranged from ten feet long to youngsters no bigger than a monitor lizard while their females quietly floated into the water looking like harmless wooden logs. Further in the center of water were two popped up eyes of a Gangetic crocodile (often mistakenly called the alligator, since alligators are not found in India). He noticed us and with a snort disappeared.

With so much of wildlife there seemed all peace but it was indeed an armed truce. At night the hunt would begin again. Tigers, hyenas and jackals would span the vista, snakes and civets wriggled through the grasses and climbed the trees in search of latent birds and their eggs. The crocodiles, awakened from their daytime lethargy, would be ready to drag down any unwary quarry as it sipped water.

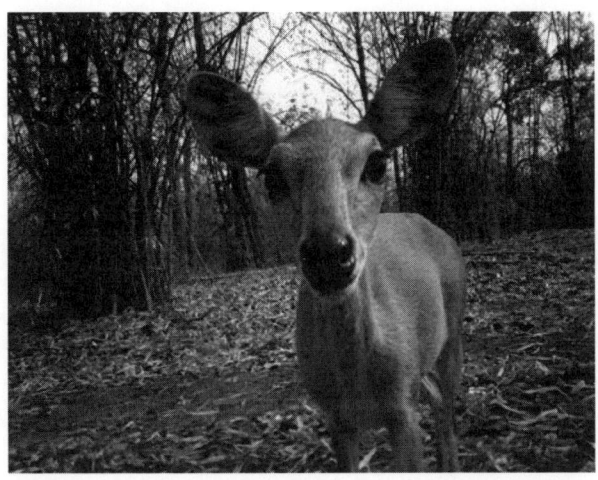

Chowsingha or four horned antelope is the only member of Bovidae group that carries two pairs of horns. Of these the front pair is always shorter. At times these are no more than bony knobs of covered studs under the skin. *(Camera Trap Shot/ Maharashtra Forest Department)*

It was no fun place for a pedestrian to walk when the predatory animals started their prowl for food under cover. There is no real peace in nature. Only a few except man, die a natural death. All others are hunted. There is no peace for them ever; only a daylight truce.

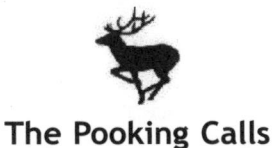

The Pooking Calls

Tiger vocalizations are mystic.

- Author in his book 'Tiger'

One early morning, a thin blood-red line of light had just marked the east when my eyes opened, and within half a mile away a clear cut metallic bell like cry of a *sambhar* stag was rising in the air. The animal belled and walked broadcasting a warning not far from the village. I judged the deer to be within 300 yards. It called eight to ten times and then fell silent. Then I heard the muted calls of a tiger on move from south to east and an answer from its partner from further east. The calling continued intermittently till dawn broke. *Sambhar* responds to potential danger more readily than *chital*. Their alarm bark termed as "pooking" or "belling" by hunters because of its resonance is audible for at least a mile in the open. They perceive danger which the other species nearby often fail to detect or simply ignore it.

Despite being in a half-sleepy state, I remember the feeling of surprise I felt to discover that the animal of dense primary jungles were also present in this farmland. Perhaps this was some individual straggler who had become regular resident of the island like tigers. It was unlikely that he had other members of his species with him.

That very day, I examined the ground from where the calls had emanated and found the pugmarks of a tigress. She had passed through the mustard field. We also searched for *sambhar* hoof marks or pellets for good two hours but observed no indications about their presence.

A week later, I was sitting near a water hole, when in a little while six hyenas appeared, with their ugly rolling walk. We crouched down behind a concealing termite hill, a hundred feet or so away and hoped to watch them drinking, but we got something better. If I had a camera I would have clicked some excellent bathing pictures. As I sat enjoying their playful antics, the idyllic peace of scene was spoiled by the arrival of a cattle herd that entered the pond to bathe and the herd boys shooed away the scavengers.

That night the *sambhar* calls were heard again, and this time the loud ringing call was answered by another *sambhar* feeding not far from the village. At intermittent break of ten to twenty seconds, the duet continued for some five minutes, it seemed that the pair of large deer was informing each other about its whereabouts before leaving the moonlit farmlands. Probably there were two or more *sambhars* on the island.

Next morning the ground as usual revealed the account of the night where herds of wild ungulates had raided crops. The marks of swamp deer hooves are nearly similar to that of *sambhar*, so it was normal to assume that the *sambhar* marks had got mixed up with no less than four or five types of ungulates. Predominantly a forest dweller, *sambhar* comes out into the open occasionally during the night but seeks dense cover within an hour before dawn. Apparently before the sun rose the shy species had retreated, seeking isolation to spend the day hours in the deep tree shades.

However, the method I had chosen to study sugar tigers was not easy. My interest was whether I am able to physically see the tiger or not, I must keep a date wise record of their geo-location data and avoid disturbing them. This process required daily input of tiger news from islanders as well as my personal input of field forays. During the month of March we came across remains of some five kills that ranged from one week to one month old. The bones indicated that all these were large animals that could be killed only by tigers and no other predators. The hooves confirmed them to be three blue bulls, one swamp deer and a stray cow. Dalbeer Singh told me that the tigers were not in the habit of preying upon animal husbandry. They better searched for wild game and feral cattle that raided the agricultural fields.

After several fruitless days with no news, one day an excited villager came running. Panting and gasping, he informed us that he had just seen a tiger's drag mark at a place called Banna Devi. The single thick line running across the field suggested

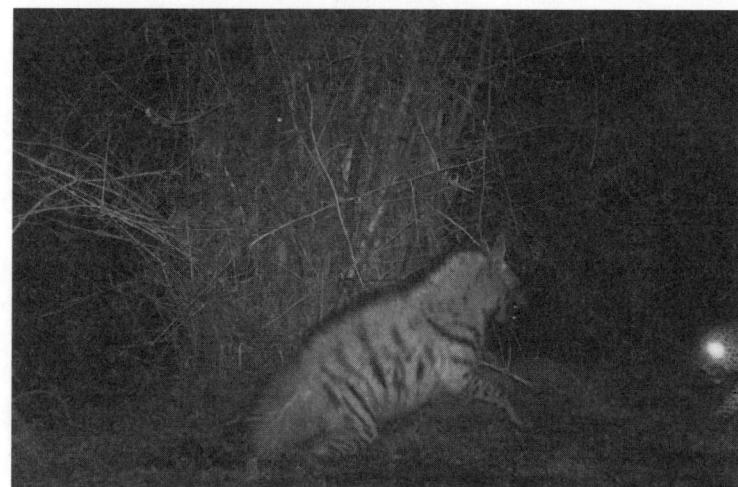

Camera Trap Shots reveal interesting interactions between carnivorous animals; a Hyena challenging a leopard. *(Photo credit Wildlife Conservation Trust)*

that the tiger having killed some animal had carried it into the cane retreat. The place was only a mile away. The Sikh had gone to Bicheya, a principal township of the district. I readied my Yashica box camera, handed Phagunia and Chhotey a spear each, whilst I loaded my .375 Holland & Holland DB and set out for the place.

Banna was a stretch of half-burnt elephant grass waiting reclamation. Its periphery was littered with intermittent plots of cane and wheat crop, which had been carved out of the grassland in the last season. I examined the drag line and found several dark hair on it. There were also drops of blood along the path. The killed animal was a feral cow. The blood drops had still not coagulated into black thickly smudge indicating that the tiger had killed the hefty cattle just an hour ago, and then pulled it by the neck while the hind portion of the victim dragged against the earth.

In Tarai farmlands, I have observed drag distances, up from as short as 50 meters to nearly 300 meters, although the average drag is around 150 meters. But this particular drag in form of a jerk-pull was incredibly the largest I have ever seen. It was little less than a mile, which proved that the beast had phenomenal strength.

A tiger moving a hefty carcass clenches it by the back of the neck, and lifting the head and some part of the forequarters as well, hauls it beside him. Small animals are also gripped in the same way by the back of the neck and walked along with the head half turned. And if the kill is fairly weighty then the preliminary momentum is generally brought on by a series of jerks with the killer facing the direction opposite to the kill. The tiger then turns round dragging, with the kill to one side or even between forearms. This process may be repeated ad infinitum to clear barriers like clusters and saplings until the tiger feels like feeding.

The trail led us to a sugar plot. We were half way when we heard a *sambhar* call coming from a distance. The unseen stag was unmistakably seeing the predator.

He never moved and kept repeating his dubious interrogative bark at intervals. I looked at Chhotey to ask what was the deer doing here? But Chhotey asked me to notice that the sound lacked that acute bell-pitch of *sambhar's* warning. It was not the deer with bad throat but could be the tiger itself, calling his partner. After five or six pooks, the call suddenly ceased and a deep silence fell.

Tigers do use different sounds to communicate but I had no first-hand experience of this kind of communication previously.

Starting afresh, we covered half the way when the soft breeze brought us the unmistakable sound of crunching bone followed by odor of the big cat, much like that of a house cat on a stuffy humid day. I drew a deep breath and moved forward tensely, my rifle low on my hip. We drifted slowly through the canes, stopping frequently to listen for the crunch of bones and a low growl as the tigress fed in the dense leafy stillness.

As long as the noise continued the tigress did not suspect our presence. Suddenly the noise stopped then we also stopped when Chhotey pointed ahead. I lifted my foot to the side slowly forward and saw the tigress standing motionless and looking in our direction; and behind her was her male, chomping the food though he was very indistinct in the matted cover. I could only see his face through the stems of canes as his jaws slurped at the meat chunks. The pair had sensed our arrival and was seemingly disturbed.

Resenting our intrusion the tigress admonished us thrice with threatening growls, came a bit forward and then returned to the male. Still giving deep short grunting coughs and her tail flapping in the air, she seemed very proud of her accomplishment for which she expected to be recompensed.

The heavy stalks of cane had made it absolutely impossible to swing my rifle sideways, and it was not the kind of cover to tackle a pair of tigers with a single gun. The situation warranted us to move away immediately.

Chhotey and I stepped backed a little when suddenly the pair left the kill and bounded off into a dark cluster of grass. Chhotey and I, with my rifle cocked, slowly retreated from the place.

That night the swamp deer called from the sugarcane plantations. Their loud trumpet blast addressed as stentorian bugling is a unique sound that commences with a loud note with an accompanying drone which is kept going all the time in the background. Next to a call of tiger and an elephant this sounds is the identity of the Tarai. Anyone who hears the call for the first time cannot help being mesmerized by the outlandishness of the sound, and few will escape without having a feeling of undefined strangeness spawned in his being. Even those who are acquainted to forest sounds, usually stop talking, listen to this call with curious admiration until it dies away.

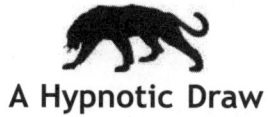

A Hypnotic Draw

"Together these six men represented close to two hundred years of hunting experience- most of it in tiger country- and yet none of them had witnessed anything quite like this."

- John Valliant

I had not been able to obtain a picture of tigers in sugarcane, which was the main objective of my trip. So we returned to the place next morning. By all probabilities the tigers, having eaten their kill during night, would be relaxing now. I discussed the matter with villagers and they agreed to drive out the tigress for my photographic purpose. A beat was steadily performed for a mile. Plot after cane plots were bombarded with stones and lumps of earth but nothing came out. We searched keenly for the glimpses of a slinking striped form but the terrain appeared empty. The beaters first stumbled upon the carcass of cow that was more than half-eaten and hundred yards from it they saw a wild boar as they called me to see it.

After the feral cow, it was the second kill of the tigers executed within twenty four hours. Having demolished the choicest parts of cow in a single day, the tigers had got this wild boar towards the past midnight and also consumed a bit of it. Different tigers have different food preferences and perhaps this pair had liking for different preys. The tell tale signs showed that there was no kill sharing this time, only the male had fed from the rump and the tigress had kept sitting away and watching him. In the very first sitting the male had consumed some twenty pounds of meat and then played around. Towards morning they had left the place for some cool and shady spot to enjoy a comfortable siesta.

The fresh kill lead to an interesting learning. It was not just left in the dense crop, which in itself is a strong cover but was carefully concealed with several pushed down sugar canes and some *pataawar* (a kind of reed). Normally, while leaving the vicinity, tigers habitually cover their kills with available material such as leaves, grass, twigs and earth, while in the closed atmosphere of grass and shady coppices, such measures are not required. But here inside the impenetrable sugarcane I for the first time saw the kill covered with bitten-off stems. I am constantly amazed by the idiosyncrasies of tigers. The signs on the ground also showed that while attempting the task, the tiger had faced away from it and also thrown a modest amount of earth over it from the middle of the furrow with backward strokes of a forepaw. The beat however ended in failure as no tigers could be found out.

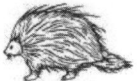

Phenomenon of Surplus Killing

Is it a pythological need of some tigers.

- Author in 'Sugarcane Tiger'

Next day we reached the place again. The terrain harbored a great number of porcupine burrows by the roadside where we discovered the carcass of two porcupines. A quantity of quills lay under a tree with plenty of tiger signs around. The critter had been caught dexterously and the quills were pulled out of its body in bunches. Having done a well accomplished job, the tigers were fondling with the carcass, when we had abruptly butted in on the scene and they had given us a chase in excitement. However, having profited by this experience in favourable circumstances I have never attempted to go near courting tigers.

The porcupine carcass appeared like the product of a ritualized destruction. It seemed that having taken guard, the creature had formed an armor of erected quills around its body. The tigers followed it for almost a furlong, attacking it in flanks, plucking out and spitting out the mouthful of quills. In an exercise that must have lasted for some half an hour, they denuded the porcupine of more than half of its quills, then one of them finally caught it by the head and in a crunch killed it.

John Daniel Joseph (1930) says, "Apparently the porcupine possesses only few of these quills that can act as darts, for tigers with expertise will first engage in feints by a few attempts at attacking the animal in order to draw off the injurious quills, when the creature becomes an easy prey."

Porcupines are a potential source of danger to tigers and possibly to other carnivorous animals. Many sportsmen are inclined to believe that they attract attention of tigers due to the delicacy of their meat. That is why in spite of the protection afforded by the pointed spines and quills the tiger does not hesitate to meet the dangers involved in chasing such an animal. But island tigers did not seem partial to this flesh. In their idiosyncratic way, they rather disliked the repulsive animals and killed them out of hatred. I had often thought why tigers should go for a troublesome creature like porcupines when natural food abounds and here the answer was hate.

Arthur Locke explains further, "Tiger will hardly ever come back to a dead animal which has been left uneaten on his own accord. It is hard to account for these apparently aimless kills when the tiger goes to a great deal of trouble to secure them but the fact remains that such instances do occur. There is no apparent reason why the kill is left."

A week later, while passing through the same area, I again came across two porcupines killed by tigers that lay some 20 meters apart. Two kills intrigued me.

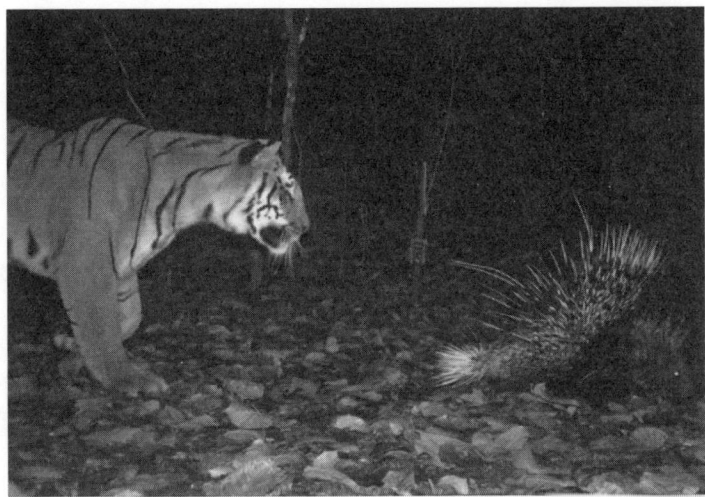

Porcupines are a potential source of danger to tigers and possibly to other carnivorous animals and they have to be more alert and way while dealing with them. *(Camera Trap Shot; Credit Karnataka Forest Department)*

Surely it was the work of two tigers done separately that had behaved in an interesting manner at the discovery of a porcupine pair. The kills were about three days old and slightly rotting in condition. But surprisingly, like the previous instance, no attempt had been made to make a meal of these, though this would have proved merely a sop to their killers' prodigious appetite. Perhaps the tigers already had eaten enough. The entire dorsal crest of these creatures had been plucked out yet a very little amount of flesh had been nibbled from one, not by tigers but by some passing animal perhaps a mouse or a mongoose, while the other was left uneaten.

This peculiar behavior amongst predators, large and small is termed as 'surplus killing' which manifests as a kind of spontaneous frenzied slaughter. Tigers, leopards, wolves, hyenas and even polar bears and killer whales are known to practice wasteful hunting, which demands a high expenditure of energy. But it is still not fully known for what purpose it is done. Similarly these incidents seemed a mixture of curiosity and playful rambunctiousness, with perhaps more than a dash of predatory urge thrown in. I have known of a leopard killing 26 goats in a pen and a jackal killing over 100 hens.

There is a great difference between a tiger out on hunting and one bent on destruction. This makes the old question crop up again with undiminished interest on the part of naturalists – that the idea of a learning tiger, killing only large game to polish its hunting skill is pure nonsense. Sometimes a young apex predator, to maintain its versatility of slaying often goes for wanton killing and tests its skills on any animal they find chalinging, howsoever unpalatable or palatable they be. This exercise increases their aptitude and expertise in killing. But so much of useless destruction of an important animal is also puzzling because porcupines are great excavators of the jungle and their disappearance from any terrain may affect the lives of a number of creatures.

Having examined over 40 tiger cadavers in cane fields poisoned by pesticides, hit by vehicles, netted and shot by poachers, I never came across any porcupine scarred tiger that might bear the signs of quills or carried any quill imbedded in its body. Porcupines are numerous in Tarai farmlands and it is difficult to believe that they don't interact with them.

The tiger's digestive system is remarkable. Sanjay Pathak, during his tenure as Field Director Dudhwa discovered porcupine quills in a tiger scat proving that big cat's stomach and relatively uncomplicated intestines can easily cope with such material. Russian studies also attest the same, showing presence of half digested bear claws in tiger scats.

However, I was exultant that a unique pair of tigers had lived in this area for over a year, which knew as how to transact business with man along with many qualities of great interest for a naturalist.

While we returned for Khariatia, the evening had closed upon the lonely island and the trumpet voices of swamp stags were calling from mound to mound. We crept along the course of a small water body and came upon a herd. Two stags stood separately on two mounds and with their heads risen towards the sky, they were slowly releasing the trumpet sounds that seemed to announce the time of the nightfall. The noise starts with a loud and penetrating *eeee-ooonn-eeee-ooonn* which is repeated in decreasing volume as the air in the lungs gradually exhausts. The landscape had assumed a strange timeless quality. Suddenly I saw all animals begin to get suspicious, and then stood staring in one direction, not ours but away, where we saw two natives coming along to inspect some fishing traps they had left at the mouth of a small stream that joins the river.

The calls stopped. The brown undulating mass of does, alert and nervous stood crowded together, moving their large ears back and forth and then suddenly split into rippling waves.

There is something fascinating in seeing a swamp deer troop startled into a gallop, as they made for a cover with the sun glancing off their rich brown yellow hides. The wild scene lasted for some half a minute then gradually faded over the skyline as the deer took cover in sugarcanes and *narkul*.

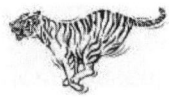

When a Rifle can be more than useless

Our guns were like toys against these incarnations of strength and fury
- Author in his book 'Tiger'

Courting tigers are vulnerable to uncertain temper. They ignore obvious signs of danger and behave in a carefree manner to impress their partners. Often both male and female become extra bold and indulge in extra-ordinary deeds of savaging, including over killing of prey or bumping into passers-by and oxcarts. Such rushes cannot be called a bona-fide charge for a real charge is made with intent. In rarest of the rare case, a pair of tigers may act in combination against humans.

A week after the Holi festival, I had a harrowing experience on this line. I was returning from Khariatia to Jasnagar in the dead of the night. I was driving the motorcycle with Phagunia sitting in the pillion carrying my .375 Magnum. As we negotiated a bend we became aware of two dark figures running to our right some eight to ten yards away. We had no proper spotlights to confirm their identity, though heavy thumping sounds of feet could be feebly heard amid the staccato roar of the motorcycle. For a moment I thought they were pariah dogs, for they have a curious tendency of running along vehicles but as the reflected glare of the headlights fell upon the runners, we could identify these were a tiger and a tigress.

My heart gave a leap as I remembered Lord Krishna! The mad race had already lasted for some seconds, without any grunt of warning from them, and they were running within striking reach. They could be upon us in a flash and in every sense we could be overcome by their sheer inexorable force. Having no wish to confront tigers with impunity I pulled the accelerator with maddening force, luckily the road was dry and smooth and soon we left the tigers behind.

Over 30 years have passed of this incident and I don't know how to define it, for my natural reaction was that of a heavily pounding heart and stomach full of bats, that precedes the horror of death. But, despite this something still tells me that it wasn't a charge, for charging tigers can cover a hundred yards within just over three seconds and here we were only less than ten yards away and entirely at their mercy. Perhaps the tigers were attracted to the motorcycle which in its staccato roar appeared to them some animal trespassing through their home-ground and their reaction had more to do with competition than with predation. One may feel seemingly secure in the protection of a noisy motor vehicle and its headlights but is necessarily not always that with tigers.

However, even if the incident is a display of light-heartedness and good humour of tigers; it stands as a unique example of their unpredictable playfulness when they court their soul mates. An impish attempt of closing in upon us had certainly created a dangerous situation.

Phagunia was a child of nature and hunter at heart, who had been on tiger trails for forty years that included gruesome involvements with them. Even he had never witnessed anything like this. In this kind of business you mug up to dredge up close calls only for what they have taught you, not for how they may possibly have turned out.

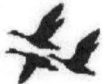

Consolidating the Venture

The job of protecting farmland wildlife and studying it is a expensive hobby for an individual.
- Author in a Foresters meeting

This point blank engagement with tigers thrilled me to the core and I decided to relax for a few days. It was good to get back home again. Although to both my daughters and even to my wife Anita, when they met me at the Lucknow City railway station, I was just a very tanned stranger with an overgrown beard like that of pirates and a haggard face. It was like returning home after a long sea crossing. The kids were most unimpressed by this stranger's earnest pleadings for attention, whose long hair curled around ears and over the collar of his sun-bleached and smelling shirt, was hardly fit for civilization.

When I looked at my face in the mirror, I saw a regular wild man of the woods. I had never realized earlier how quickly men deteriorate without razors and clean shirts. A single day's growth of beard makes a man look careless, the stubble of two days makes him look polluted; and four days' growth sure makes him appear dilapidated. As for the facial vegetation of more days than this, the resemblance would be potted plants that go to weed unless they are pruned and tended properly.

The children refused to be friendly. The sweets and chocolates failed to do the needful till I had shaved and bathed.

A day later my camera reel was processed. My first attempts to get tiger pictures from a fixed focus camera were very poor. I was not careful in cutting down the grass and cane leaves in front of the lens and the distance of the subject from the camera too had remained a crucial factor. The consequence was that the waving grass and leaves had blurred my shots and distance had made the subject insignificant.

While in Lucknow, I wrote letters to the Forest Department, reporting the presence of tigers as well as of swamp deer and other kind of wildlife on the island. I demanded that these should be declared as important study animals for the understanding of sugarcane wildlife phenomenon and be given immediate and rigid local protection in addition to legal protection the animal already has. Otherwise, it was unlikely that the isolated population would survive.

All this appeared to be a cry in the wilderness; a remote or unlikely event. However, my wife's father B.K. Avasthi was then a mid-level IAS officer of Uttar Pradesh cadre holding double charge of the Director of Land Acquisition and Managing Director of State Brass Ware Corporation. He was close to the then Chief Secretary

Mr Girish Mehra. He motivated members of the civil services fraternity for the noble cause and took me to his boss. I had already met Mr. Mehra quite a few times with Ram Advani, a legendry personality of Lucknow and the owner of the well-known Ram Advani Book sellers shop in Hazaratganj Street which was a meeting point of city intellectuals. Luckily the chief bureaucrat had seen me on television a week earlier and was therefore aware of my interest in farmland wildlife.

He took cognizance of the matter. Reports were sought from the Divisional Forest Officer (DFO) and the District Magistrate of Lakhimpur Kheri to confirm the existence of tigers in farmlands. Furthermore a four-member committee was constituted to investigate cane tiger phenomenon and monitor the "straying predators" as they referred to island tigers. I was appointed a member of this committee which unfortunately never held a meeting. But one of its members, a secretary-level officer, despite restriction on giving public statements, was recorded as saying with whimsical rigidity that a special team of experienced shooters should be employed to clear such tigers before they start claiming human lives. Apparently his concern was not scientific but managerial as how to safeguard villagers from danger.

There were no proper management strategies to protect wildlife outside the forests. The foresters, in their ecological ignorance continued to show signs of confusion about the status of these tigers, which had continued to live quite comfortably amidst human activity. It was definitely surprising that big cats could on their own hold on in a rural landscape that was hemmed between two thickly populated townships of Bicheya and Tikonia and even people not disturbing the quiet of their lives were glad to pass on unmolested.

Regardless of the scarcity of natural prey in some areas of Tarai, livestock losses to predators are never high and almost everywhere in the Tarai farmlands, unwanted feral cattle top the list of natural prey for tigers. To my mind this lot also works as a cushion against the predation of livestock. Furthermore there are dogs in every village. Though the predators avoid the area where guarding dogs are patrolling or barking loudly but these too serve as staple food for tigers, falling victim when off guard.

Tiger movements in farmlands are more governed by their wandering instinct and stereotypical behavior of avoiding humans than the search of prey as they do in the jungle. William Baze's assertion that "the local game begins to move out of the area as soon as a tiger moves into it," is a factor that keeps the tiger moving. True, the life of a common prey of a tiger like *chital, sambhar* or swamp deer is focused on avoiding being eaten. Therefore they are not easy to catch. In jungle a tiger is extremely lucky if it can kill one deer a week but sugarcane zone offers a greater collection of prey base.

Evidence suggests that despite the presence of a variety of easy prey they leave the area easily due to human avocation. This shows that anthropogenic pressure is a bigger controlling factor of tiger movements in farms than the movement of their prey and tigers do this with a decision of safety issues that under the circumstances would necessitate extraordinary restraint or caution. It may be a far-fetched possibility but perhaps farm tigers are capable of sensing men who are likely to worry them.

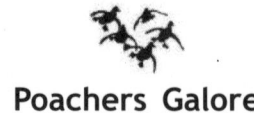

Poachers Galore

"Hunters tend to range into carnivores' habitats with firearms... Few wildlife agencies have the wherewithal to prevent such illicit killings and must depend on the goodwill of farmers and hunters."

- Adrian Treves, Conservation Biologist

Two and a half years had passed but the tigers seemed to lack cubs. The area was well stocked with game and therefore reproduction should have been high as many young ones could be successfully raised. But nothing of that sort was being heard. In spite of high reproductive potential of females, the low percentage of litters in tigers is largely attributed to the failure to conceive and equally proportionally to high prenatal and post natal mortality. It was natural to conclude that something of this sort might have happened. We didn't pay much attention but later to my ineffable sadness, learning the reasons for this not only confirmed my suspicions but increased my natural sympathy for them.

During mid 1980s, the WWF had revealed through its field investigations that Katarnia Ghat forests and its adjacent areas were facing poaching pressures from both sides in India and Nepal. Occasional trigger-happy *nouveau riche* from Kanpur and Lucknow were joining hands with Nepalese ex-servicemen. Some organized gangs were also suspected to have entered the scene in a clandestine manner and market-driven hunting had reached a flashpoint. Such hunting is invariably focused on high value products. Consequently many tigers inhabiting sugarcane fields, known to locals (not to foresters), had been poached and most of the cubs had died because their mothers had been wiped out and they were hardly strong to survive on their own. The carcasses of two young tigers were found near a water pond when their mother was trampled by a logging truck. Skeletons of five tigers were recovered from the possession of Kanjars, which were to be sent to the markets in the Far East for the mumbo-jumbo smirk of ancient Chinese medicine.

Unfortunately in an environment where the very existence of hunting is often marked down or even negated, there have been very few attempts to assess its forces and its biological impact on wild residents. Furthermore sycophantic officers were declaring tigers as man-eaters on the least pretext of man-tiger conflict and

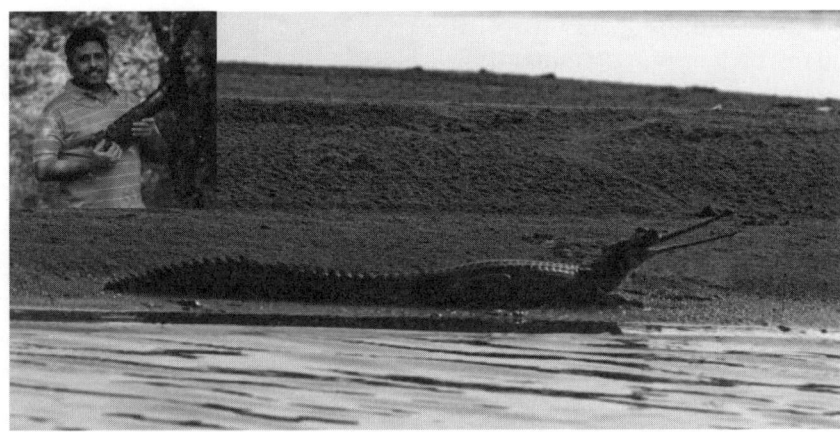

When the winter sun is high in the sky, Gangetic crocodiles (so claled alligators) arrive on sandbars to sun themselves. *(Photo credit : Praveen Rao, IFS)*

using it as an excuse to cover their failures of management. The solution was: a problem tiger should be removed from the scene, and there is nothing wrong even if it is poached.

By the summers of 1984, when I visited the place again, I got the news about a band of opportunistic poachers that had repeatedly ravaged the area. They had targeted wider variety of prey species and posed a serious threat to the stock of local wildlife. The number of swamp deer had drastically declined. I came across only one stag whose antlers had shed and the knobby orange stumps on his head were growing as new antlers. There were some five does, whose summer coats were tawny, looking thoroughly harassed. A structured estimation of herbivores in the area had not been undertaken.

A steamer named *Shark* used to pass through the river. People recognized it as one of the oldest boats on the river. No one knew from where it came from and where it went, but when it came close to the island it always issued forth a series of whistles. It also sometimes passed in the nights sweeping flash lights on river banks and looking for game species feeding close to the terrain as it passed by them. Recently a new development had taken place as opportunistic shooting had also started from the steamer. Many unfortunate animals fell and got wounded by the thoughtless firing from unknown men on the swaying deck of the steamer. The wounded animals survived having received painful wounds from rifle bullets, for it is absolutely impossible to put in a vital shot from a moving vehicle unless it is pure palpable fluke.

It won't be out of context to underscore that vital shots are purely a question of angle and this matter of angle is the best reason why long shots should not be taken. It is the thick front sight of the gun that often creates the problem in shooting the object. Apparently at a distance of more than 150 yards it is impossible for the human eye to discern the angle in which an animal is standing. A small antelope at that distance, nestled into the 'V' of the express leaf, will be blotted out if the front sight is large; so for really good work, a foresight should not be larger in diameter than the head of the small pin, which will be found to be one-fifth of an inch.

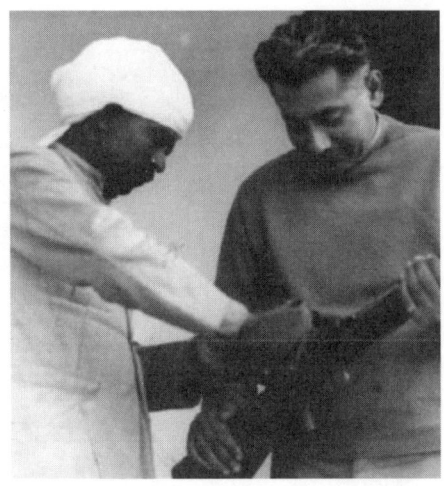

Some may find these details to be out of place in this narrative, but I would remind readers that during my teens I had been a student of active hunting, and in attending camps of Indian Shikar & Tours Pvt. Ltd., with professional hunters like M. Haider Mamman Khan, I assisted some highly sporting American big game aficionados like Fredric Smith of Nevada, Jim Lion of Houston, David Bo Henen of San Francisco, Lauren D. Stak and Sam Antonio of Texas, William Hanson of Los Angeles and Bum Garner who came to India seven times and took away nine tigers.

Mamman Khan, professional hunter of Shikar& Tour outfitters at the height of his fame in 1971. Honored by American Professional Big Game Hunters Association, he had given 132 tigers to his clients.

Hitherto, in my passion for shooting, details such as the action of bullets in the body of the game, were of great interest to me. Over the years I had accumulated and still possess an assortment of soft and hard nose bullets in my collection framed in a butterfly box with a glass top, artistically designed by Ravi Grover of Halwasia market, Lucknow. There are partitions inside for different game, and there are 22 distorted bullets from different rifles that I collected from dead tigers during *shikaar* camps including one of 450/500 that was extracted from a carcass blasted with a bomb and found in sugarcane fields near Paraspur village in 1984.

On one hand, because of maturity stemming from my present age, I do not dither to say that of all the stratagems which humankind has originated and introduced sport hunting is most debased action. It is the most dubious, and the phoniest feat which is diametrically opposite to civilized thinking, whereby man relishes massacre of living beings for his personal recreation. The supposed natural law of might is right, by which the human race has appropriated the world which he increasingly claims as his own, is a great factor for the mass genocide of animals. Killing for pleasure is conflicting to the verdict of live and let live which normally prevails among wild animals.

On the other hand, of course I naturally know many interesting things about game hunting circles and sophisticated firearms, their range and ammunition, about wild animals that offer a good mark for a rifle if properly stalked as well as ethics of the sport, much as I know about the conservation of wildlife, so I often expose that knowledge too. Not surprisingly my earlier firsthand experience as a hunter-naturalist is now my most accurate tool of safeguarding wildlife that consolidates my conservation ventures more sanctimoniously.

Well, having sought my Holy Grail as a deer stalker and a killer of pot game, I have run the all-inclusive gamut of wildlife matters; from a cognizant observer of sugarcane tiger phenomenon to an environmentalist, conservationist and ultimately a preservationist, who as a wildlife warden also savors a gratifying feeling of fighting battles with well-armed poachers and compulsive killers of jungle life but that is another story.

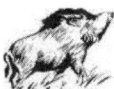

The Insensate Massacre

It is not possible to exercise the immorality of taking the life of an animate process of evolution for the sake of individual pleasure.

- Billy Arjan Singh

On June 15, 1984, the steamer was noticed moving in the darkness as the sounds of gunshots echoed. The silence was disturbed only for a few minutes as the trigger-happy poachers collected trophies and quickly slinked away. A week later the rotting carcass of a swamp deer was found near Banna Davi grassland. It was infested with maggots and green with heat and dampness. Its skin and head were full of holes and there were several SSG pellets still sticking to the skin. Perhaps owing to long distance firing these had failed to crack the skull and none had penetrated but the larger LG's had found the heart and lungs and destroyed the animal.

When I reached the island, even I had had my full share of this disastrous scenario. The animals were restless. One unfortunate *chital* had fallen foul of poachers' shots on his back that had left his entire posterior ridden with SSG pellets. He had survived but was in such a bad state that it was almost impossible to approach him for the smell of numerous gangrenous wounds. Blue bottle flies were feeding on the open sores in hundreds and even speedily depositing their eggs. It is every bit as serious an affliction as is cancer to the human being. At the time of our meeting, the stag was starved and must have been suffering this deadly agony for days. A slug from .318 Accelerated Express in his brain must have come as a welcome relief to him.

We examined the awfully smelling carcass. "These devils do not even follow wounded animals. Their shooting spells trouble for poor creatures. These wounds impregnated with infections turn into masses of worms," said Vishnu Narain Singh, as he went on an abusive spree against the poachers.

Next morning when the light had improved we went out photographing the crocs. We crept along the banks using a trampled down route – a game trail – that the swamp deer had used night after night. During the day the crocs lazed around in deep waters, floating on the surface at a safe distance from the shore with their heads just sticking out, and eyes on the land to keep a watch on enemies in form of man. The crocs had moved to a huge mound in the river about five hundred yards away but our approach alarmed them and they quickly submerged in the water. After a few minutes their eyes, nostrils and flat of the head just broke the surface, letting out their peculiar snorting. While walking back home through dark, green reeds we came across a defunct carcass of a giant saurian. A fair size of the croc's skull lay inside a reed patch, which we left and went ahead but the Sikh farmer accompanying me picked it up and brought home. It is now amongst his collected trophies that he has consciously picked up from the wilderness around.

However, the area was too large to investigate, yet by studying the signs I could tell how matters were going. The sight of vultures and marabou storks circling in the sky always called for investigation. No beast is allowed to die in the fields without the scavenging birds knowing its location. They soar like distant specks far up the azure sky, perceiving the dead by rising thermals and drop from their airy heights, like stones, to their kill. The crows, the kites and the hawks follow them; thereby denoting that something has died – possibly from natural causes but also possibly because of the activity of poachers.

Soon three more carcasses of blackbucks were recovered through vulture activity and all had shotgun pellets resting in their bodies. Little we understood that the bug of fun-seeking hunter had arrived in the region, the trigger-happy rascals that put the whole nature into jeopardy and destruct the environment.

The summer had set in, crops had been harvested and the agriculture fields lay bare. It was this phase when the poachers eyed the tigers and made regular forays on the island. One night a Jeep arrived, equipped with flashlights and combed the vista from one end to the other in search of game. The lights flashed on the open terrain and happened to catch the tigress standing in the middle of a freshly cut barley field. The tigress' stomach was heavy. She seemed fully pregnant and perhaps was about to lay a litter within a couple of days. Upon sensing the danger she turned and begun to run for a cover. The shooting party, insensitive to her condition set the vehicle in chase. The chase lasted for some five minutes. The tigress ran slowly in cumbersome bounds, her bulging stomach swinging from side to side and the jeep chased it over the uneven terrain. A volley of shots was fired but it kept missing the target till the harassed animal neared a mango orchard and disappeared in it. The hunters searched her for entire night and then went back home towards morning.

After this incident they came looking for her at regular intervals, perforating wild animals and even giving wounds to village livestock. Once, a farmer picked up the flattened buckshot from the head of one of his pigs that had strayed in the field that night. The pellet had just got under the skin and stopped against the hard

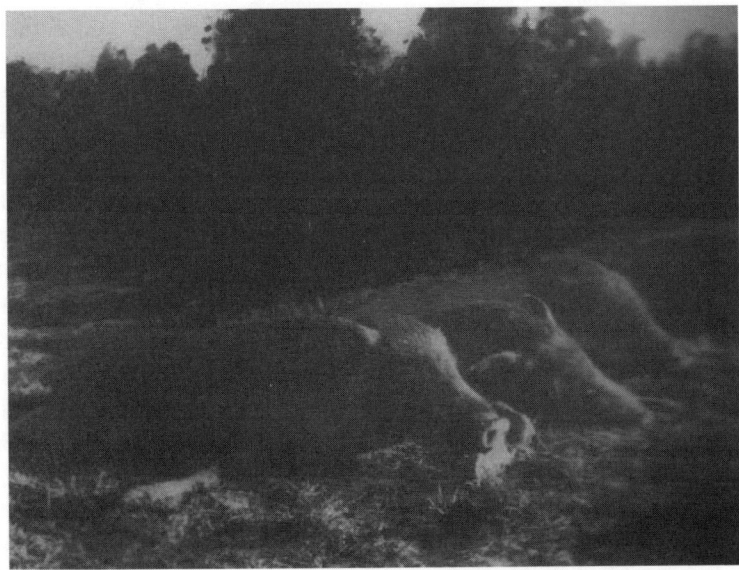

Wildboars killed by poachers bullets in a nightly massacre were later collected by villagers *(Photo credit : Sardar Kuldeep Singh)*

skull of pig and the fat animal had survived. The tigress, however, seemed to have disappeared for good; the poachers did not spot her for the second time.

Possibly the excessive strain of running to protect life in advance pregnancy had cost the tigress with her litter. A wretched islander, Hari Ram, who had guided the opportunistic scoundrels for a paltry sum of 10 rupees, told me later that the litter either got aborted or was born dead. During the latter part of pregnancy, tigresses are often unable to kill their prey, and just before laying the cubs face semi-starved conditions. In such crucial times if they are compelled to undergo strenuous physical drills, the weak litter dies inside the womb and is born dead. In such conditions the starved tigress does not hesitate to eat the dead new-born along with consuming the afterbirth placenta. I don't know what had happened to cubs but aggravated by their loss and driven on by her unfulfilled maternal instinct she called continuously for a week all through the days and nights.

That night as I lay in my tent Hari Ram was in his elements, giving the events of the previous days a through going over. "The water level was low enough to allow the vehicles to cross the river so they came regularly almost every day carrying arms and hunted throughout the night. They never gave me money for the second time and disgusted I tried to inform the police and forest guards but no one appeared keen to take any action. The outsiders held me at gunpoint and warned against opening my mouths. We have no security. They looked like devils from hell. Though Sardar Ji has three guns, even he was not ready to open a confrontation with them."

"Where did these poachers come from ?" I asked.

"From Kanpur city," was his answer.

"And what did they kill?"

"Swamp deer, wild boar and tigers as well."

As I heard the story, I felt sick with all the bloodshed. I could almost hear the sharp crack of rifles and perceive the sweep of spotlights. "Is this not a cruel amusement?" whispered my conscience, "does not their savage nature relent as they saw the graceful creature relent in his own blood, and in the last agonies, bending his eyes on their face, as if asking, what had I done to deserve this?" I felt an ineffable sadness, ashamed of my race. The story of the incident was pitifully short. On the night of July 30, the hunters spotted the tigress again in search lights, they fired and she escaped wounded into thick sugarcane before others could get a finishing shot. Then one of the poachers got down to follow it. Inebriated with heavy dose of alcohol, he went alone after it with his double rifle. The tigress lay under the cane growth, she watched the hunter coming and charged from there but before she could knock him flat several shots rang out from the Jeep and as the luck would have it, the poacher who had walked up to her spun to run away, and was shot down in the face by another inebriated poacher. The firing was halted immediately and in the meanwhile, the tigress managed to escape in the darkness. The death of the partner created a bad omen, grieving the poachers loaded the body of their partner in the jeep and since then, they stopped coming.

Tigers have evolved to respond to direct physical attacks from other animals. But they haven't evolved to counter remote threats like those of firearms. They do not naturally understand what a gun is or how it works. Thus, it is difficult for them to be able to make the distinctive connection between random explosions in the air, followed by an acute pain in the body that they can feel, and an abrupt gush of blood they often cannot see. The attacking humans may be a hundred yards away, but it definitely gives the tiger a strong perception of danger from this agency. While many animals of higher intelligence are capable of making this association, there are very few who, if threatened or attacked would respond like a tiger.

The tigress was injured and there was no news of the male. Having returned from his long range patrol the male was last seen with her a week before the unfortunate incident took place and after that it had disappeared. Since then people had no clue of him. Perhaps the male had been previously poached. There is big money involved in such things and so are its players, who are often desperate and dangerous individuals. All tiger parts are sold separately, parallel to drugs by their weight in grams and bones in kilos. A 400-pound tiger in international market is a mine of money. While most people poach animals to survive but there are some amongst them that poach tigers for money.

A week after the incident the tigress unexpectedly returned to the island alone. A Thanait fisherman was smoking a *bidi* when she passed by outside his hutment, hobbling across a drain and the native happened to notice her wounds from close quarters. She was injured in the rump, where the blood had coagulated and rising stench from the wound was perceivable. She halted periodically to nurse her wounds, trying to soothe her incessant searing pain. He even claimed that her wounds were infected with maggots. "I saw the leech-like white creatures crawling upon her wound."

This was promising news for maggots are not slow killers as is wrongly thought. They are the creatures that keep injured wild animals alive. They are rather excellent cleaners of rotten flesh and wounds that prevent gangrene and blood poisoning. Cats are in the habit of licking their wounds avidly as their saliva contains a strong antiseptic element which heals the injury quickly. But as this female couldn't reach her back the maggots were doing the same business. Once the wounds are healed the maggots themselves drop down from the body and die.

The tigress was emaciated and thin and looked exhausted but the more serious problem of damage to the cubital (the equivalent of human elbow) or shoulder joint, which could impair her movement didn't seem to be there, only her walk was slightly malformed.

It is important to realize that a wild tiger has only to get injured critically to become temporarily incapable of hunting. Death by starvation, gangrene or other infections may quickly follow. They are often the ultimate agents that kill wild tigers that escape hunters.

In order to assess her condition, it was essential for me to have at least one close look at her. Evidence suggested that she was rendered disabled by her injuries; which indicated that there was a chance of normal recovery, provided she is properly supported.

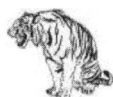

Dealing with a Wounded Tiger

"A tigress is most likely to demonstrate but is easily turned away and if a tiger once demonstrates he is more likely to charge and charge home than tigress."

- A.A. Dunbar Brander

Dealing with a wounded tiger is more confusing for a naturalist than for a hunter who aligns him in the rifle-sight and inflicts the initial wound. I had plenty of time to reflect on the quaint stories of hunters I had heard so often. In the rule book of big game hunting, a tiger is not considered to be dangerous for about 24 hours after being injured. In case of a light flesh wound it usually moves away on being approached whereas with a painful body wound that stiffens after 24 hours, it might continue to be dangerous for several days.

It was over a fortnight since the tigress had been shot and there was no blood trail to follow. We spent three consecutive days looking for her without success.

The trail proved to be too tiresome and disappointing, as each day we were never sure if I would find her dead or alive. Then one morning after breakfast, news came that the tigress had been sighted entering a pocket of termite-land, towards the north of the island, which was littered with several humps of anthills.

A bumpy ride carried us to the landscape but seeing the grassed terrain up to six feet high we lost heart. We were fully aware of the consequences of dealing with an injured tigress and there was no thought of reckless foolhardiness. It is a mistake to think that tigers or any other dangerous animal is going to charge every time you cross their path but it is an even greater mistake to assume that they would not if they are wounded. Faulty interactions with humans contribute to the uncertainty of temper, leading big cats into more stressful conditions and this makes them a potential engine of destruction. And a big cat inclined to blame its wound on someone, is the source of an out-of-control dangerous fury.

We entered the grass with caution. My sensibilities and reflex mechanism had never been turned to such a pitch before as on that moment. The Sikh family, moving in the grass with me was seeing, hearing and almost tasting the tigress every moment as the foliage became dense. Moreover, rifles in their hands, with safety catch off, were pointing haphazardly in every direction including at me recurrently, so that I had to physically push the barrel flat down to the ground. I would have saved myself from a wounded tiger from the front but the risk from these mishandled firearms seemed greater. I asked the Sikh and his sons to keep out of this affair for while. He agreed without the slightest hesitation while Chhotey and I entered the thick vegetation.

Fortunately it was dry season and there was little foliage. The few leaves remaining were dry and yellow, a sharp contrast to the tiger's hide. I slipped the safety-catch off my .375, and followed. Although I felt Chhotey should have taken a rifle from the Sikh and two rifles would have been better for such a work but we were already inside the cover, which had closed around us like a great yellow fog.

Owls, grasshoppers, butterflies and mosquitoes flushed continuously as we took some forty long minutes to advance that short distance of 200 paces. I caught the glimpses of a *gutaria*, the little mouse deer that compare in size with a normal hare. The little animal shrieked in alarm and bolted out of the scrub like rabbit. Just then, there was a flutter in the grass, and a menacing growl as the tigress took note of our presence. Anticipating an antelope, she had got up to catch him but perceiving human presence she retreated in the cover, admonishing the intruders from there. For a brief moment she even rushed within grass as if coming towards us, but remained unseen. We sensed her deeply through harsh snarls in that claustrophobic environment.

When the grass is higher than the standing tiger, then the odds are definitely against man. I stood my guard with my rifle pointed in the direction, expecting her to break cover. The night sight of my rifle, an oversized bead of wild boar tush

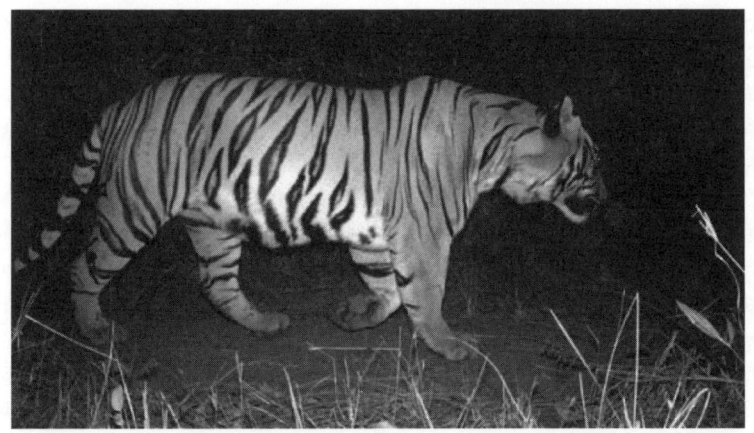

An animal that kills a 800 pound bluebull male with a single bite, easily sorts out a mere human in one slap. (*Camera Trap Shot-Photo credit Wildlife Conservation Trust*)

which doesn't yellow like elephant ivory, was flipped up for sighting in the deep shades. But the self-preserving animal did not advance close enough for me to see her. Only grass strands waved at the top pin-pointing her location within them.

Wild imaginations raced through my head. In such a closed environment the tigress had an edge over us. It was hard to quell the thought that the wounded animals do often resent their injury on the first human they meet, who unfortunately is not always the person who deserved the attention. But it is often the way of life that innocents suffer and culprits escape – for examples politicians in a war.

We retreated a few yards and broke out in an open plot. At our full view she suddenly lay flat on her stomach in crouching position with her head on the ground and her tail waving perpendicularly in the air. Saliva dripped from her mouth as she watched us intently.

At the moment, a small flock of red-headed *sarus* cranes flew low over the vista crying their loud trumpet chorus – when their calls were abruptly drowned in a deep throated growling – not unlike the purring of a cat, but amplified a hundred fold.

I stood facing her without batting an eyelid. The grip of my gun went slick with sweat from my palms as the growls continued with their ultrasonic effect which paralyze the brain, literally making one stupefied. These were one of the most dreadful, blood curdling booms that even hardboiled hunters don't hear throughout their intense tiger times. The sounds proclaimed convincingly that why hunters tumble down from *machan* and why deer appear benumbed of their faculties; and that thing called sportsman's nerve which temporarily provides you power to endure such nasty times, gives up after some time.

I marvelled at the power of her voice – so much of life and energy was pulsating deep within that wasted body. The roars rumbled as much in my chest as they thundered in her. The sorry creature appeared famished for weeks, and yet was a match for all of us. I wonder if these sounds freeze the flight reflexes of prey species during the final seconds of charge.

A trice later, the point of her tail came into view, swinging from side to side. My heart beat like a sledgehammer for a disturbed tiger contains all the qualities of a load of dynamite and there is always a premonition of death in such explosive situations; a kind of animal horror that is genetically inherent in human takes control over you and makes you feel nuts.

Usually an accurate bullet, the punctuation of life, is the imperative solution, and Chhotey, who had tracked many injured animals under the most uncompromising conditions was telling me constantly, "When there is no shooting Bhaiya, then why this risk?" Finally deciding that discretion is better part of valour, we wasted no time in moving back.

Having attained a hundred yards from the grass patch, I halted in suspense. The spectacle had lasted for around 40 seconds but it had proved to be most realistic and terrifying. The growls had sent an alarming report around the vista, worrying the Sikh family. Soon I heard the sounds of tractors. Having collected workers from the field, they were coming running to help us or perhaps collect what was left of us. My name was being shouted when I ended their anxiety by shouting back. The Sikh was mighty happy on seeing us alive. Although the events had become exciting and a reliable observation of the tigress's condition could not become possible, but there seemed no need to try such 'crazy proceedings' again just to set my eyes upon her. The last picture of the tigress in my mind was of her fierce and decisive intent. However, she was alive and this was enough.

That night as I lay on the bed her roars seemed to return and reverberate in my mind. My mind went to the three tiger charges I had faced earlier in my ventures – that jerking of the tail tip, the paralyzing roar and an incredibly fast low rush which is bound to knock down any trespasser. Even injured tigers have been known to cover a hundred yards in just over three seconds. This can give you some idea of the nano-seconds we had at our disposal to escape if a charge had come from twenty yards. A tiger can cover that distance much quicker than one can pronounce his name. There would have been no time to halt her and my one-sided affair with her would have concluded within a blink of the eye.

Furthermore the colliding impact of a tiger charging home can be compared to that of 300 kg automobile, moving at 30 kilometers an hour or a Victorian five-seater sofa thrown down upon you from the third storey of a building. A hunter possessed of calm judgment and unshakable nerve may shoot the tiger dead in the way but once that 400-pound body has taken a start there are no bullets made to stop its great momentum; for it is made for the very purpose of attack, the collision impact of which was of some 10,000 pounds, is enough to deflate a hunter.

Maharaj Balrampur's records mention a case in which a tiger's region of diaphragm and his heart were half blown away by double shots of .505 Gibbs yet unstoppable like a torpedo it covered some fifty yards and collided head on with the hunter who was literally thrown some 15 feet back. The tiger died in this effort and so did the man, bleeding from his mouth and nostrils. His body from the navel region up to rib cage, where tigers head had rammed with full drive, was all blue and black. It was as if a Land Rover had collided with 30 kilometer speed, indicating severe rupturing of internal blood vessels.

Well, the era of great sea captains is gone; the era of great pilots is gone, Berlin wall is history and so is time of big-game hunters. Yet, such incidents bring back those forbidden memories that do not exist in our minds, but were there in the hunter's blood. They are proscribed but they are there to span a chasm whose other side we cannot see.

As I tumbled on the bed and sleep overwhelmed my tired limbs, my mind played recklessly with unconstrained imaginations. The fact is, the more you know about tigers the more they get into your imagination as you learn to respect them.

News travels with the speed of radio in Tarai. The word had gone around that a college-teacher-turned tiger-researcher from Lucknow had been killed. Next day a police team and rangers arrived to collect my remains. They even carried a local newspaper that had published the obituary, albeit the deceased was named Rajesh Shukla. They sat at the Sikh's house and inquired about tigers. We listened to them as snacks were served. A search was about to commence for the dead Shukla's remains when I ended the suspense. I asked the inspector with a smile: "Won't you ask the remains to tell the details?" There was a startled look on the faces of the cops as I revealed my identity and narrated the incident. When my explanation was over, I got the tongue-lashing of a life time from the police inspector who told me that my funeral procession would soon follow if I continued to behave inconsiderately with the tigers. His assistants very professionally told me that I could be jailed for attempting suicide.

Anyway, it was a strangely satisfying experience to read my obituary with a different name – such a howler is traditionally considered an auspicious omen for the person wrongly described as dead, and it blesses the person with long life. Reading one's own obituary removes the bad spell and you don't sign off early.

That very afternoon we found that the tigress had emerged at the far end of grass-field but had turned back on her tracks at daybreak. Her right leg was injured; enough to make the animal reluctant from venturing into the open.

Tigers do not have social bonds like lions to help each other in difficult times. Even invalid starving lions get food to pull through and get better while the pride hunts for him. It has been said that an individual organism is gene's way of making more genes. Society is one aspect of this, for the ultimate function of sociability is to increase the chances of survival of member individuals.

If a solitary beast like tiger is hurt, it has no providers of food for him. He must starve and die or kill cattle or frogs or at worst, attempt to snatch some other tiger's food. The last option is full of hazards, for the owner of the kill may be a powerful opponent and his aggression may further injure the already incapacitated beast. After all, this is the trait of their tribe, the standard way the tigers eliminate their aged and injured kin so that the population control is maintained.

The nature of animal's injury is important. It matters whether it is superficial or hard-hit, recoverable or not, whether the animal has been shot by a powerful-enough gun, the distance of effective shooting, whether some important tissues has been put out of business, whether vital bones of limbs and shoulder have broken and whether the rifle ball has crossed the body or the nickel jacketed part is still inside the body. A weak load of homemade buckshot often does more damage from point blank range than a tightly concentrated factory load from a distance. Not having the same wallop, the pellets lie inside the muscles and sooner or later may lead to septicemia, causing a lingering and painful death.

There is need for collection of data regarding the recovery of injured tigers because records show that hardy beasts often miraculously recover from frightful wounds, including compound bone fractures and multiple perforations in internal organs and carry the deflated lead, sometimes up to 500 grains, all through their life in their body. If the lead gets adjusted with the body, inside skin, fat and muscles then they may behave normally, but if it generates agony then they turn extraordinarily troublesome.

There are many who question an injured tiger's competence, for it is a heavy-bodied animal with thick short legs, and its injured paw must prove a great handicap to him in hunting his food. My answer to them is that even if one leg is limp, the other three still remain favourable for catching foothold in soft earth and possess enough power to control a moderate-sized prey. This way the injured tigers, whose wounds are painful without being fatal or incapacitating, survive in the wild. The diet that keeps them alive is something of an accomplishment.

However, these were vague conjectures and one thing was sure that the dice was loaded heavily against her. The main problem of an injured predator is as how to obtain food, and even for the managers, with the imminent prospect of human deaths, lethal control of injured carnivore is the only practical option. Treating a wild tiger's injuries for a resource-scarce naturalist like me with no technical skills was a wishful thinking. I knew of no text book which dealt with this impossible subject. All my aid to her survival was reduced to a narrow compass of easy food and if this sponsorship worked then it would be the best reward.

Suddenly it was a holy war. A new agenda had been added into my sugar-tiger study that temporarily transformed my programme and focused my hard toil upon the recovery of an injured tigress. Convinced that there was still a fair chance to save her, I decided to deliver her with weekly baits.

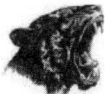

Crowded against the Wall

"For reasons impossible to explain, the impulse to console an animal in distress is equally as compelling to many human beings as is the impulse to console another human being. To many it is more compelling."

- Cory J Macham, Environmental Activist, California

Since the tiger had been eliminated and the female crippled, a leopard had begun to frequent the island. At times lying in bed and feeling the oppressive stillness that reigned the area in the night, I heard the 'spots' calling, a repetitive, rasping cough, not unlike the sound of someone sawing wood. It would be answered by a sudden explosive bark of a *chital* herd then a throbbing drum like sound of their feet as they ran away. Then invariably the shrieking and barking alarm of *langoors* would echo for a few minutes as they shifted uneasily among tree tops. Then silence would settle down, reminding me how the agrarian floor of Tarai like its jungles gets cloaked with blood in the nights and how uneasily the ungulates and primates sleep in that darkness.

During this phase, Billy Arjan Sigh was clandestinely baiting Dudhwa tigers to localize them near his residential territory of Tiger Haven, within a small patch of forest that he fondly called as Tiger Haven Range. His aim was three fold; first to draw the tigers out of precincts of the park and hold them in his Tiger Heaven range; second to take the pressure off the wild prey population as during prey scarcity baiting can also be used by tigers to live through lean period and third, to attract foreign tourist and make commercial films on tigers of Tarai.

But our reasons were different. While Billy was conducting his activities inside the premises of a National Park without necessary permission, my plain and simple purpose was to abet an injured tigress to overcome her crisis of survival outside the protected area. While Billy's target was to earn money by offering photographic opportunities to his foreign clients, mine was to produce life-sustaining results for a dying animal. For after all, an injured tiger, unable to kill wild herbivores, doesn't lose its right to live. Hence my programme had a clear conservation target and presumably a well-defined path to get there based on effective implementation of baiting.

Baiting for a tiger is widely misunderstood, though it had been practiced for hundreds of years. Providing live bait to tigers to lure them at a given spot is part of custom that was once preparatory to great Indian *shikaar* events. There is nothing like pain and agony that the tied animal must endure in suspense and fear, while it awaits its fate. In comparison to swine herds who butcher pigs in barbaric ways, tigers are quick killers. They approach silently and finish their job within seconds. Evolution has given them the ability to do their work with utmost efficiency as their very existence depends on this. David Livingstone was severely mauled in his early years by a lion he had wounded in Bechuanaland. The cat grabbed him by shoulder and shook him until he felt no pain at all. A.W. Strachan of Indian Police who lost one leg to a tiger attack, says "Before an animal attacked by a tiger can feel pain, it is dead."

The fact is that I have never been chewed or seriously injured by any dangerous animal. I don't even have any experience of body touch attacks by animals. Hence I am no expert as how it feels on being chewed by a predator. Furthermore, man has no natural weapons of offence hence I believe that all animals are dangerous for him. As a teenager, I recall witnessing the capture of a black buck doe and her fawn by natives. I was standing and watching the scene when the male came bounding over to chastise us and hit me with full thrust. Luckily, my thin profile came between his cylindrical horns, as his head collided with my stomach and I was knocked down but before he could trample or gorge me someone hit it hard with a lathi on its legs and I walked out without injury.

Well, predators are dangerous but if any member of antelope or deer family gets a chance, you are just as dead from their pointed horns as from an elephant's stub tusks. The horns of even domestic cattle can punish you severely. That is why big cats strategize in hunting and respect the armaments of their prey. The fact is when some people show their assorted scars with pride, like military decorations, I feel ordinary of my clean skin. However, three villagers I know who have survived tiger attacks namely, Shiv Shanker of Ghola, Rajiha Pasi and Anita Raidas of Kaanp Tanda, who got more than 300 stitches, claim that the pain inflicted in such attacks is excruciating. It won't be out of the context to quote hunters such as Paul Nielssen and Willy De Beer, both African professionals who faced serious lion attacks and were badly chewed up. They also claimed the same feelings.

Buffaloes have very low intelligence and it doesn't matter to them whether they are tied to a peg inside the cattle pen or anywhere else. As long as water and cud is available, they are relaxed. They chew the cud complacently and remain oblivious of the quick and skillful death that awaits them as an alternative to a walk to the slaughterhouse. I have seen domesticated buffaloes, standing insensitive and tranquil in their sheds even on the approach of predator, while the same animal when pulled into an abattoir is highly agitated and terrified.

There was an alarming plethora of domestic stock on the island that was consuming much vegetation. I chose to use some of these redundant cattle to save the life of the more valuable animal. That afternoon a buffalo calf was taken to the river bank area and picketed between a *jamun* tree and the river, while towards evening I and Dalbeer Singh sat on a *machan* on our decisive watch to take an appraisal of her condition.

The scarlet upper tip of the sun soon slipped with arresting swiftness below the horizon, leaving the grassland that lay parched and aired before us, smouldering with the wavelets of pure orange touched by the strokes of sea green.

All around me was the vast savannah of sugarcane, where the deep silence of the evening was being emphasized by the multi-timbered notes of countless insects. I half lay on the *machan*, listening to the calls of herons and fish eagles and watching the heavens where countless luminous jewels had emerged.

A pair of fox trotted to a small water hole near the river bank. They lapped up some water then raising their heads towards the sky, let out a synchronized chattering bark. It exploded in the stillness of evening like a funeral song. The sharp yelping was repeated three or four times that pleasantly relieved the tedium of waiting for tiger but seem to bear a typical weird kind of agonizing and fear-laden expression.

I wondered what the foxes meant by it. Perhaps they had got some inkling of 'stripes' when the dolorous wailing note was taken up by a frightened *chital*. It barked in its hoarse and throaty blares from Banna Devi grasslands. The ghostly atmosphere of island suddenly became tense and charged with expectancy. Come on, come on, I thought. I knew the lesser beasts were charting the route of the great cat and I would be able to meet her on the fresh site I had set up.

As my eyes grew accustomed to the gloom, I got an impression that I had seen something swaying stealthily. A rustle in the tinder dry leaves warned me that my quarry was arriving. Some minutes lapsed then the tigress came out from the corner of a sugar thicket.

Her first impression touched my heart. She was in a state of gruesome starvation and had dwindled down to a mangy condition, a little better than a mere bag of bones. I marveled at her tenacity that in spite of her wound and her foodless condition since that night nearly a month ago when she had run into trouble, she was not only alive but still active and going about.

Our *machan* was at a low height and there was a strong chance of being detected by an animal that has the sharpest ears in the wild. A tiger makes a slow, deliberate approach to bait but she did not approach the heifer. She rather perceived our presence on the *machan* and uttered a pooking call possibly as a surprise, and then began to roam about the tree, swishing off the canes and grass as she pushed through them. Suddenly an animal bolted past our *machan*. I could not see it properly as the tigress roamed the vicinity, unseen around my tree, silent and attentive.

Needless to say I felt thoroughly frustrated on my part that I had got the *machan* made so low. It was not a hunter's or a photographer's perch where the distance is critical to prevent distortion for the flashlight or shooting, which if done well off the ground it is not likely to achieve its target. It was a naturalist's perch, which must be located reasonably high to allow him to keep an eye on his subject from a distance.

The stars twinkled serenely in the clear velvety sky as the tigress sat nine meters away from our tree, half-hidden in a ditch and watched the *machan* as well as the heifer from there. Finding a heifer standing ready for a dinner had apparently made a great appeal to her, especially when she had suffered many foodless days. This explained her reluctance to move away from there. Yawning and looking at us she vigilantly observed our behavior for around an hour, after that she felt relaxed of our presence.

The dumb heifer was happily chewing the cud and made no reaction to the predator's presence. The tigress watched it intently for some minutes, got up and half encircled it and then seized it in an orthodox style from the side. Like lightning, she caught the throat and pulled down the prey, as the grip on the windpipe lead to the strangulation. She retained the throat hold for some five to six minutes. The dying animal lay on its sides, its legs moving rhythmically in the delirium. I was deeply impressed by the power she displayed in her killing method. It gave a conclusive proof that despite being injured with a foreleg slightly twisted, her art of killing was in no way impaired.

The natural spectacle of the world's greatest predator, going about its lawful business undisturbed was a grand sight! It was notable in the sense that the victim died in a perfect grip that no blood dropped on the ground, whereas a butcher's barbaric cut on a jugular vein makes the wretched goat squirm to its death in a welter of blood and imprecations.

She did not make any attempt to shift the kill and began to feed right on the spot. Having stayed for more than an hour, she knew we were harmless. Ravenously hungry, she chomped a substantial dinner, not hurriedly, but utterly absorbed and with relish, though making a hollow growling in between as if in some resentment. Hungry tigers can consume a prodigious amount of meat readily eating the hindquarters of the prey and even switching over to forequarters for more food. They require one or two hours of uninterrupted feeding to become satiated. Her contented chomping was music to my ears for it meant that my strategy was right. Eventually when the tigress stopped eating; all the edible portion of the heifer had been consumed.

We sat silent like a statue, as if belonging to the old school of sportsman-hunter, watching the proceedings while she got up, loitered around aimlessly and sat down on her haunches like a dog. Once again she steadily ate a good deal more from the kill. She then picked a bone scrap for cursory gnawing and went back in a bush. After a long time her belly looked round and finally when she slipped in the undergrowth, there was very little of vestiges left. The hundred-pounder calf was reduced to a 50-pound relic comprising rumen contents, large hard bones, head and all the hooves. The edge of the scapula, the ends of ribs and even the nasal bone had been eaten off.

It was nearing midnight when we left our tiny *machan*. The tigress had been sitting hidden close by and when she saw us climbing down she moved away in the cane thicket and disappeared.

Our two-mile walk to home in the tiger haunted sugarcanes was accomplished at a slow pace. Far away in the solitude of darkness, jackals let forth their weird-howling amongst which the shrill choirs of cicadas' zithered. The dull moon beams had created an impression of mysterious phantoms, which seemed to have awakened to hunt accompanying the carnivore. The strong scent of tigress left behind by her for a long distance mixed with that of the lily of the night was noticeable. A transistor playing loudly at a *jhala*, ricocheted a popular song of Kishore Kumar "*Yeh Sham Mastani*", and all this cumulatively gave a weird background to the still and tranquil sugar grasslands.

Despite being shadowed by the spectre of financial ruin and encouraged by the success of my strategy, I spent some 1500 rupees of my own and provided her with six heifers. This was nearly my full salary then but a worthwhile expenditure. She often spent quite a lot of time around the kill, snacking on it from time to time and showing the signs of rapid progress in health. By then she depended largely on the weekly baits, making visits twice a day to the kill-site and when hungry enough she hovered around the place for longer times.

One day Kuldeep was tying a heifer when he looked back and saw the tigress sitting in a covert, vigilantly observing his behaviour. She yawned repeatedly and stayed calm. Perhaps it was her friendly gesture for a man who brought her presents and gifts. Without losing his nerves the man accomplished his business and then slowly backed away while the tigress stayed at her place yawning, allowing him to move away.

The man was hardly away from the scene when he heard the death bellow of the heifer which meant that the fate of animal had been decided. Having killed it, the tigress seemed to eat it rather half-heartedly and left much of it covered with leaves. Next day when she returned a stray dog had discovered her kill and was busy gorging the leftovers. She ambushed the dog and pulling it in a covert ate it out completely. This happened even while during all these nights she returned to the heifer and finished each scrap of it.

It was one of the hottest months of June I can remember. To get an idea as to what she was doing I and Chhotey spent much time patrolling the area on foot during the hottest part of the day. We came to an area that had with over a dozen pools. It was surrounded by crowding *jamun* trees; hence called Jamunhiya. We had tramped a good five miles and were rather fagged with intense heat. Some one hundred yards away from Jamunhiya was a rise locally identified as Dhamar, with a plexus of tamarind trees standing on it. I went there to rest for a bit. The rise was some twenty feet above the surrounding country, an excellent place to keep a look-out over the great vista of the river.

A dried snake skin lay low on the grass, where I rested. It was a seven-foot rind that might have once encased a venomous snake. Chhotey recognized it as that of a king cobra, "The diabolical ingenuity of Nature" whose venom comprises heterogeneous toxins, made of 90 per cent protein. Its power of strike is acknowledged as having speed of lightning flashes. Towards the east some peacocks were pecking grit on the low grounds making a sound like cats mewing loudly, and many other birds could be seen including two ospreys fishing in the shallow waters of Baghar. Still further away, a wild boar standing near a cluster had dug his snout in the muddy slush and was ploughing through it as they normally do before rolling leisurely on their back in the manner of their kind. At our sight the peacocks took to flight shrieking and the boar vanished as if by magic.

The summer heat was terrific. I had barely sat down in the shade with my hat over my eyes to keep the glare away when Chhotey tapped my shoulder and said "the tiger is in the pool." I got up to have a look. The tigress lay a hundred meters or more away in the west, in a stagnant stretch of water and was clearly visible through the gap of *jamun* trees. She was doing something which the tigers do at midday, resting in the watery slush, but her motionlessness and indifference towards us was worrying. While resting, tigers spend much of their time in the fastidious process of grooming themselves, their coarse tongue moving along the inner edge of paws, chest and every part of their body, cleaning blood and tiny scraps of meat that attract flies or roll in the dust or sludge but she seemed all doleful. Perhaps what had caused the lethargy was the extreme heat, and undoubtedly it was exceptional at that time.

The silence was captivating that I had no desire to interrupt. The binoculars allowed me to examine her properly. She was watching me intently. Her paws stretched outside in the cat fashion. Once the food situation had eased she had gained weight and her body, seemingly flexible, did not apparently hold any conspicuous mark of injury.

Then onwards we saw her several times in the same pool. She would see us and then turn away casually. Perhaps she recognized that we were acquaintances who shared the same range and had often also fed her. She now seemed to walk without a limp and the twist of her right paw had also smoothened. It may have been my imagination but her rich coat appeared healthy and glossier to me, its colour suddenly showing bright as her lost strength had returned. Once when she got up covered with slush all over her stomach and sides, she rubbed herself vigorously against the edges of an anthill. Then she got further and did more rubbing against a tree, which I had noticed before being covered with mud all over it and where she must have repeated the exercise many times in the past. It was clearly a ritual activity as the practice helped her to clean her body.

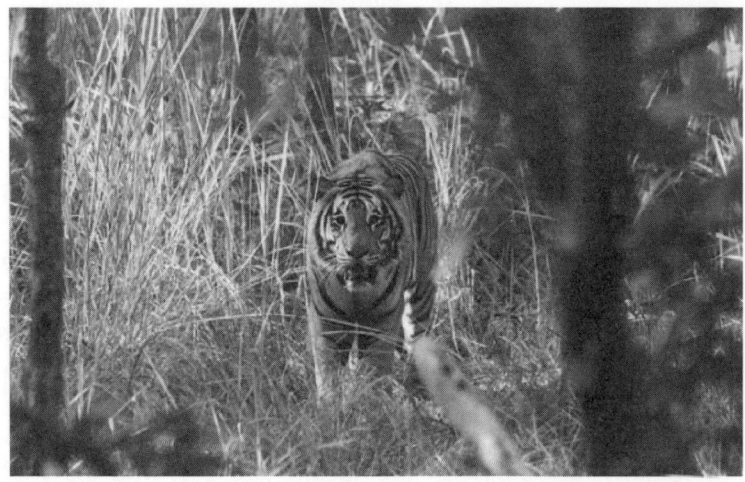

Tarai is mind-bogglingly large where tigers disperse properly. In theory they travel hundreds of miles to settle away far from their natal range where often they are not related to new tigers they meet hence Tarai males are more violent and aggressive. *(Camera Trap Shot; Photo credit Govt of Nepal)*

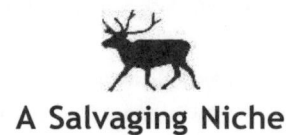

A Salvaging Niche

The man made shelter of sugarcanes, with its reassuring ease of food, water, cover and space had precisely played a critical role in the survival of this tiger.
- Author in 'Sugarcane Tiger'

A day before I was to leave for Lucknow, a big storm swept over the island. The sky dramatically darkened in the mid-afternoon and rain broke, accompanied by violent thunderstorm and strong wind. The relentless power of cyclonic gale did an awesome lot of damage in a short space of time. It uprooted some trees completely, broke many stout tree branches, and lifted the residents' huts as if they were built of card board and shattered them on the ground. There was something fascinating in witnessing that violent storm. It is quite impossible to face such speed of wind that was succeeded by heavy hailstorm, with hailstones as big as lemons.

The rain came down torrentially as the blinding flashes of lightning and clouds seemed to open just over the village until the ground was heavy with water logging.

Such tropical storms, luckily, don't last long and are rapidly over. I went up the rooftop when the rainfall stopped. The country seemed to hold all the water that had collected in pools and assumed the appearance of a lake. A strong wind was still blowing and birds apparently killed by the hailstorm lay scattered around. Just then I descried a small herd of gregarious swamp deer splashing through the inundated paddy fields. I stood on the roof and taking a grandstand view of whole proceedings, watched the scene with engrossed intent.

The western sky was heavy with the blanket of rain clouds but a damp and moist sun shone through the gaps in them. The whole country was bathed in dramatic storm lightning and a rainbow lurked in the eastern sky. A flock of white egrets shimmered against the slate grey clouds as if being tossed about the wind like torn leaves. Suddenly a vivid flash of forked luminosity gave the trees and grasses a viridian glow and the moving swamp deer looked like the ghostly shadows imposing their beauty, boldly and irresistibly on the landscape. It looked as if the nature's artistic license had gone crazy after the sheer perfection of things. The harmonious togetherness of water, drizzling, paddy crop and wild life, in the imposing background of greenery and the powerful reflection of gorgeous sunlight on logged rainwater, with some lovely reds and its delicate tints, was a sight of priceless colors and shades.

I am sure no photograph could have done justice to that scene. It was something simply to admire with absolutely no bindings in mind and heart. It was the most dazzling combination of colours and shades I had ever seen. Such times truly establish that nobody can catch nature's elemental essence in whatever respect it may be.

The gale raged for some minutes and when it slowed down, the nervous calls of swamp deer fell into my ears. They were looking intently towards east perceiving some danger. I shifted my glasses there and through the blades of intertwined grass, I caught a fleeting glimpse of a reddish object that was moving swiftly, rather gliding like a sun-dappled wave, which abruptly lay down as if in wait.

When viewed through a magical lens, reality, perspective and space are suspended. It was then that the bonus sight of the day emerged on my binoculars. The tigress had been hiding behind the trunk of a silk cotton tree and watching the herd from there. The great animal crept forward in a low-shouldered crouch, taking advantage of some heavy patches of scrub and after about twenty feet stopped again. I held my breath as the spectacle unfolded. The stalk was true to text book. The wind carried the molecules of feline smell to the deer and they perceived her presence. For a brief moment, they deliberately advanced towards her roughly covering some ten feet through a thicket, as if to confirm her location and then abruptly turned and ran away in the opposite direction.

The tigress made no effort to chase them because once the element of surprise is lost the tiger invariably retreats in every instance. She coolly got up and walked out of the cover like an indolent queen as if nothing had happened. She watched the running deer that were already a hundred yards away and then walked towards Banna grasslands. She seemed to move smoothly without any limp. I was amazed to see how quickly she had put on the bulk.

Her attempt to hunt was a great indicator that her injury had healed and her predatory drives were back. This present maneuver may have flopped but these would soon bear fruit. Tiger survival depends on their killing expertise, and they

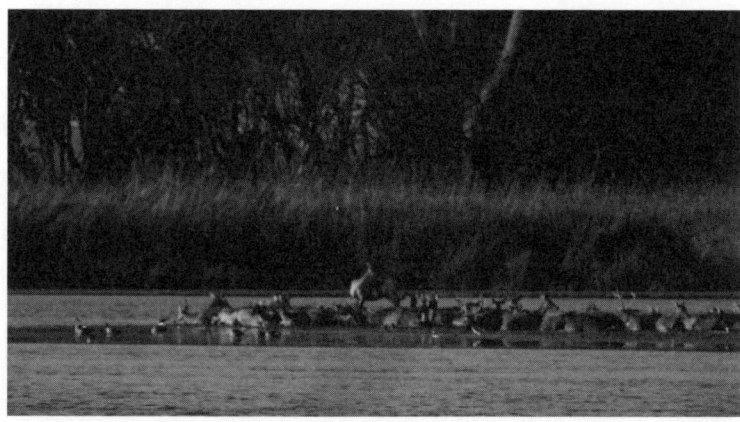

The evening had set in as the swamp deer called from the banks of Girwa. *(Photo Credit : Sanjay Pathak, NTCA)*

never allow it to become degenerated. It also proved that getting easy prey through baiting had yet not changed her mind and by inherited instincts she still preferred natural prey.

The shining sunlight went off suddenly and the grey somber looking shades quickly descended on the landscape making it dismal and depressing. While returning I pondered over Sanquist's assessment that only one tiger attack is successful in twenty attempts. If this statistics is applied upon an injured tiger, it may bounce out of proportion to a hundred energy sapping attempts without success. That would rather drain out the pursuer by enhancing its starvation levels instead of sustaining it.

Indeed the master predator does not make its kill easily and an injured one, compelled to seek food from human resources, often goes for livestock that invites trouble. Thus baiting has its moral and practical considerations in favour of invalid predators.

I stayed in Lucknow for a month then returned to island again on week days. The tigress was living in Banna grasslands and still unable to kill her natural prey lurked around human settlements through day and night. In the silence of nights, the plaintive wail of peacocks and the throaty alarm coughs of *langoor* monkeys from high up in the tree canopies often advertised her presence in the vicinity of human settlements.

By this time she knew where her prey came from. One evening she reached her killing site and not finding the bait tied there, picked up the old remnants of bones, took them to some ten meters away into bushes, where she chewed them. She then walked towards the Sikh's house, reaching up to his vehicle parking yard and spent her time till past midnight. The watch dogs begun to bark raising a nervous din that continued for over an over. I woke up and looked out of the windows, throwing the torch light around to know the cause. In the gloomy shadows of trees, fireflies gleamed as they flew pulsing their jade green misty lights. The remains of the kitchen fire that the servants had built to cook their food, glowed like a patch of garnets at the edge of the wall. Perhaps the unusual clamour was due to the ego tiff of some pariah dogs, I thought so and slept.

Next day the evidence on the damp soil indicated the visit of tigress. She had spray marked the tyres of a tractor trolley and then sat under the trolley for some time, watching the house from hundred yards away till midnight, perhaps wondering as why the man had forgotten to bring her meal. I am sure she recognized Kuldeep personally and knew that from where all the juicy presents came to her. Another time she came upon an abandoned hutment and finding it isolated and undisturbed walked inside it and slept for whole of the day.

One evening she killed a heifer and ate more than half of it. But then the remnants lay there for good four days and nights and she did not return. After this she began to disappear over longer periods on hunting missions of her own and twice pointedly abandoned the bait. I could clearly read the telltale signs as she had walked right past the tethered bait. She had passed so close to the wretched animal that it had to move to the other end of its peg to remain unhurt and unmarked, and yet the tigress overlooked it. This assured me that she was self-reliant now and there was no need for my intervention. She had begun to make kills of her own and was on her way back to her normal diet, which was gratifying. The last bait I tied remained there for good 10 days and was unfortunately eaten alive by hyenas that until then had stayed out of the scene. They knew that tigress had stopped frequenting the area and as a natural corollary the bait was theirs.

As a young and vigorous tigress she had now taken to making dinner of feral cattle, the mainstay of a farm tiger's diet, besides blue bulls and pigs. Her confidence had apparently returned and she was no longer nervous of tackling full-grown animals. All the kills had been seized by the nape of the neck; an efficient form of attack that is generally used by powerful and confident tigers since it paralyses the animal by crushing the vertebrae. While the grip of the windpipe leads to strangulation, the expedient nape-bite brings death instantaneously.

On October 16, 1984, while driving the jeep on a usual look-around in the evening, we halted the vehicle close to a dead blue bull. The grown antelope lay flat on the ground with fresh blood oozing out of its mouth and nostrils. Superficial signs of mauling made by fangs and claws were clearly visible on his body as the base of the animal's neck had been crushed by the jaws. I marvelled at the power of the vice-like crunch. As I put my hand on neck and belly of animal, its body was still warm. The kill was freshly made, perhaps hardly a few minutes ago. When tigers put down their prey they don't leave it but show a proprietorial attitude towards it, snarling and growling at intruders. But here the killer had heard us arrive. It had left the kill and shifted in the grasses, where it was probably crouching, resting from the struggle and instead of demonstrating waiting for us to depart.

While looking at the kill that weighed close to 400 pounds it was obvious that it required great energy in handing. I could make out that her prey-selection had again reached her supreme capacity as her almost-lost powers of hunting had returned to a fair degree. Somewhere deep inside me was great satisfaction and admiration about the way she had nursed herself back to strength with her speed, agility and ambushing traits. Like zoo tigers recognize their keepers as providers, I trust she recognized us, especially Kuldeep Singh in a similar vein; she didn't consider us any potential trouble, and never issued any admonishing snarl at us.

The evening was drawing in. Horizontal rays of the sinking sun streamed through the clouds. We did not disturb the kill and took to riding the vehicle onwards.

In my immense hours of observation I have spent after farmland tigers I can safely vouch that she was a unique sugarcane tigress. Despite a potential punishment lesion received from the master race, she had not developed a sweet tooth for humans, and did not leave the place completely. She preferred to stay in her old haunt, where she felt fully naturalized and secure and when the tiger is truly naturalized anywhere, in any environment and terrain even if it is physically retarded, it never exhibits an abrasive behavior whatsoever because the physical surroundings and baseline ecology, as is of sugar farms, is complimentary to its life pattern.

I didn't say *Eureka*, I didn't see fireworks cracking in the sky, there were no temple bells ringing for me but precisely this was the answer that the man-made sugar farms with their reassuring ease of food, water, cover and space had played a critical role in the survival of this tiger. Precisely it had worked as a medicine, as an elixir of life, striking home the fact that only a potential habitat, where optimum conditions exist for a big cat's survival, can produce situations conducive for convalescence of an injured predator. Though scientists believe that the impact of human activities on tigers and their prey base is largely negative as was observed earlier, but human intervention also proves positive in many cases. If people are a part of problem then the best way is to make them a part of solution too.

Some pseudo-experts uphold the idea that man must not interfere with the natural process of life and death. To this my answer is that care-taking and medical intervention has increased the life span of a human to more than its double in this very century and even helped his pet to not to die untimely death. Then, why should wildlife be deprived of care-giving? Humans have already tampered seriously with natural systems in their quest for animal meat, skin and bones. Their greed for forest products has degraded the tiger habitat so thoroughly that a positive human intervention is required. We lack such management programmes that support injured predators to put them back on the track until optimum condition of their health have been restored.

Next day the real monsoon broke. The dark clouds flashing with lightning rained over the vista and made the forest totally inaccessible. Within no time tall rank grass grew everywhere and visibility turned low. Animal life went on higher ground and as there was abundance of water everywhere, hence it no longer needed to stay close to ponds. The deluged country and muddy roads turned into virtual ribbons on the wheels of passing carts and as the waters rose to flood level proportions, the low-lying baiting site was first to get inundated. I knew that monsoon was liable to be a particularly lean period for her but as she hadn't touched the last bait, so there was use to continue baiting for her I and Kuldeep decided to leave her to fend for herself.

I returned to Lucknow. I was happy that I had played a small role in making a tiger naturalized once again by supporting her in her vulnerable times. It was my very personal but triumphal flagmarch that she could now return to free living.

A Reorientation of Management Principles

The onus which develops on a single bureaucrat pressurized by political superiors, needs to be amended.

- Billy Arjan Singh

It is not known what happened to this tigress afterwards. The Sikh family in my absence continued to carry out my programme. I give full credit for its success to them as they had in fact enjoyed the entire exercise, its thrills and adventure, getting an opportunity to interact with the legendry animal that the people fear. It dispelled the notions that the unpopular blood-curdling canards, generated by quintessential Victorian writers, have created in their minds.

The tigers themselves cannot solve their problems, it has to be solved by man only and the solution does not lie in fearing or eliminating these creatures from the face of earth. The pragmatic solution essentially lies in maintenance of an intricate ecological balance where both men and animals could thrive in a symbiotic relationship. Here, human endurance and sagacity count most.

Providing baits to wild tigers is a punishable crime. In accordance with regulations designed to prevent cases of poisoning anybody indulging in it has to be arrested and prosecuted. To this my argument was that the Forest Department should better punish poachers who impair the wild animals and catalyze the making of man-eaters rather than to question my intentions. Moreover, tiger is a protected species in India and that when the department concerned is unable to control poaching, particularly in the farmland areas, and lacks skillful plans to treat sick and injured wild beasts within their habitat, then any effort to protect tigers by enlightened preservationists and nongovernmental groups, where conservation rules are properly observed, should not be frowned upon.

Moreover, when conservation itself is defined and understood in so many different ways, it is perhaps simplistic to believe that there is any single overreaching agreement on what constitutes effectiveness in conservation. For example feral cattle are a nuisance but from predator conservation point of view, feral cattle are an asset. Once held responsible for degrading the habitat of forest areas and potentially out-competing wild prey, these cattle have now been arbitrarily elevated to the status of buffer prey by scientists in recent reports.

Schaller, the father of modern scientific study of wildlife, was first to highlight this fact. He wrote 50 years ago: "Taking India as a whole, domestic cattle and domestic buffalo are the most important items in the tiger's diet. With the wildlife in most forests decimated or eliminated, the tiger has taken partly or wholly to living on livestock, which is easy to kill and readily available. At least 10 per cent of the cattle grazing in Kanha Park and on its fringes are killed by tigers each year."

So what are the finish lines in this conservation in the context of tiger conservation and how does one read this example of increase in feral cattle population in farmlands abutting jungle – as success or failure?

In a meeting with foresters, I took the responsibility for the whole affair and declared that my law abiding team's action from the viewpoint of ethics and conservation was justified to ensure the survival of the afflicted tigress, which bore a bullet in its festering flesh for over a month and still endures the same. The only difference is that the bullet has been absorbed by the body and the wound is healed, though the exuding scar left by the wound would follow throughout her life. I therefore consider that the cause is a worthy one as the animal is expected to behave more comfortable.

After a long harangue the managers and ecologists did agree that the project was a huge success, due to effective implementation of home work and well managed network. But it was difficult for the foresters to understand that the reassuring ease of sugarcane shelters, the food, the closed environment and the universal solvent – water – had precisely played a critical role in giving her a startling recovery. It had worked as a medicine, striking home a fact that only a latent habitat – where optimal conditions exist – can produce situations conducive for the recovery of an injured predator. We need to understand how tigers legitimately utilize the resources of the large sugarcane plantations' ecosystem and come to live in rural landscapes fully naturalized. It is sad that scant or no effort has been made by any capable cadre of biologists to corroborate these facts with on-ground scientific assessments.

This example highlights how the narrow disciplinary confines or spatio-temporal limits of our inquiry influence our ability to understand processes that help maintain a high representation of wildlife even outside defined conservation landscapes. We must scientifically establish natural conservation gains in rural landscapes, where villagers are living materially better life and where no human agency is consciously involved in protecting wildlife. Yet, a complex biota of life is happily established in the region. In many farmland areas of Tarai, despite identified disturbances and pressure on resources that the natives and livestock impose on landscape, wildlife populations, like wild boar, blue bull, Iguana lizards, monkeys and peafowls (all substantial preys for a tiger) have recovered tremendously. Such natural achievements are rarely articulated by media or foresters because they don't interest people much.

I even took this opportunity to raise this question: "Was the conservation of sugarcane tiger a lost cause against the beasts of the protected areas and whether the presence of tigers in farmlands, who never touch a human being and who clear the area from the menace of feral cattle, be only seen as detrimental to man?" I even added that all the farmland tigers, some 30 in number, I had so far reported to forest department had either died of poisoning or were poached. It is sad that when the state grows complacent about stewardship of its bountiful wildlife no tiger in farmlands lives to a ripe old age to die a natural death. Like so many others even this tigress would have died had I not initiated timely intervention. We need to drop our anthropocentric approaches for farmland tigers and preserve such animals.

The then Chief Wildlife Warden of U.P. C.B. Singh though had his reservations on the subject but he was a right person at right place at the right time. On the request of Padma Shri Ranjit Bhargav, Chairman WWF UP Chapter, he understood the emotion behind the entire effort and withdrew the Wildlife Act violation charges against us. It was sad that Billy Arjan Singh remained initially skeptical to this affair. He wrote several complaining letters to Project Tiger authorities and personally came to meet the then Forest Secretary Kamal Pandey in Lucknow along with local Member of Parliament. He held a press conference in which he reprimanded the Forest Department for its policy about baiting, for which Billy was blamed and I was pardoned.

The old doyen of Dudhwa, who was once hugely and ridiculously gratified by the department and was the chief beneficiary of its largesse had lost his stardom in their eyes, due to his pet tigress Tara turning man-eater and baiting inside the park. Tara's rehabilitation programme had disastrously flopped and instead of turning into a wild creature she had turned into a feral critter. In the last months of her life her appetites were purely anthropophagous. She no doubt preferred the flavor of better-nourished flesh of man. I am sure that at some moment the human kills of this case-hardened offender were also shared by her wild mates and that had generated a series of man-eaters in Kheri district. .Now for this reason, the doyen was being treated as *persona non grata*. To all intents and purposes his role in the frenzied scenario was all tedium and pain and a confused promotion of his personal agenda.

Tara was dead, shot by foresters yet Billy maintained that she was alive. He knew it very well that having the doubtful honour of being mentioned in Parliament Tara episode had brought him into limelight again and he would enjoy this revived controversy for years to come. He knew which side of his bread was still buttered, while foresters had no intentions sailing under false colours..

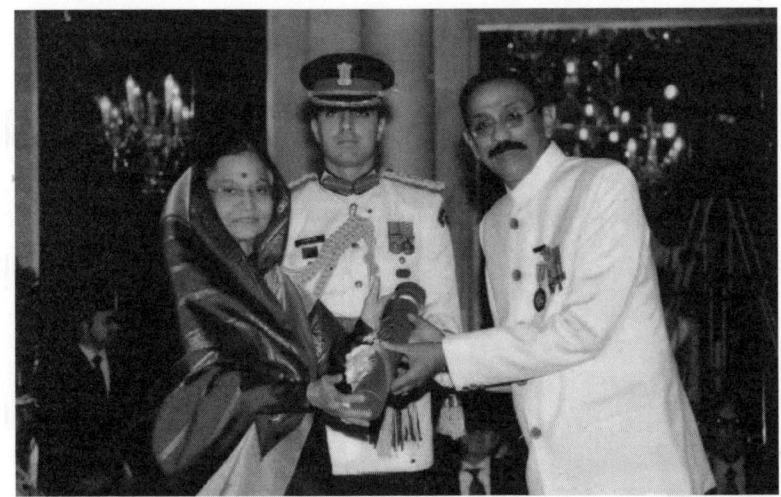

Ranjeet Bhargav,
receiving Padma
award from
HE Pratibha Patil, the
then President of India

He was highly critical of R. D. Gupta and Vijay Bahadur Singh, both senior foresters, but concluded the conference with a positive note telling, "While this example illustrates problems in judging success of a conservationist against the impediments posed forward by a system but it certainly plays a crucial role in problem identification". Ashok Kumar of WTI said: "When Rahul's conscience did not permit him to desert the injured tigress he did what he deemed fit." Ranjit Bhargav was of opinion that "When many poachers slaughter animals and get away; and the Forest Department still advocates pumping wounded tigers full of lead, Shukla's crusade to save a tigress without permit is ethically and conservationally all right which needs to be understood in emotional way. I consider him a valuable protagonist of better methods of wildlife preservation that draws many people into the working field of conservation."

It was a bold comment, fully and cynically justified by history because in pursuit of successful conservation, we have miserably failed to highlight the importance of acknowledging failures and documenting them properly so that they may never be repeated.

To find out a clear cut definition for conservation is a great problem. It will continue to mean different things to different people. Given the nature of conservation community, it is perhaps naïve to expect that conservationists of different schools will step away from their strongly held ideological ideas to attempt a dialogue on a common front. It is interesting to note that at every stance such debates are backed by an equally compelling rational and no party is right or wrong when viewed through different ideological lenses. However effective conservation is ultimately about creating and maintaining negotiated spaces for meeting ecological targets in human dominated world.

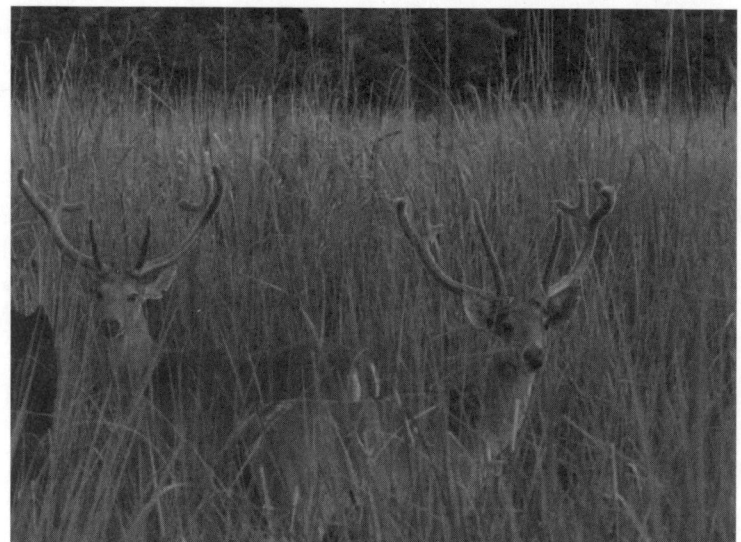

Swamp deer in velvet
(Photo credit : Gaurav Mishra)

Authors note

I personally rate this chapter as the central story of my book. To fully understand the plight of sugarcane tiger today it is necessary to take an excursion into yesterday. We need to review the making of Tarai, for the decline of its wildlife paralleled its growth. If there are no such places left for sugar tigers to live in pinch periods, the best conservation programmes and the goodwill of mankind will avail him little. Even if entire mankind decides that the tiger should be saved for posterity ultimately his fate will depend on whether or not human population growth is checked and checked soon.

Though swamp deer have been virtually wiped out from this region but as recently as ten years ago, one could see scattered black bucks and large herds of blue bulls still itinerant in the area. With such a base of prey animals, and since the observation of Island tigers no less than a score of tigers have frequented this island in winters. In 2012, I was not surprised to learn that a tigress with a single cub had again appeared in the area. The river course provides an easy access to this island where tigers find great cover of continuous sugar farms and their off springs return to it repeatedly considering it their key wintering area and their parents' favorite hunting grounds.

Appendix to Chapter 6

"There are never victories in conservation. If you want to save a species or a habitat, it's a fight forevermore. You can never turn your back".

- George Schaller

The prognosis for the survival of swamp deer in the island was grim. During winters of 1988 in Bahraich district some farm labours caught a pair of tiger cubs in the cane-fields that were abandoned by their mother. When I learnt of it, I immediately managed to send them to Lucknow, where they were raised as home pets by the Zoo director Rashmi Kant and his wife Mallika, while I myself favoured to return via the island. The area had suffered more from the depredations of outside hunters than most other parts. Poaching had been exceedingly heavy and the population of swamp deer having run the gauntlet of errant floods and poachers' bullets was nearly exterminated. I did not come across any male or fawn. Only two does had survived and as battered remnant of the past, they had joined a small heard of *chital*, eking out their precarious existence. They had attained a respective hierarchy in the herd and were seen leading some 6 *chitals*. Perhaps two *chital* antlers in the herd had courted swamp deer hinds in estrous and they were pregnant.

Chital bucks make no attempt to collect and retain a number of does, nor do they establish or defend a territory. Stray *chital* bucks practice different sexual behavior pattern. They are often freelancers, having no qualms in courting females of other deer species, which may correspond to their physical size. They join a succession of different herds in search of a receptive doe, and are known to court even with swamp deer and hog deer hinds. The buck is apparently able to determine the hind's state of receptivity by her odor and when the master bull's attention is diverted elsewhere, the *chital* enters the herd and copulates with the hind in estrous very quickly. The doe doesn't avoid the buck because she is in heat and the heat in both the parties synchronizes them physiologically, making actual coitus very brief.

To say I was let down at the dastardly elimination of swamp deer population is to put things mildly. Despite my repeated letters, the Forest Department failed to take any cognizance of this isolated population and slowly these declining remnants had already reached the point of no-return. I wrote several letters to people in authority querying the status of the species on the island and never got a reply. One officer was courteous enough to call back and his reply was "Never heard of them being there." (Incidentally in animal count the population of swamp deer is rarely counted due to the inaccessibility of wetlands.) The man had no recorded data of petite deer populations in his area. Apparently with such unwillingness of the department to take on poachers, no hope was left for the survival of swamp deer in this isolated pocket. Last time in 2004, while driving through this area, where I used to see dozens of animals, there was an incredible sense of life missing from the landscape that was so recently defined by these animals. The scenario was just hollow.

As regards pooking calls that I had often heard in the nights, I discovered it quite late that there were no *sambhar* inhabiting this island. *Sambhars* cannot restrain themselves wallowing and also create regular stamping grounds in the area they come to live. Chhotey and Phagunia had travelled the island quite regularly searching for these signs amidst rank grass and shrubbery, but found none. So it is safe to assume that the calls were made by tigers. I remember the loud clear pook, somewhat flatter in tone and lacking the resonance of the deer call, is a kind of vocalization that tigers often make to communicate but I had heard this kind of communication for one and the only time in life on this island.

I am thankful to Dr. George Schaller, who personally took care to send me the causes of such vocalizations by tigers that have been reported in a number of specific circumstances.

1, by a captive while ejecting urine (Boswell 1957)

2, just after a tiger had relieved (Champion 1927)

3, while walking near kill (Powell 1957)

4, just before approaching a kill (Anderson 1954)

5, when disturbed at kill by man (Brander 1923)

6, on seeing a man sitting on a tree (Perry 1964)

7, by a male accompanied by a female, when noting a person climb a tree in the distance (Lewis 1940)

8, when shot at or disturbed on a kill

9, when approaching a kill already occupied by another tiger (Schaller 1964)

10, by a male (?) tiger in response to roar of a tigress at a kill about a quarter mile away (Schaller)

11, by a male tiger when approached by a cub as he lay 20 feet from kill (Schaller)

12, mother calling the cub. A call which seems designed to communicate a mixture of alarm and suspicion (Arjan Singh 1984)

13, my observation tells that the tigers in pair, normally courting male and female, when separated in their forays often communicate this way to join each other. It is a moody communication, a sex call that suggests that the sound serves to advertise the animal's presence to its partner. The fact is that pooking has also been reported in conjunction with scent markings and relieving nature, both of these are behavior patterns for self-advertisement among cats. Dr Schaller and Dr Ullhas Karanth lend support to this contention.

It was the result of my reports in newspapers about farmland wildlife that I became involved in a long and acrimonious debate with the Forest Department as well as the editor of a famous wildlife magazine *Chital*, issued from Dehradun, now in Uttrakhand state. This eventually led me to writing my first book *'Killing Grounds'* spanning my years of tiger adventures with a chapter on concept of Sugarcane Tigers.

Conservation seems invariably a compromise between the need to protect wildlife and the aspirations of the local human population. The study showcases that the inevitable shunting of tigers in Tarai sugar fields should not be seen as detrimental to man; and with just a little motivation even hardened unwilling men can have the change of heart and help in protecting the magnificent iconic animal.

Book 4
MAN-EATERS CALLING

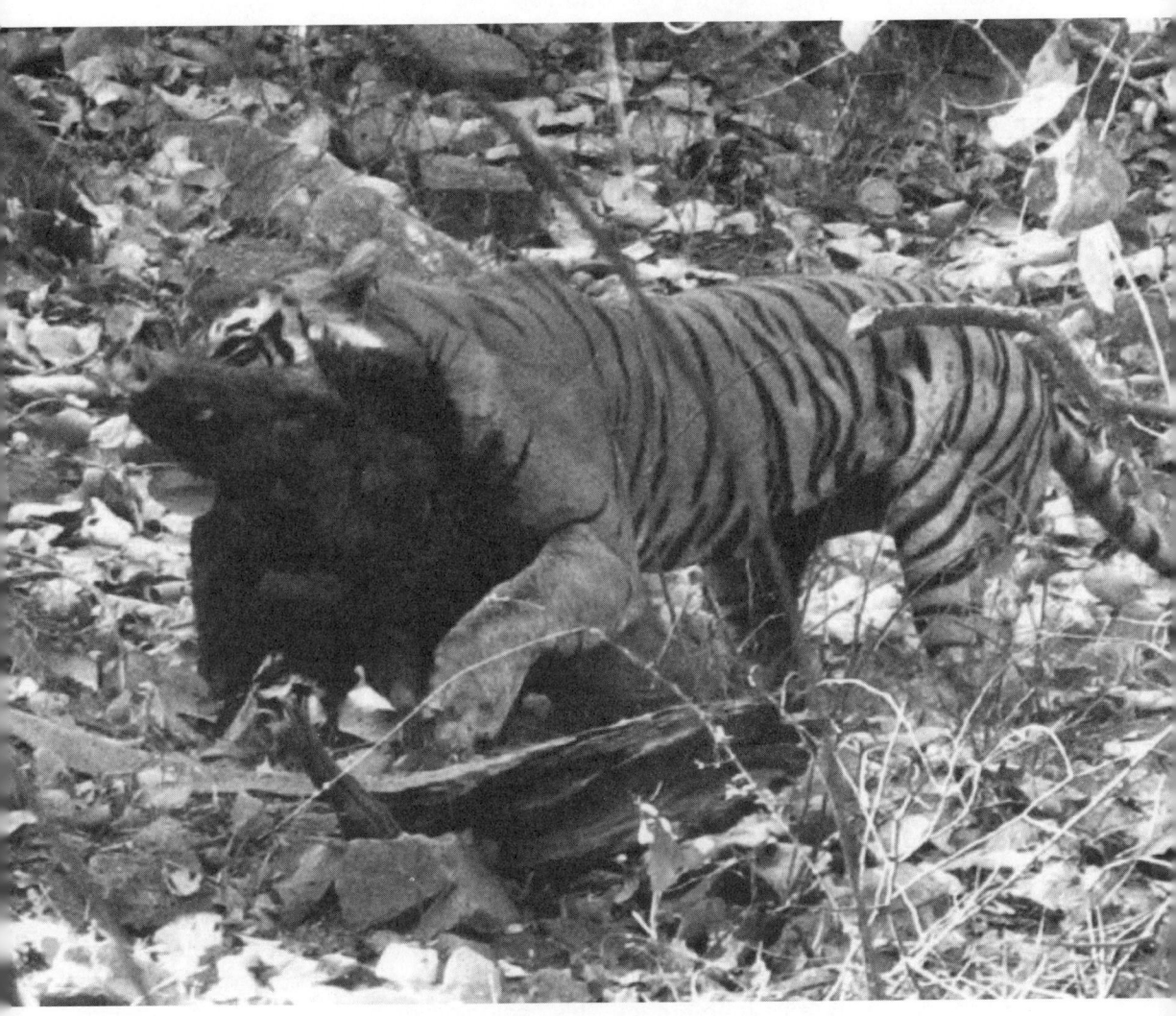

CHAPTER 7
THE KAANP TANDA MAN-EATER

Chapter 7

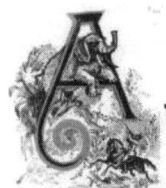

uthor's Note

Feeling no need for false modesty, I can say that after an exhausting and hazardous search for tigers in Tarai farmlands, spanning forty years, I have come up with a new milestone in tiger research. On the basis of uncommon knowledge base installed in my brain which, in fact, is the result of the exploratory desire to understand farmland wildlife. Academic at best, this book, (as what it entails is microscopic in nature) is also written to address my self-perceived intellectual need of revisiting the phenomenon of man-eating, which still continues living in nature's secret nature as its inner essence. The new light of modern ethology tells us that predators are not instinct-driven androids as presented in hunting literature of British Empire but are complex beings that need not be sequestered to a limited set of prototypes.

Authors from the past explained man-eating only as an act of a deformed animal incapable of hunting and thus unnatural. However, differing with them, I strongly feel that a new interpretation for causes of continuing man-eating is badly required. Hence I have attempted to provide an alternative picture by putting animals in a set of circumstances that may lead them to man-eating without moving away from natural flow.

Tiger being a symbol of the apex of the biotic pyramid can feed on anything live. Nature has decided for more than one food chain in each eco-system of the earth just to maintain its balance.

Ecology is inter-relationship between abiotic (physical) elements and biotic organisms of the land. If an organism does not get its natural food then it may abandon the eco-system meaning thereby the native shifting out in search of natural food. Alternatively, it will derive its food from the second-option food chain – the natura-naturata or the other contents of the nature and thus will not leave. This means preying on God's First Creature is not an aberration or a rare event. It offers advantageous circumstances when necessities of survival determine instincts where more and more large cats might accept humans as a regular prey species and become compulsive man-eaters. This ecological demand of any large predator might be interpreted as an ecological crisis but in fact in natura-naturans, which is an active and vital process of nature, its real empirical definition is very difficult to arrive at.

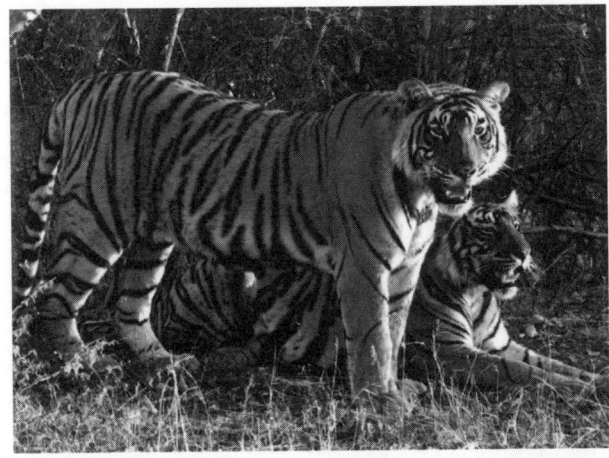

Tigers potentially become sexually mature at about three years of age, but they are not likely to breed untill they have established a range for themselves as residence, where they feel confident. *(Photo credit : Wildlife Conservation Trust)*

Man-eating does not belong to an era; it is just a natural phenomenon that will emerge in various circumstances. The country may be swarming with prey animals yet there are predators that deliberately come down to human neighbourhood and commence man-eating. There is no explanation.

The practice of early *shikaris* to consider all man-eaters as mangy brutes was rooted more in psychology than in reality. Perhaps humans still don't entertain the thought that they are food for a predator and any large carnivore would want them to eat for the very purpose. Unfortunately if anything like this happens, humans will be in a real precarious position for not even the plethora of other prey will prevent their deaths and there would be no explanation then whether it is the law of nature or the lawlessness of nature.

It is important to realize that just while you are reading this book, somewhere on the mindboggling expanses of Tarai, there are bound to be booby traps laid for a tiger and somewhere, the scourge called infernal man-eater is on the move; and I am inclined to believe it.

The Kaanp Tanda Man-Eater

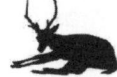

The Tiger Hurricane of Uttar Pradesh

"Carnivore management is as much a political challenge as a scientific one."
- K Ullas Karanth, Conservation Scientist

IN THE ANNALS OF U.P. WINTERS, THE PHASE FROM OCTOBER 2009 TO March 2010 would stand as unique forever, when far away from true jungles, no less than six tigers were reported at large in the rural landscape of six districts. A pair reported in Sitapur district (addressed as no 1 and 2) was perhaps a strayer from Katarnia Ghat sanctuary of Bahraich district. A single male tiger (no 3) was reported to be loitering at Ambedker Nagar, no one knew where he had come from. Another (no 4) was operating in Azamgarh district, probably a strayer from Valmiki wildlife sanctuary of Bihar. A young magnificent tigress (no 5) had arrived on the outskirts of Lucknow city. It was believed to be a strayer from Madhavtanda jungles of Pilibhit district. The last tiger (no 6) was an established man killer. Creating gore and mayhem in the sugar fields of Lakhimpur Kheri district, the audacious beast having eaten four people, had come to be known as the man-eater of Kaanp Tanda.

The conservationist community was aghast and the Forest Department was least equipped to deal with the problem of this magnitude that had so abruptly and simultaneously erupted in so many districts. In fact it was a crisis of sorts with an acute shortage of competent field staff. Their poor infrastructure with no experienced team leader, no solid operation strategies, no tools like tiger roar CDs or even tiger dummies, lack of proper cages (as most of cages were small in size and fit only for leopards), lack of reliable knowledge about tiger biology and so on made it worse. They had just three dart guns and inept marksmen who bungled even at point blank range. There was only one technically qualified darter who was a zoo vet by profession and who couldn't be everywhere to save the flagship species. He was rather in a fix as to from where he should to start and waiting for the marching orders to arrive.

The case of tigress no 5 that had started from Pilibhit, crossed through Shajahanpur, Lakhimpur Kheri, Sitapur, Lucknow, Barabanki and reached Faizabad district, had been completely mishandled. Since the tigress had strayed, it had been constantly on the run. Alarmed by the continual pursuit and disturbance, the 350-pound predator had killed four human beings accidentally, presumably in reflexive defense action. Despite being driven by hunger she did not accept them as food, and left the entire carcasses uneaten. Every day she journeyed some 20 to 30 kilometers across open fields through an area which had no wild prey and where a conflict with human interest was inevitable.

There are certain parameters an aberrant tiger has to qualify before being declared a man-eater. Circumstantial evidence suggested that this tigress had not degenerated into a man-eater; it had rather avoided many confrontations and adjusted to human malpractice. Yet, shoot at sight orders were issued. The short-sighted pretext was that it had become dangerous for humans.

The conservation buffs were stunned by the emergency of order. Articles appeared in press questioning the decision and several rescue schemes were suggested. A city conservationist remarked in a newspaper that "the way problem is handled it seems that the job has been given over to municipality and the 'Safai Karmcharis' have failed to catch the smart dog. Hence the orders are given to shoot the dog and soon others may also follow."

What ensued next was a chaotic phase in the state's wildlife. The newspapers followed the developments on day-to-day basis, analysing the events and making many a bad manager and poor masters a 'hero'. Photographs of conventional DFO sahibs with a sun cap and a rifle in hands were published that looked momentarily worth watching. A bizarre scenario ensued whereby, lured by an interesting stroke of fate, I too had become a part of it for some time. My intention was to renew my engagement with wild tigers, trying to control chaos, trying to bring things in order.

❖

The telephone bell chimed. Uma Shanker Singh, the then Field Director of Dudhwa National Park was on the line. "Rahul, I have just finished reading your book – Tiger! Your faith in old timer's credo – the will to face dangerous challenge with caution and fearlessness and use of rifle with deadly effect – are the great merits I come across in you without a doubt," he said on the phone line and waited to get my reply.

"You have many boosters up your sleeves, buddy; that make my day, anything special?" I asked.

"Yes, very special. A tiger has turned man-eater here. I want you to tackle it immediately. We need men like you who can stand up to this moment of challenge without blinking as we go after the man-eater."

"You need to gauge me carefully. I don't like close encounters with man-eaters. Anyway I am coming," I said and hung up.

Uma Shanker, tall, fair and ruggedly handsome, had a contention that aberrant tigers should not be destroyed out of hand. They should better be caught alive and be transferred to some more suitable area so that they may have another chance to live normally. The result was that the director had invited me to his area where killings had suddenly erupted.

In contrast to my city routine as a teacher, where my movements are regular and cyclical, the schedule of my tiger enterprise had always been random. However, presently it was a doleful phase, where due to overriding urgencies to solve some pending problems, my wildlife expeditions had virtually come to a halt. But a desire for adventure was very much there. For me losing contact with tiger is analogous to a Buddhist monk who has lost his contact with Nirvana.

Knowing that man-eating tigers don't get sorted out in a day or two I applied for a long leave from the college, packed up and the next day, I was off into the ominous pocket of terror to pitch in for the hunt of the errant animal.

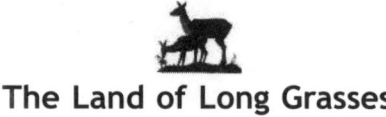

The Land of Long Grasses

Here I am, where I ought to be, because here I belong...

- Karen Blixen

January 10, 2009 was a cold, bleak and biting day. I stood on the rising escarpment of the Kishanpur sanctuary where the vast banks of Sharda river lay sprawled before me. The mist was floating in its forlornness over the land, choking the road that lay before me. The darkness and the deep silence of the place were very solemn as death had been hovering there with abandon.

A strange sensation surged into my veins spreading the warmth of endearment to enchanting pictures around. This very lonely area of South Kheri still retains the effervescence of the past. Here one can see the vast complex tracts of sugar grasslands stretching till the end of the horizon with endless monotony. For untold millions of years, the huge lowland savannah has been a paradise for deer and wild boar and therefore a favorite hunting ground of tigers.

This had been my boyhood playground. The very feeling that I owned this savannah, not materially but emotionally was still heavy on me, for I had come to possess its every *nala* and water pond, every anthill and burrow and every broken and dead tree in my heart. From 1996 to 2003 I had served as honorary wildlife warden for this Sanctuary, having a tempestuous time. I had acquired the reputation of being a fairly average Joe in confronting poachers, patrolling and responding to calls of natives against potentially aberrant animals, hence the confidence of foresters in me was prompted by their experience with me. I was not only familiar with the terrain but I felt I could interpret its moods and vagaries, predict its winds and seasons.

Far off a small herd of swamp deer splashed in the river. Behind the deer, a flock of marabout storks paced up and down on grotesque skeleton legs. Their bodies looked like hunched undertakers with their hands behind their backs.

The huge tract, distending before my eyes, was the territory of a young and lusty tiger, which had no alleged inability to subdue a virile prey yet it deliberately sought humans as food. It had taken refuge in 10,000-acre expanse of sugarcane, cultivated illegally on the river bed. Here it had killed and consumed four cane-strippers; all from a single village of north Kaanp-Tanda.

For many years the great carnivores had lived quietly and peaceably close to the village paths and the line of huts, undisturbed by the villagers and domestic animals. Yet, they sought their meat from nature. It was a world as ancient as time but as new as human foundations had made it; an agrarian landscape was as much a tiger land as it was of my race.

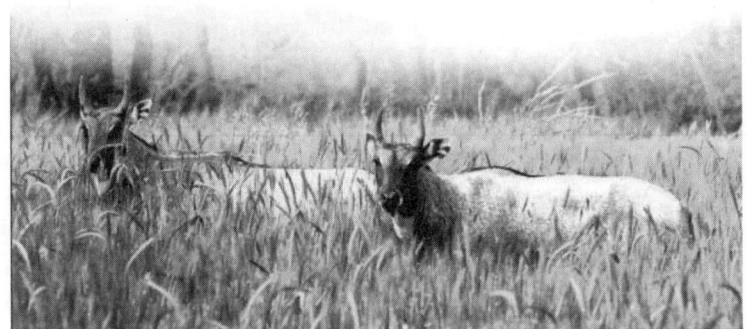

Nilgai is a great ungainly animal somewhat horse like in built, with high withers and low rump. In many parets of India they enjoy complete immunity, being regarded as a near relative of the cow and therefore sacred.

❖

The peaceful settlement of Kaanp Tanda was little-known to people prior to the advent of the man-eater. This juvenile tiger was possibly a little over three years old and had started his dreadful but short career on January 5, 2009 by killing a boy stripping canes in a field. The boy named Pinto was smashed to the ground as the great cat pounced upon him, pinning him with his steel-sinewed body and weight of 300 pounds, the way a bull terrier demolishes a rabbit.

As the news of the incident reached the village, its chief Ishwar Chand organized a group of men to recover the victim's body. The killer had dragged the boy inside a cane pocket and was eating it at leisure when the rescue party arrived. The tiger came out, issuing warning growls. His appetite whetted by what he had eaten, he then crept into a reed-filled ravine across a stream, from where he growled constantly, voicing his objection to the interference in his feeding routine. By the time the case was reported and forest guards arrived darkness had fallen and they fired a volley of shots in the area but were unable to find the carcass. Next morning the body of the boy was recovered and it was a horrid sight.

Uma Shanker told me that the tiger seemed to have initially hesitated at the unfamiliar carcass which it had got by accident but the smell of blood and predatory hunger proved sufficient inducement for the animal as he tasted his first human meal. The quantity of flesh eaten from the body was hardly some 20 pounds, which was just a small snack for a tiger.

"But now I have no doubt about the tiger's motive. His last two assaults are calculated and intentional, which means he has learnt about human vulnerability," said the director worried, "acquaintance has generated condescension."

In man-eating cases, generally the first human kill is largely a result of mistaken identity and the reluctance of the predator naturally applies to its eating out. Moreover, tigers are puzzled as to where to begin on a human body, because human contour is unfamiliar to them. They often abandon the carcass or encouraged by hunger and smell of blood, which is a sufficient stimulus for a meal they just make a snack of its projected parts, like genitals in a man or breasts in women. Later depending on the degree of duress, this acquaintance generates disrespect and man is included in the prolific prey species available.

❖

Although there were many qualified trackers in Kaanp Tanda who were ready to help me follow the tiger but my first preference was always for my old companions, so I decided to seek help from them. Unfortunately Chhotey and Phagunia were no more but old hands like Neta, Bajjaney, Dilli, Shripal and Joginder were still around. All these men – the last embers of my boyhood crew, my half brothers – were the stalwarts of tiger trail and the best companions for any challenging venture. I had learnt to tread the dark, cool *sal* forests with them, learning the ways of its inhabitants. This company was sure to make a world of difference for me while I looked for the master predator.

Larti was only 15 kilometers from Kaanp Tanda as the crow flies. A wireless message was flashed from the D.D. office to Mailani Range. The ranger officer personally went to Larti to convey the message and towards late evening my men arrived on the troubled turf riding on their bicycles. Now well above fifty and sixty years in age they were still full of bonhomie and energy. It had been more than two years since we had met last and many years since we had seriously gone after tigers together.

I told them about my plans for next few weeks and they all agreed to drop everything important in favour of this operation.

A recent hailstorm had caused much damage in the area and the village itself was a sad tumbled-down affair. We were given a two-room building of an abandoned dispensary where my crew seemed quite pleased to make their headquarters. They cleaned the place and immediately unloaded their stores on its ramshackle verandah. Dilli is a competent housekeeper. He set pressure lamps and folded table ready for the evening and kept my night-vision and binoculars, my rifles, Jeffrey .400 HV double, made by Thomas Bland & Sons and .416 magazine by Rigby that had tiger teeth marks on its barrel, which my men had brought from Larti for use in the hunt, were safely placed in a corner.

It was already afternoon, we surveyed the sugarcane fields where bated cages were put into various plots. On a narrow footpath we came across a day old spoor of the man-eater. Nose to the ground, he had deftly traced the path of a wild boar, picking up its spoors as surely as a blind man reads Braille. As my men gazed at them, we felt the first real qualms about catching this beast. The spoors seemed to make our business a very different proposition from the way it had appeared to us earlier. Neta looked at spoor intensely, "*Bhiyaa, yeh sher acchha bum katega, taiyar rahana hai.* (This tiger will offer a good battle, we must keep ready)," said he as he guessed the size of the animal to be a little over 8 feet and its weight around 300 pounds.

Old hunters, incidentally, used to measure tiger forepaws, specifically the relatively narrow heel, which is called *gohna* in Tarai and which the Russian biologists of Taiga call *pyatka*. The value of *pyatka* measurement lies in its uniformity, for physiologically, it is constituted of a single heavy pad so it won't stretch or clinch from step to step and thus leaves the most profound and clear impression. A large Tarai female will have a *gohna* size from two and a half inches up to three and a half inches across the back of the heel while males will start from three and can go as high as four to five inches. Five inches onwards is, at least by standards of Tarai tiger data, a giant.

The fact is that when you pick up a rifle and take the first step against a fast deadly animal you are aware that you are taking a fair chance of being damaged or even killed.

A marsh harrier called, a lone voice in the stillness, proclaiming its territory. We returned as the darkness shrouded the landscape. Foresters R.C. Jha and KK Singh, both DFOs holding charge of North and South Kheri forest divisions arrived in my camp. They introduced me to a ranger named Om Prakash who was to associate with this hunt. Om Prakash was a fine, courageous and essentially simple man who later proved a great asset to me. We sat around in chairs, more wood was added to the fire, and for the rest of the evening, there was but one topic of conversation — the man-eater.

The sight of sport arms had brought some peace of mind to the villagers. They felt certain that soon they will celebrate the demise of their arch enemy. Singh whispered in my ears, "we are being blamed for not taking serious steps to destroy the man-eater. It is difficult to convince these men that we need to protect even those tigers that have developed a proclivity for humans. These are important animals." Besides snaring, trapping and lethal control have been the traditional methods of conflict mitigation but the idea of saving this tiger was unpalatable for many.

Vigilance teams were raised to patrol the village periphery in the night. People agreed to keep a look out for the tiger but for a financial consideration. Their belief that every villager is essentially a labourer and is worthy of being hired is very firm. It left me wondering about native psychology. They were living on a man-eater's turf, ever exposed to his violence but we could not preserve their miserable lives without being expected to pay them handsomely. They will allow themselves to be eaten but 'no pay, no work' was stiff policy. The payment mode was decided through National Rural Employment Guarantee Act (NREGA), including an additional one hundred rupees by the Forest Department.

I did not think the man-eater would kill again that night as it had feasted on a big-sized pig the night before. Still my men knew of cases where tigers having had substantial meal went killing as frequently as twice or thrice the same night. This surplus killing is even followed by man-eaters. It recalls me of a single pride of

Najombe lions in Tanzania that between 1932 and 1947 killed approximately 1500 people till it was exterminated by George Rusheby. In his book "No more Tuskers", George records the pride to have killed an entire group of twenty travelers within a 200 meter area. They ate a few and left the rest showcasing a collectivity of feline mayhem. Though such cases are extremely rare but I asked my men not to ask me to reflect my bookish knowledge at such unfortunate times; for it worries people unnecessarily, making their mind play with wanton unconfined.

Finally when the foresters had gone, I kept my Jeffery .400 HV-2 double under the mattresses, thinking that my solitary parking place could not be deemed as safest because man-eaters have an uncanny way of showing up at the least expected places. At such times, a powerful firearm is very comforting thing to have under your pillow in case the killer chose to strike yet again in the night.

I was tired and sleepy, listening to the background music of nocturnal birds, punctuated by a flurry of jackal calls rising from the sugar vistas. I soon dropped off into deep sleep and dreamed of the gory predator, while local watchmen patrolled our camp and four of Colman's pressure lamps burned with roar to light their way.

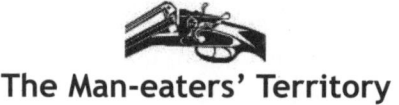

The Man-eaters' Territory

The more diverse the food of the animal the more developed his intelligence is..
- Sergei Sokolov

The next day, long before the sun was above the horizon, I awoke to the misty flights of parakeets and was surprised to see two hog deer standing near the dispensary. I watched enthralled as they suddenly galloped at incredible speed, crossed the fields and jumping down the knoll like steeplechasers plunged into the sugar cane fields.

During the night Ishwsr Chand's pet bitch had made way into my quilt with her two puppies and lay across my feet with a puppy on each side of me. I did not drive her away. I came out carefully, covered the puppies with my quilt and called Neta for the morning tea.

The boy Pinto's death had created panic in the area and as a result the ludicrous exercise of find-and-kill had been initiated. A number of forest guards and armed guards from adjoining districts had been called upon the scene, enlisted as trackers and asked to monitor the tiger's movements. Four Jeeps and more than 10 tractor trolleys had been pushed into service. There were ACFs, SDOs and no less than six rangers and 20 deputy rangers, all on their tenterhooks and fluttering in various stages of excitement and frustration. Overnight, the village had been transformed into a quasi-military settlement.

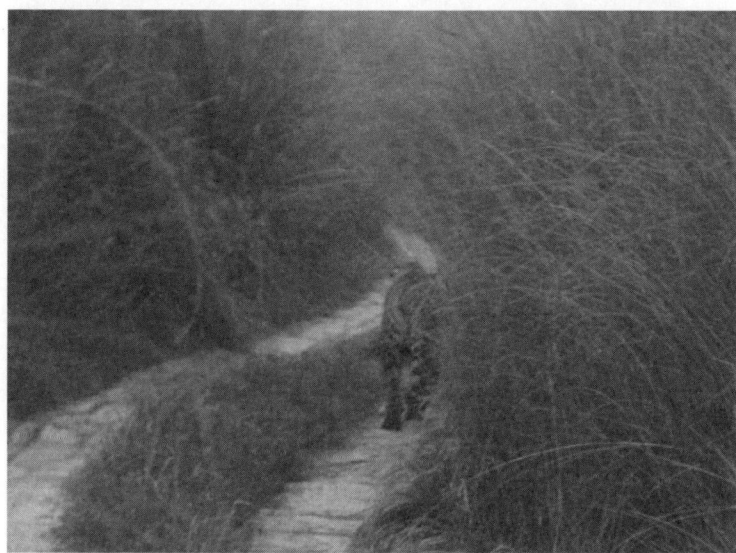

There were no less than three tallied tigers living within and around man-eaters operational area that were occasionally encountered by trackers.

Examining the record of three kills I found that the tiger had not used any special method to kill his victims as they do with standard prey in order to break their neck. Given that a young tiger weighs some 150 to 180 kilograms and is many times stronger than a WWF prizefighter, their ultra-fast reflexes are devastating. The corpses of victims carried evidence as how man-eaters behave in killing humans whom they carry off as easily as a cat takes mouse or a dog carries a squirrel. Tigers are obligate killers of prey in the 20 to 600 kilogram body mass category and for all practical purposes a 70-kg man in the jaws of a tiger is almost like a weightless rag-doll. When a tiger catches a man trying to run away, it clutches him and a full bite in this clutch anywhere on the human body, save hand and legs, is enough to kill the victim within minutes.

Though the force of a tiger's forepaw strike has never been measured but it is a great instrument of destruction. Brander cites a case in which a tiger had driven a man's skull with a blow from his paw delivered on the top of his head. Many years ago, I had examined the carcass of Dubar, Ram Adhin and Tauley, killed by the Katna man-eating tigress and Sarju Jatav of Sitarganj, their necks were completely broken by the stroke of the tiger's barbed sledge of paw and their heads loosely hung to the body. The last victim of Kaanp Tanda, Rinku had been killed the same way.

The man-eater's operational area covered some nine hamlets and three villages namely Uttar Tanda, Dakshin Tanda and Maharajnagar. Instead of directly embarking upon the hunt, as the old-timers did, I felt it proper to first counsel the villagers with an awareness campaign as to how they could protect themselves from becoming a victim. The very thought of wildlife preservation did not seem to hold any charm for many and there were practically no apostles of this new faith. The presence of carnivores does threaten human existence, as in general animal husbandry and agricultural practices affect vulnerability to predators.

There are six situations when man is likely to fall victim: Coming between tiger and its fresh kill, inadvertently surprising a tiger; coming between tigress and cubs where she is compelled to adopt a protective attitude; squatting or crouching for long time; encountering an injured tiger; and provoking a tiger unnecessarily. Awareness of these situations was badly needed to reduce risk to the villagers.

I had brought along the pamphlets of *'Saving Men from Tigers'* campaign which mentioned practical guidance for countering man-tiger conflict. Based on real world lessons that help enhance understanding of the predators' behavior ecology; these rules of self-protection drew upon collected empirical knowledge. When exercised by public with care, these measures augment the public's positive involvement in wildlife protection management.

I held a brief meeting of locals and gave them hundreds of these pamphlets along with fire-crackers with instructions that these were not to be boomed for pleasure-seeking but were to be used only in emergency moments.

(These non-lethal, aversive techniques for preventing predatory attacks are preliminary.

'Show No Fear' was the introductory foundation of the campaign followed by:

'Do not plough your field alone'

'Move in groups'

'Keep to the main roads'

'Talk loudly'

'Wear colourful clothes'

'Some people should always stand on guard with labours who work in the field'

'Do not sit on haunches for long hours' (A tiger may mistake people for a quadruped as the silhouette of a hunched over man from a short distance looks surprisingly like a browsing deer)

'Take a dog along'. Even if it does not possess enough courage to bark at the tiger its behaviour will forewarn of the big cat's presence or in the event of attack tiger will prefer it to a man

'While moving alone beat an empty tin can or rattle stones in it'

'Play a transistor'

'Play songs loudly on your mobile'

'Guard your cattle by erecting a thorned fence around.'

One more important method is to 'Wear a mask behind your head.' The backward facing masks are expected to deter tigers, which are behaviourly attuned to avoid frontal attacks on prey, this situation specific innovation developed by a forester of Bengal, some Sanyal when put to test in Sunderbans is claimed to have been effective in mitigating man-tiger conflict)

To intensify the operation, at least one vigilance team of ten members was formed in all the villages. Their work was to keep watch over fields, collect information about the place where the tiger was sighted most recently, and apprise the villagers. With spears and guns, they were to patrol the borders of their village in the night, with special alertness between dusk and dawn. If there was a slightest suspicion of the tiger, they were to beat tin cans, fire crackers and shout at the top of their voices, warning the villagers. This constant night watch was the most tiring task but the men accepted it as their foremost duty.

An old man told me that a regular ring of man-eater's footmarks was found around his isolated settlement and it had not made any kill for last five days. "This tiger is seemingly working with calculated audacity," said the man fearing the consequences.

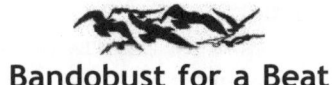

Bandobust for a Beat

"If you rile a tiger, he's going to show his claws."
— Rob James-Collier

The man-eater was a concessionaire of about 100 square miles of human-controlled terrain as his hunting ground. Every morning, two qualified teams of foresters went scouting for the signs of tiger in all the directions, that could be anywhere in that great, 20,000-acre sugarcane plantation, including sandy embankments of Sharda. It was a gargantuan, sometimes most exasperating undertaking'. The jeeps carried the parties to places where the trackers got down combing the ground, with the vehicles following slowly.

As soon any spoors or kill was found the news was flashed to camp and then the capture team would move with all the paraphernalia. Generally the place would be five to six miles away and most of the kills would not turn up to be of much importance to us except to reaffirm the fact that there were no less than two other ordinary tigers operating in the area.

During night we prowled along the edge of huts; backward and forwards along the different paths leading to the village in the hope that if the man-eater was anywhere around we might contact him. The vehicle moved along slowly and its every occupant intensely scanned the edge of sugarcane forest. The night jars and owls went around their business. We made brief halts at focal points of water ponds and glades and found scattered animals sitting, drinking or grazing but no tiger eyes reflected the spotlights.

A stern chase of a wild animal is always likely to become a long-drawn affair. You spend more time on the trail when there is no blood trail to follow. A week later on an afternoon, Neta struck upon the fresh spoors of tiger in a mustard field. The tracks were superimposed on the tracks of a wild boar that had gone in a sugarcane plot, with the predator following it. There is always something exciting about coming on fresh spoor, no matter how much you have hunted. The sight of those imprints makes the jaw muscles tighten and chills run up your legs. The prospect of action lies ahead and that is always thrilling.

After an arduous going an hour, the tracks emerged into a big open plot. It was a special piece of land, some 10 acres in extent which had been cleared of entire agricultural yield and lay threadbare. Right across it was an isolated plot of dense sugarcane with a clear rain water channel flowing behind it called Sutia nala. Bordered with dense and shady reed grass, it was certainly a fine natural retreat for large predators. The spoors imprinted on the powdered earth didn't cross the plot meaning the tiger had finally discontinued its journey here to sleep off the effects of his protein packed meal.

This was our first real success, after days of uncertainty and frustration and we all knew what we were up to. Though tigers are heavy sleepers and may stay at a place for hours but owing to continuous pursuit man-eaters show exceptional powers of calculation and knowledge of human habits and keep changing places thoughtfully. Their ways are certainly different than those of normal tigers so much so that even I had begun to look at it as something special.

To avoid many alterations on our map, I asked my team to draw their notions on the sandy ground with a stick and then after usual discussion decided the course of the beat. The nets were brought on the scene and the trackers unrolled them to set them properly. The nets, far bigger than normal and made of tightly twisted *moonj* rope, were knotted to an eight inch mesh that measured 30 feet long and 6 feet high. These were a part of the historical legacy of Larti poachers. Many years ago at Lohangapur forest, I had witnessed a tiger and three deer caught in these nets and in the ensuing commotion, the tiger had not only killed all the deer but broke the ropes and escaped. *(See author's Tiger! Chapter 4, Way out Savannah)*

Now lying unused for decades the old ropes had been thoroughly repaired for the event.

In view of the dense sugarcane, where visibility was less than five yards, there was uncertainty as to where the tiger would choose to make his bid for freedom. And if trouble started it would be at such short range as to leave very little time to take suitable action.

It was certainly no easy undertaking. The whole art of beat lies in anticipating the probable line of retreat of the tiger and by judicious use of the stops on either side, bringing the animal up to a single point. Six nets were firmly extended on the ground and their ends tightly fastened to the trees. Shambhu collected cane leaves and grass, raised several heaped piles, making fire points that flanked the crop from both sides in two direct lines. These were to be ignited with the start of the beat to prevent tiger from diverging.

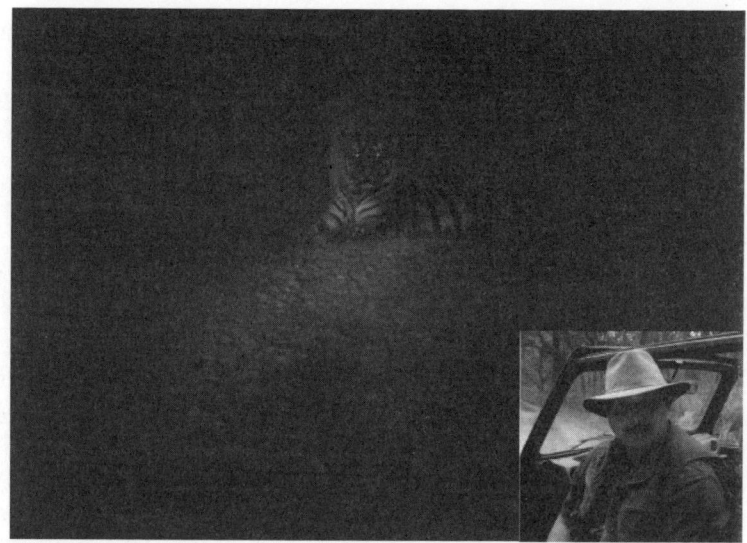

The beautiful beast kept staring at us, composed and tranquil, yet we knew he was a vicious killer. Says Sanjay Narain, a wildlife resort owner near Dudhwa who took this first photograph of Kaanp-Tanda Man eater. Inset the photographer

A probationer DFO watching the scene felt sick in his stomach. This operation had cast a purgative effect on him. Every few minutes he visited behind a tree with a score of armed guards around him who stood surrounding the tree and he relieved himself within a yard of them.

When he returned for the sixth time, he looked all haggard. His breath catching him in throat, he told me how insanely dangerous all this work was, in which a novitiate forester like him had been called upon to participate. The man had never seen a live tiger outside the zoo and admitted that the man-eater had had an unnerving effect upon him. I reminded him that I was a temporary leader and as the operation was under the orders of Forest Department, he was the authority here in absence of seniors. Hence regardless of any purgative or laxative effect of tigers upon him, he must bear that and stay like a solder till his last breath.

Since tigers don't climb straight trees I picked out a straight trunked Neem tree, where he could sit and command the operation. He went up the tree like a squirrel where his gut-wrenching amazingly stopped. He even took a guard's gun fancying he may likely have a hot time with it. I didn't want any inept marksman to bungle a shot in nervousness; I bade him to hand over the gun to the guard which he hesitantly did. Shripal presented him a thick stick telling that it will be useful if worse came to worst and the man-eater managed to come on the tree, the officer must give him something to chew.

After posting stops and arranging for the conduct of the beat I took my position at the top of an ant hill. I broke the action and checked the big Kynoch solids, slipping them back into the chambers with the peculiar metallic drainpipe sound that only a double barrel gun makes, when the beat started. The light conditions had already gone bad yet the natives and the forest guards keeping together with their packs of dogs, marched in a long column like a battalion of infantry supported by four tractors. The silencers had been detached from machines so that the sputtering sounds had magnified manifold.

Tarai is a drunken country that lives in a drunken state. The tractor drivers were high with local brew, their faces hot with alcoholic rubescence, while in view of man-eater's reputation beaters behaved timid, they advanced in irregular lines first and then bunched up into groups. The beat flushed out many jackals. A peacock with six feet of burnished tail glittering fuzzily in the glow of lighted fire, flew past on whirring wings, a pair of large brown fish owls rose giving ventriloquistic quivering *boom-O-boom*, sailing over us under a gibbous moon. A sloth bear also took to sprinting. Nets were quickly lifted for them to pass away, but no tiger came out.

I was surprised at the variety of animals that can be driven out of a single compact cover like sugarcane. They feel safe because of the density of closed environments where stillness and silence helps them avoid predation. Then suddenly a few growls were heard followed by a commotion that scattered the beaters in every direction.

The nets were stretched for some 30 yards along the sugar field and my crew behind them was wielding spears like ancient Stone Age hunters. This was the moment of greatest danger, but also the most likely opportunity to capture the man-eater that may land up in the nets during the confusion.

Beaters again bunched up on every side, enclosing the animal in an extensive sugar thicket. The tiger did not come out as expected; instead it issued some coughing roars that were soon drowned in the loud barking and wailing of dogs. It was a tense moment because the beaters had crowded together that prevented him from breaking out, and an accident resulting from the rush of the beast seemed imminent.

Finally the tiger chose to take his chance for freedom through the burning piles of dried grass. Regardless of high flames, he burst out galloping from the sugar plot, crossed a fallen tree, hurled himself tangentially into the air and like a greyhound clearing the hurdle, literally leaped his way out of danger. The treed DFO saw it broadside hitting the dirt some 30 yards away and thought that he was looking at a wild boar! By the time he perceived its stripes, the man-eater had already made up to Sutia Nala, where it disappeared in the brushy growth.

We had failed to anticipate this most improbable line of retreat. The tiger had evaded a death trap and my confident, experience-based knowledge of beats had literally been shattered at this point. Only circus tigers are known to perform such deeds with fire and that after being rigorously trained for a long time. By nature a tiger does not crosses a burning line and it works as an effective stop, bringing the animal up into the nets. My experienced men simply could not believe how easily and daringly he had made this manipulation.

Anyway, we had come with a firm determination to flush the tiger from its hideout. We ran further up the stream banks, hoping for another glimpse so that we could immediately conduct a reverse beat but it was too late and the odds seemed heavy against us; when the tiger was spotted again in a *narkul* patch.

Man-eaters and Man-tiger Conflict in Sugar Farms

Recovering human kills is a disgusting and insanely dangerous work

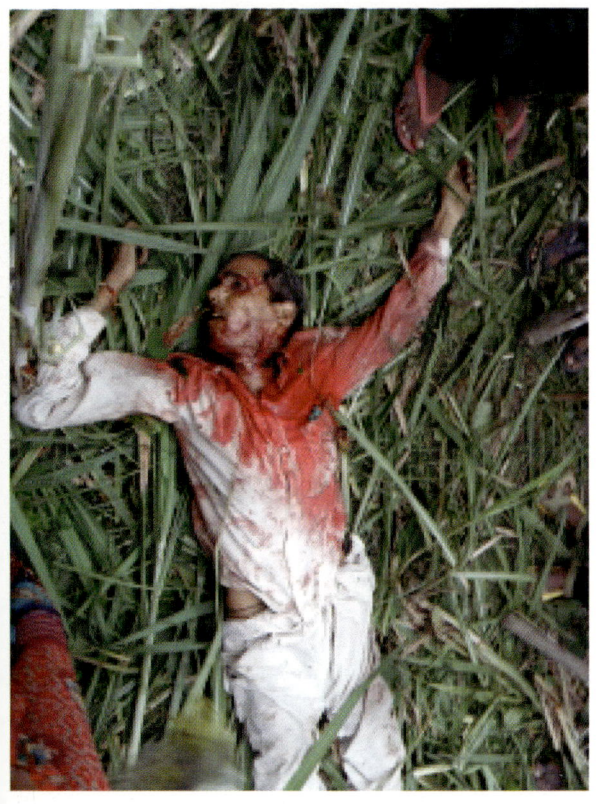

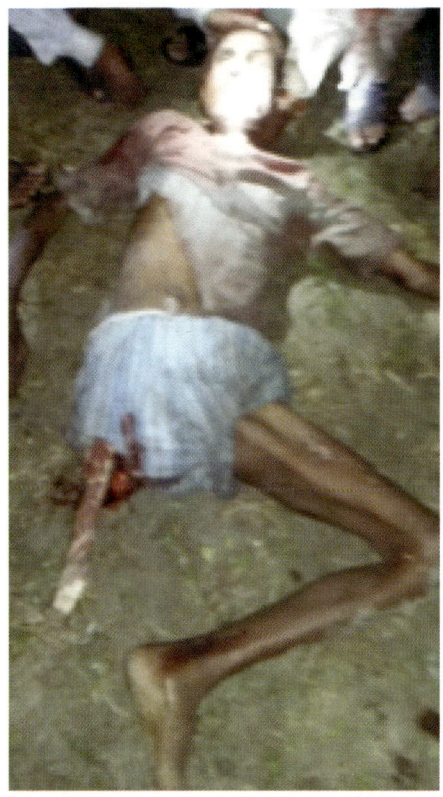

Janaki Prasad was quelled to ground by the Mailani man-eater, the way a Bull Terior holds a jucy bone.

The killer struck and dragged Tikaram inside sugarcane. He had finshed eating left leg when rescuers drove him away.

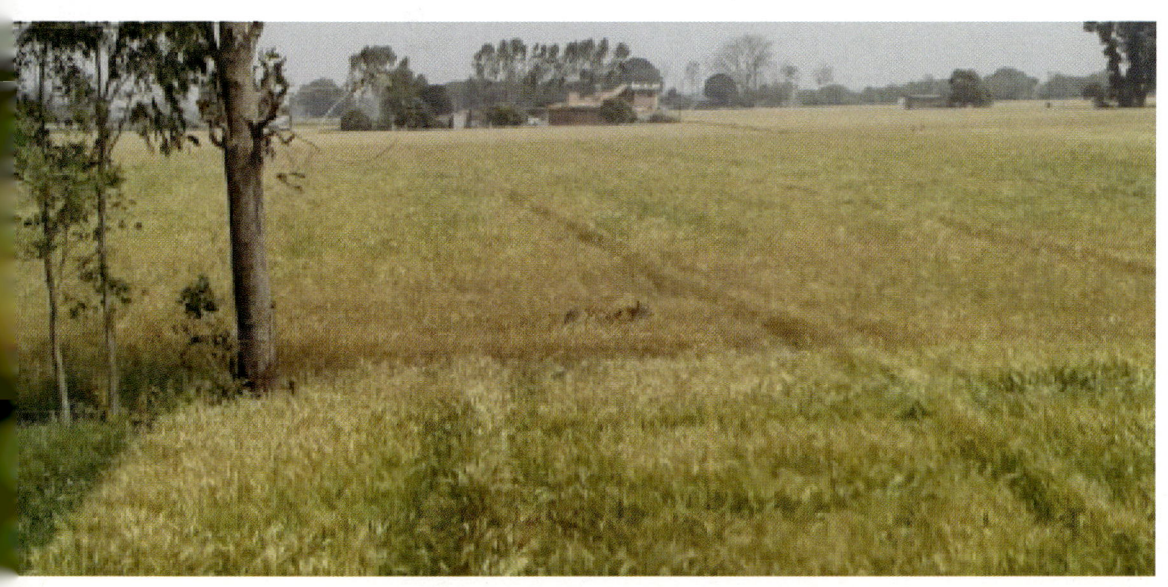

The Bankeyganj killer in a wheat field, April, 2016.

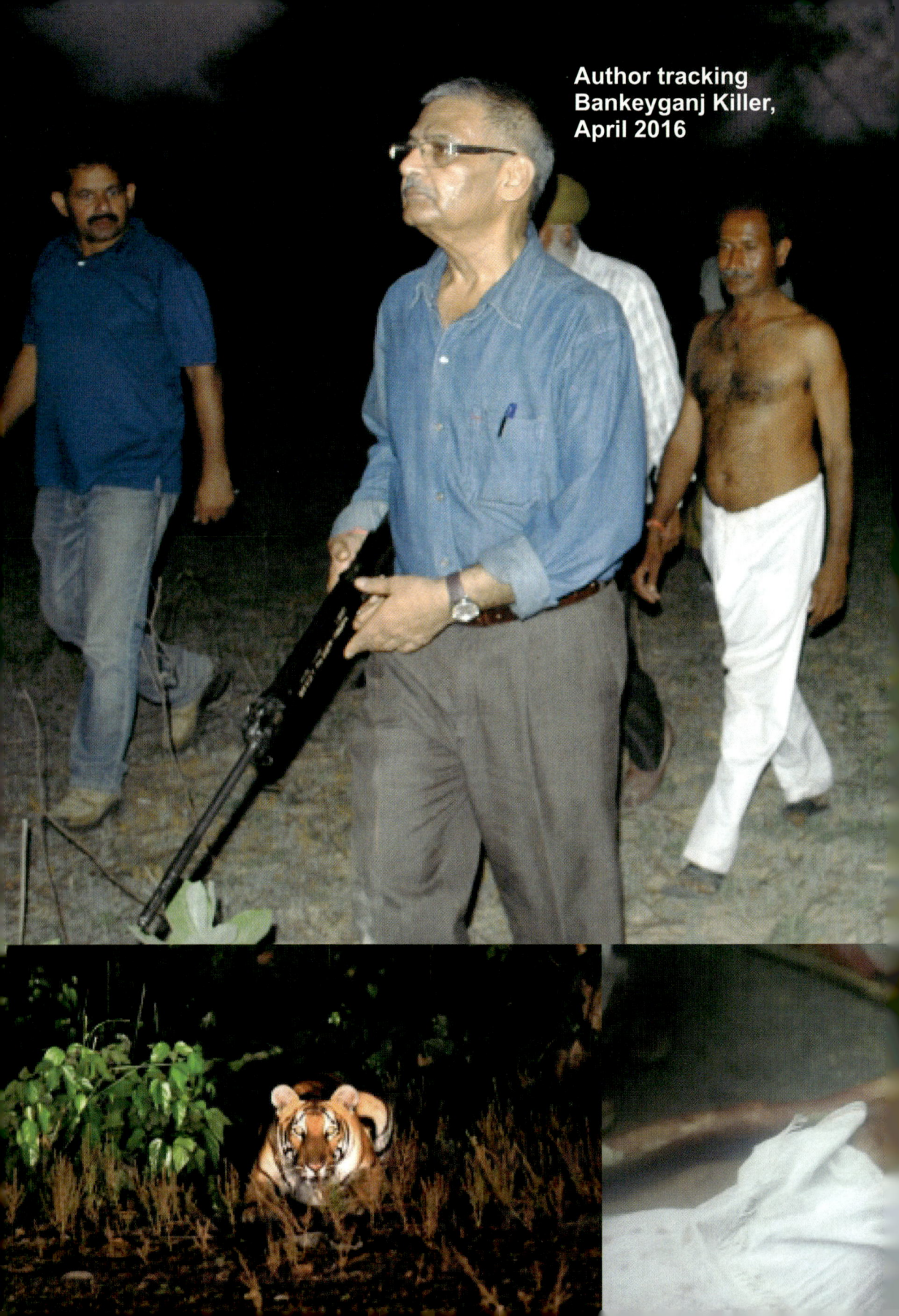

Author tracking Bankeyganj Killer, April 2016

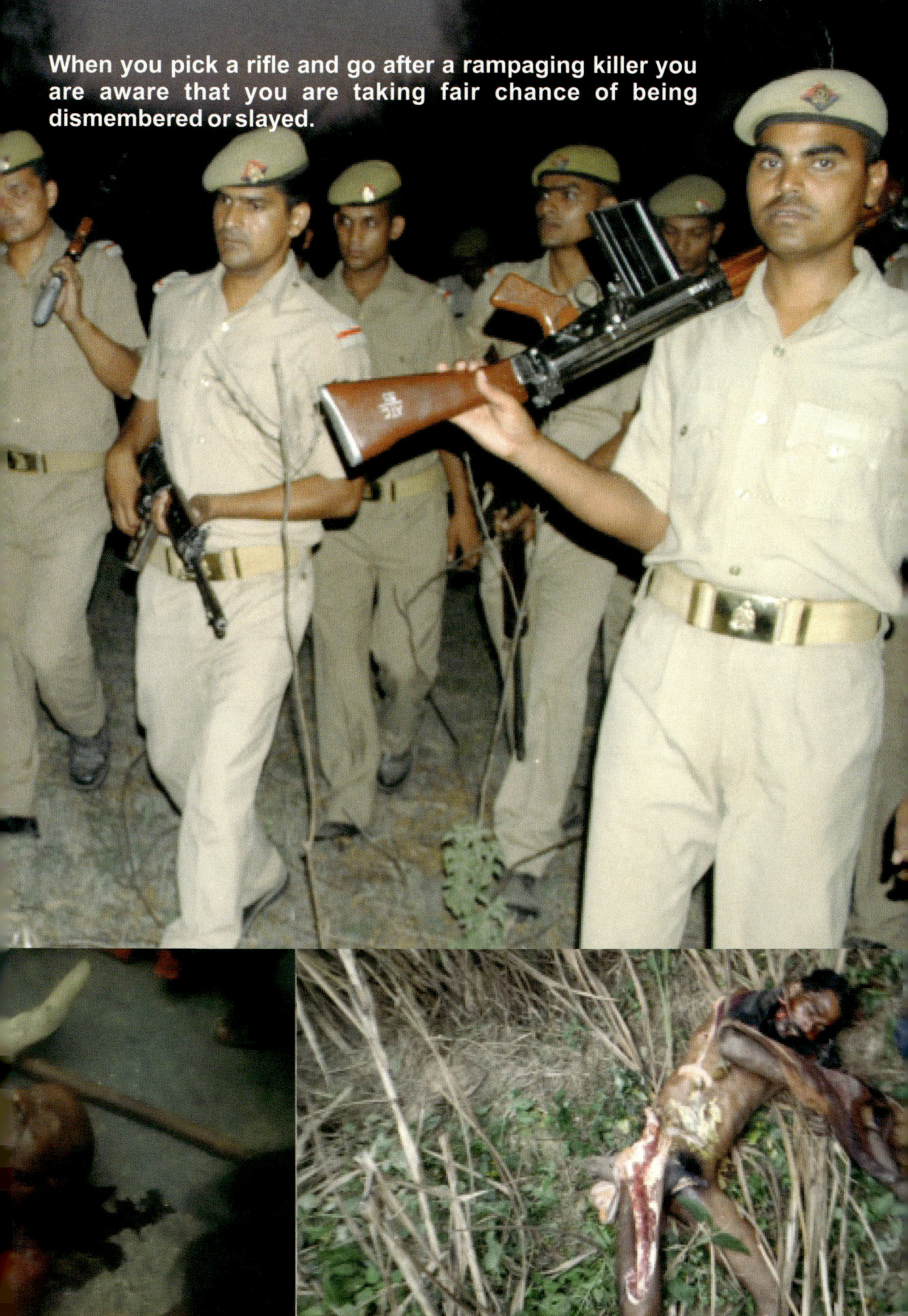

When you pick a rifle and go after a rampaging killer you are aware that you are taking fair chance of being dismembered or slayed.

The author during Moradabad man-eater operation.
Inset - Recovered human kills

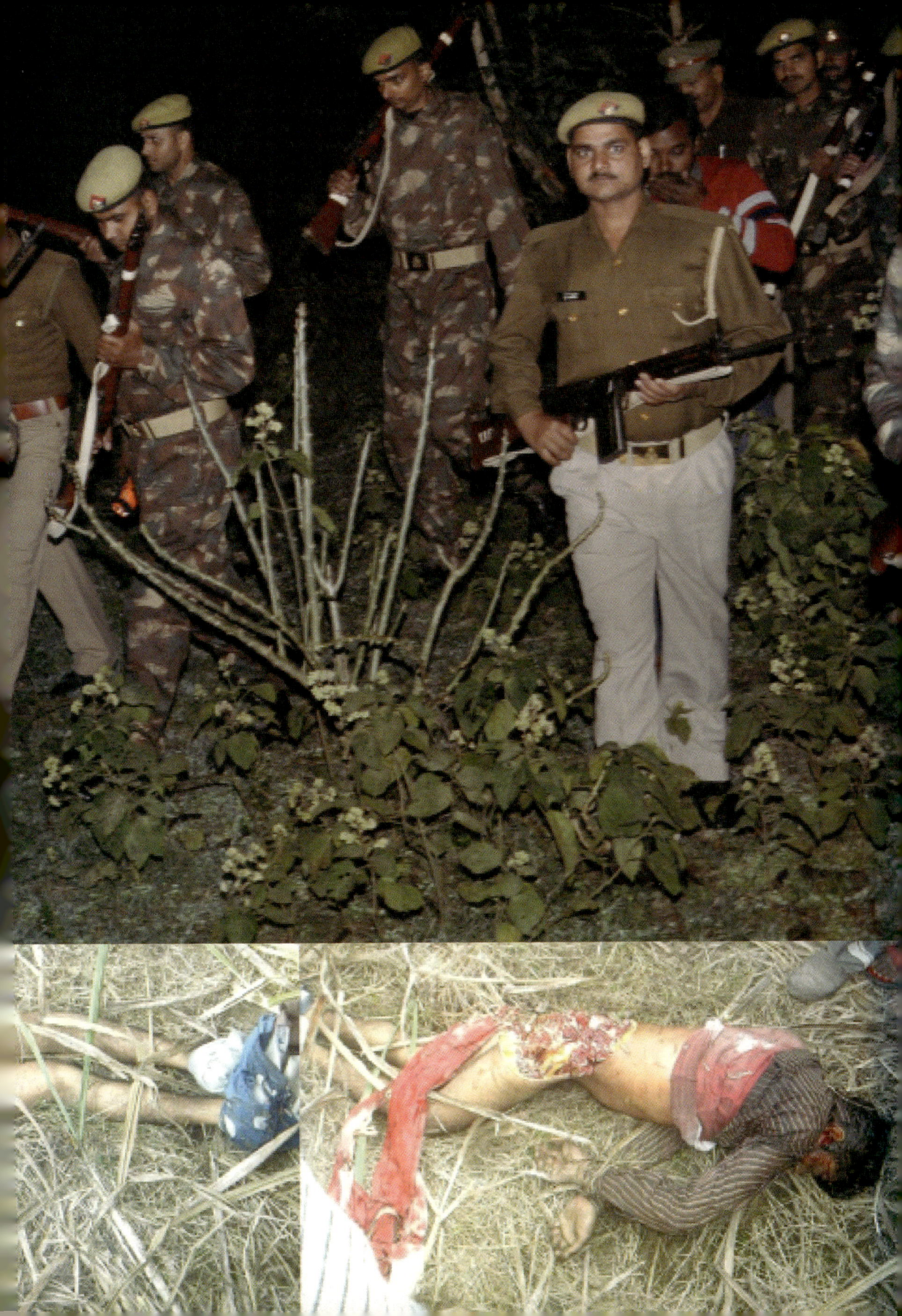

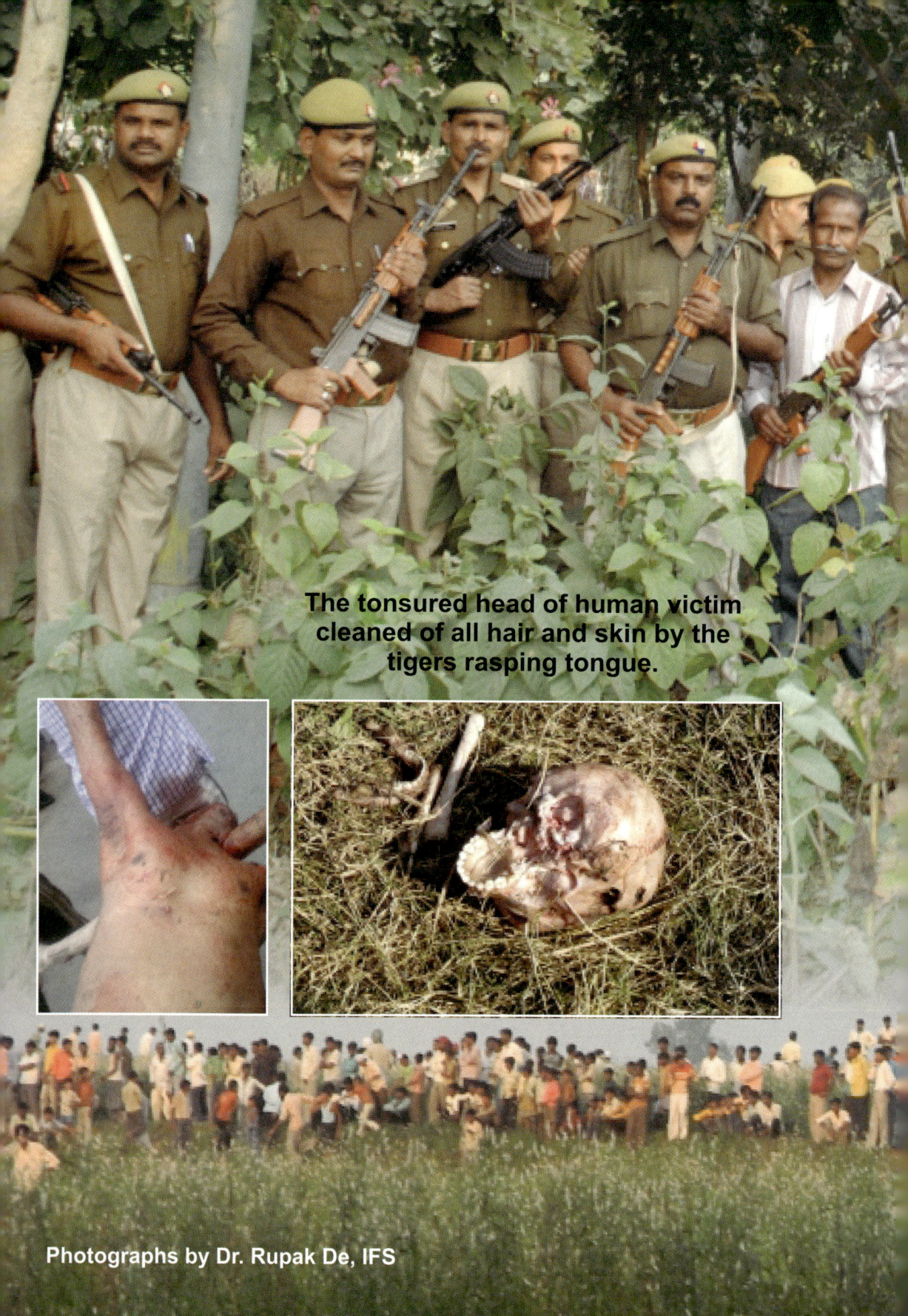

The tonsured head of human victim cleaned of all hair and skin by the tigers rasping tongue.

Photographs by Dr. Rupak De, IFS

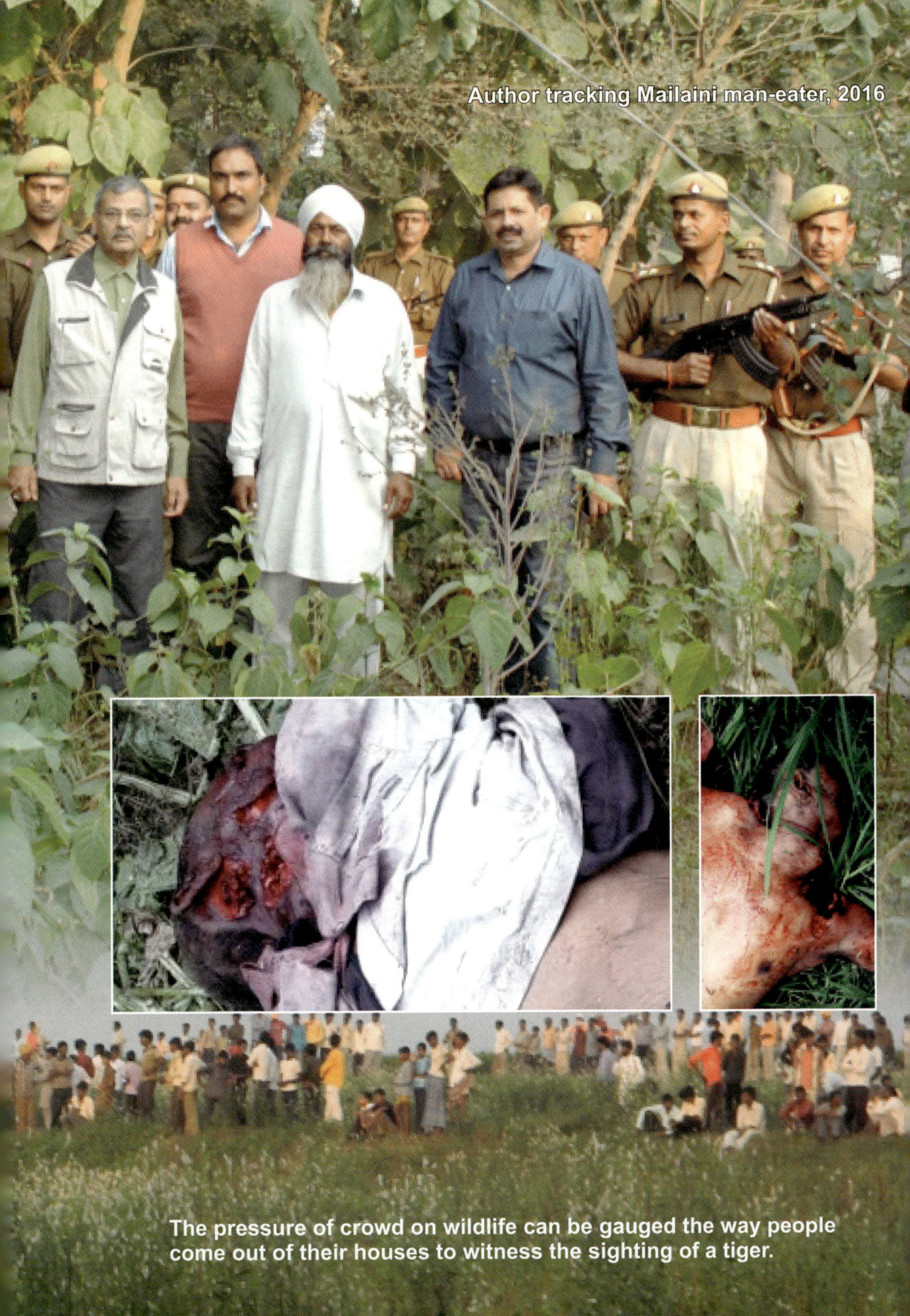

Author tracking Mailaini man-eater, 2016

The pressure of crowd on wildlife can be gauged the way people come out of their houses to witness the sighting of a tiger.

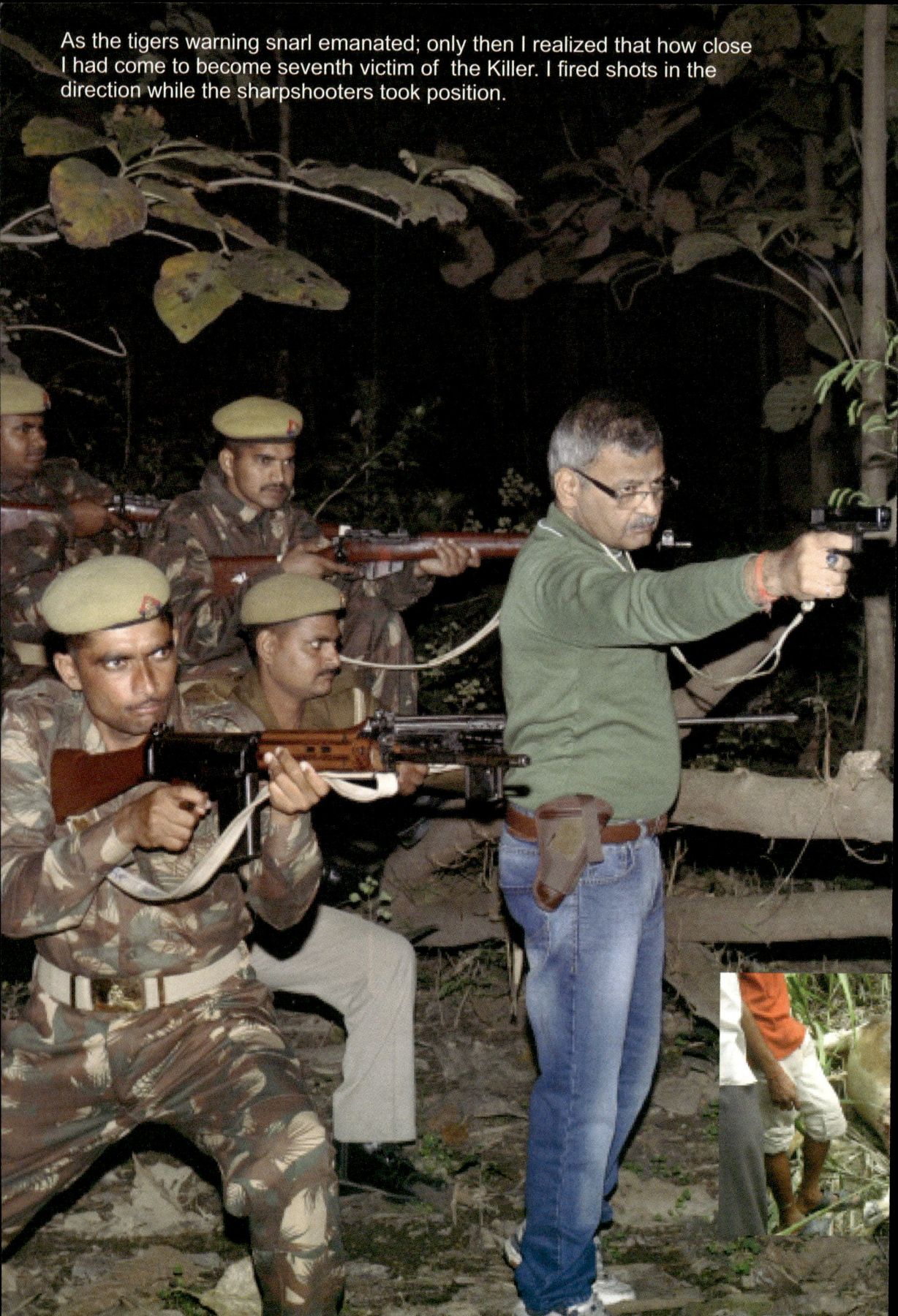

As the tigers warning snarl emanated; only then I realized that how close I had come to become seventh victim of the Killer. I fired shots in the direction while the sharpshooters took position.

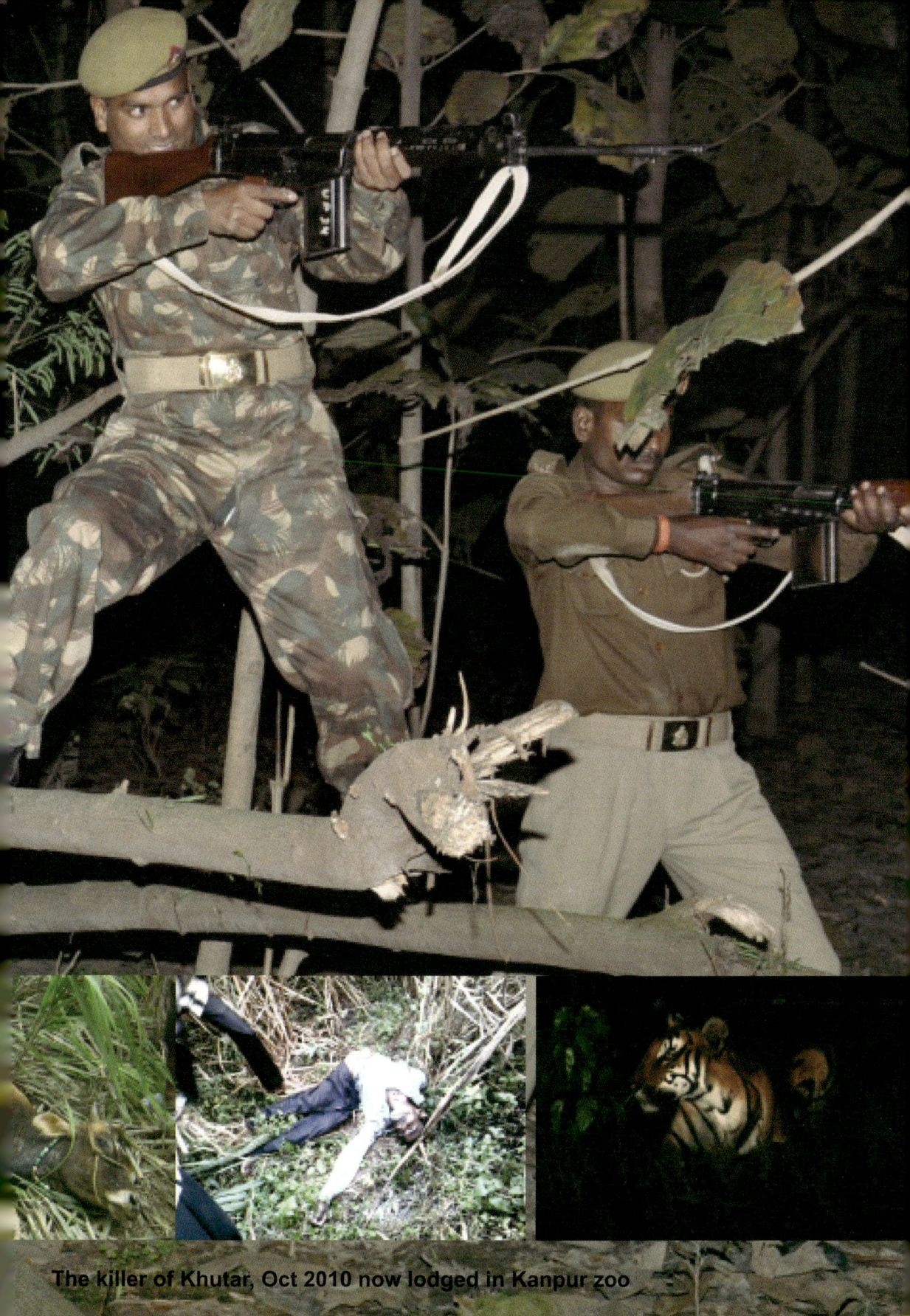

The killer of Khutar, Oct 2010 now lodged in Kanpur zoo

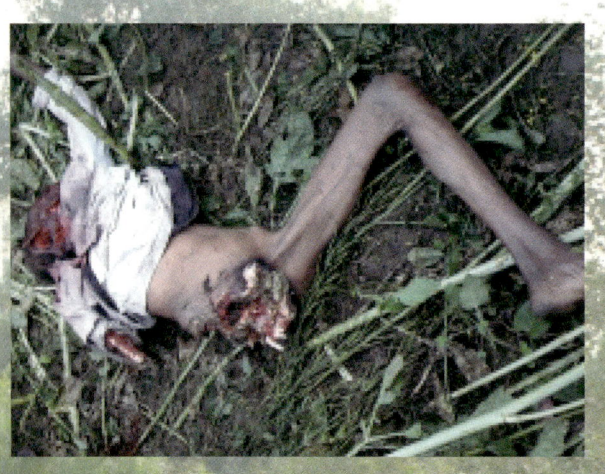
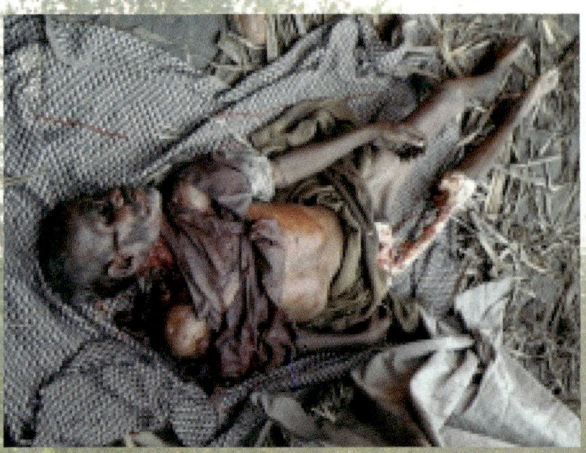

A tiger only becomes a man-eater either because he has been wounded by man or incaptiated while hunting his natural prey, or because the prey is so depleted that he has no other choice but to eat man.

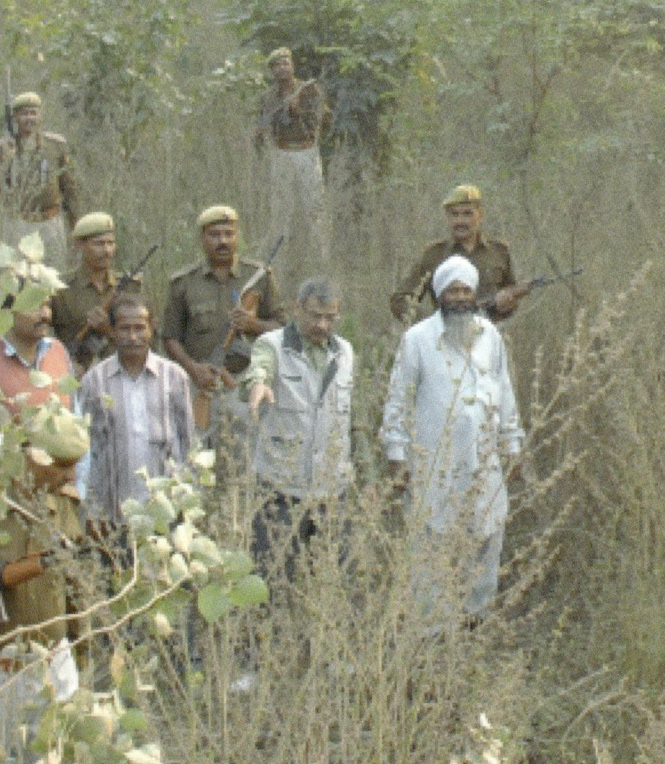

Tracking Nivedia man-eater in Pililbhit District - 10 February 2017. Nivedia falls 3 kilometers to the north of author's ancestral village Phatteypur.

Photographs by Dr. Rupak De, IFS

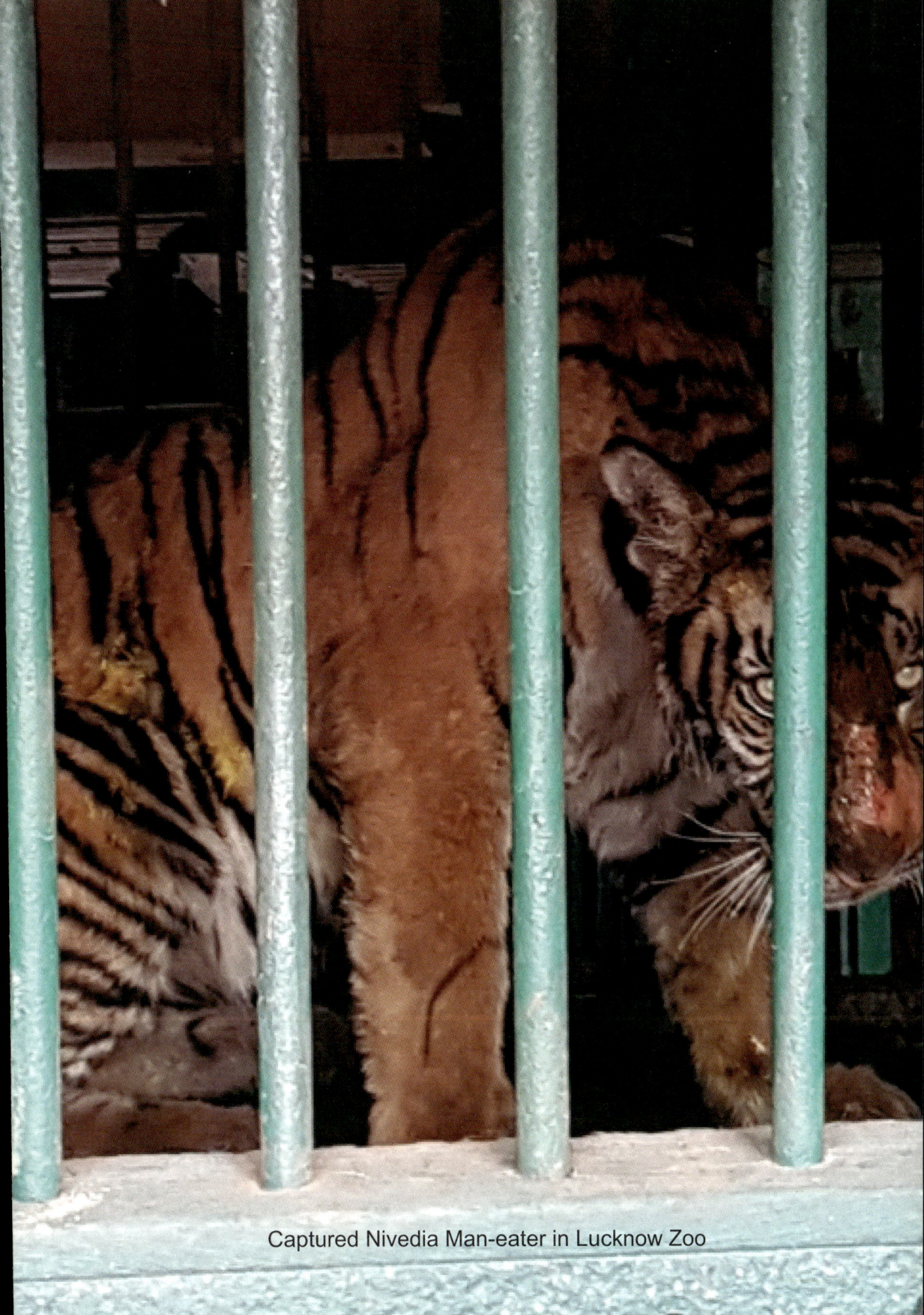
Captured Nivedia Man-eater in Lucknow Zoo

A tigress tranqualized near Palia township, January 22, 2017
(Photo credit : Mahavir, IFS, Deputy Director, Dudhwa National Park)

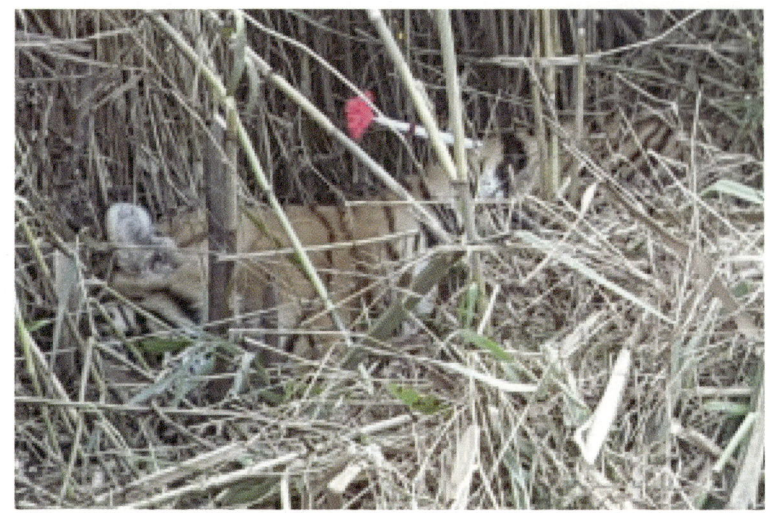

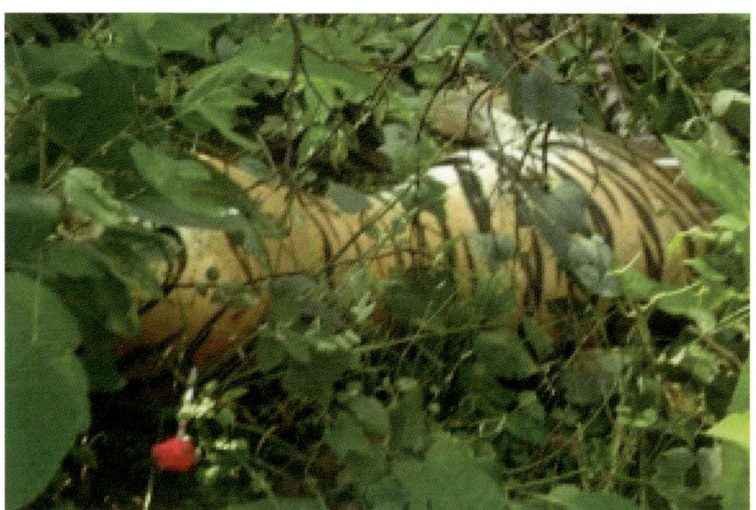

The Mailani man-eater darted on 31 August, 2016
(Photo credit : Sanjay Biswal, IFS, DFO South Kheri)

A leopard darted at Misrikh, Sitapur, June 2016
(Photo credit : Abhishek Verma)

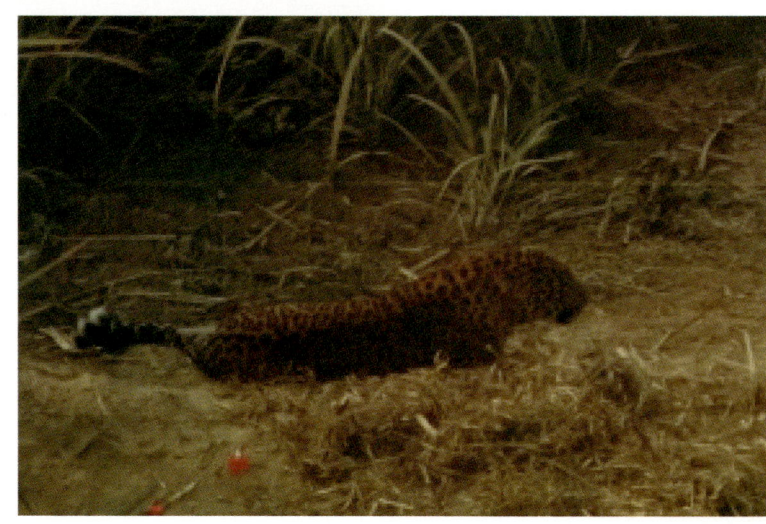

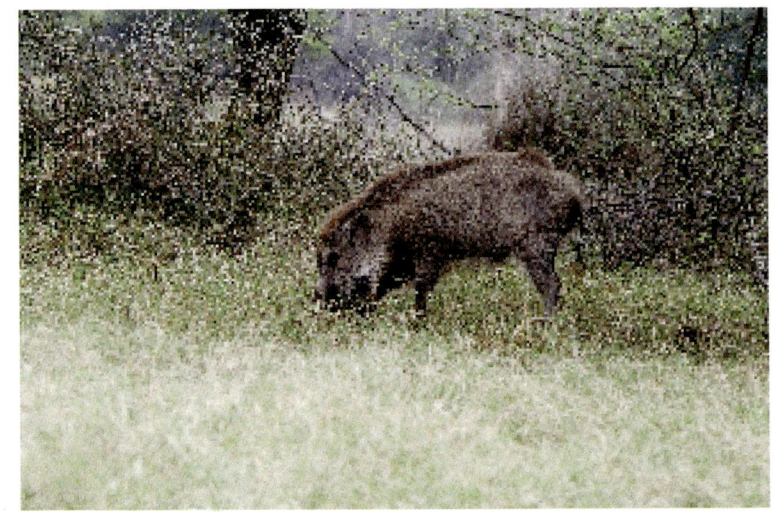

A wild boar in the Kachaara of Gomti, Hardoi district. *(Photo credit : Praveen Rao, IFS, Principal Chief Conservator of Forests, UP)*

A tigress near Sampurnanagar farms *(Photo credit : Sanjay Pathak, NTCA)*

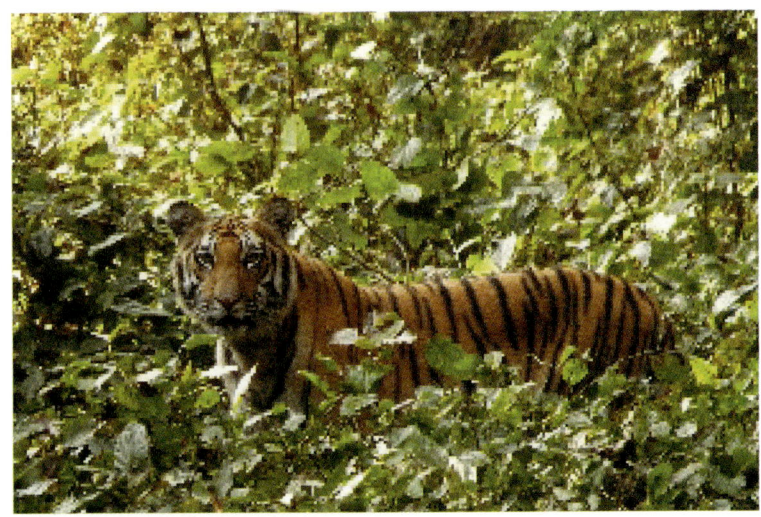

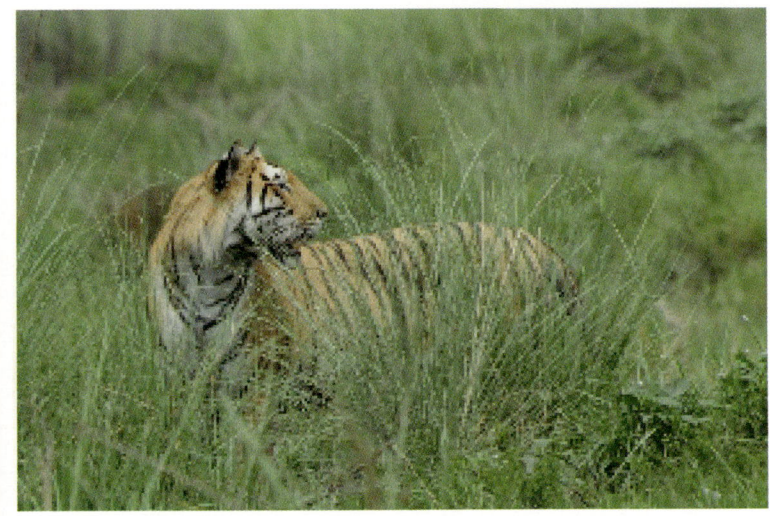

A tiger in grasslands *(Photo credit : Sanjay Kumar, IAS, DM, Allahabad)*

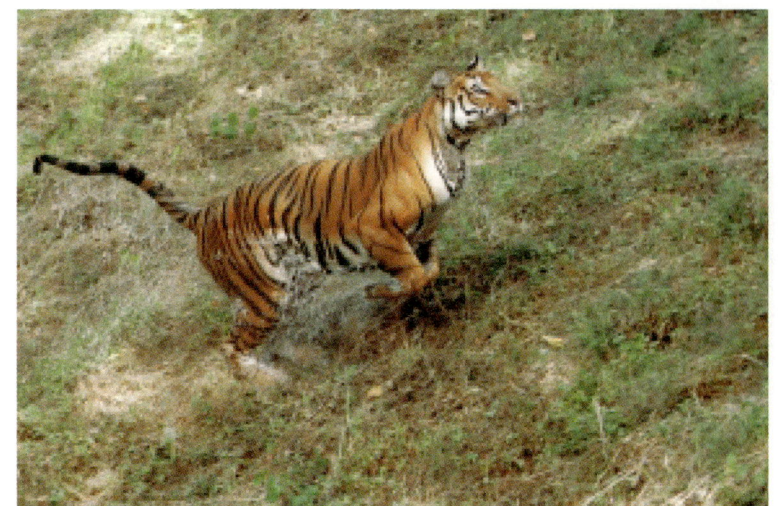

A tiger threatening viewers at near Bela village *(Photo credit : Sanjay Singh, Director, Dudhwa National Park)*

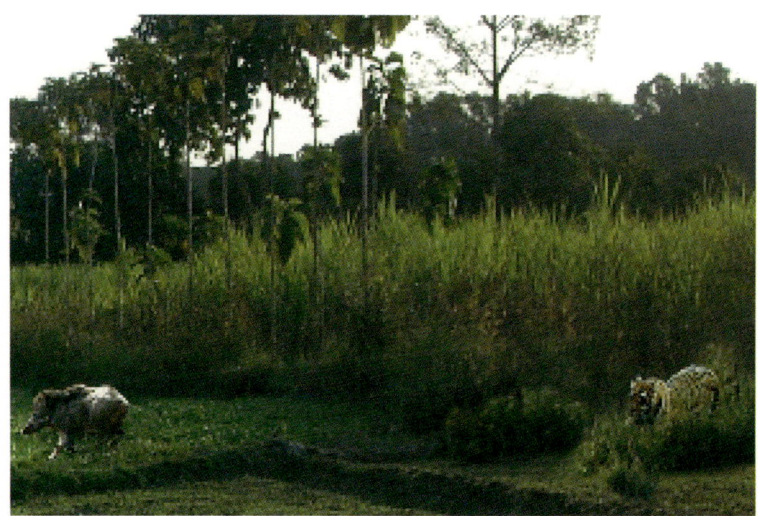

A tiger hunting a wild boar at Bhujia farm, near Palia *(Photo credit : Shrivridhi Shukla)*

A large tiger found dead in fields *(Photo credit : Madhya Pradesh Forest Deptt.)*

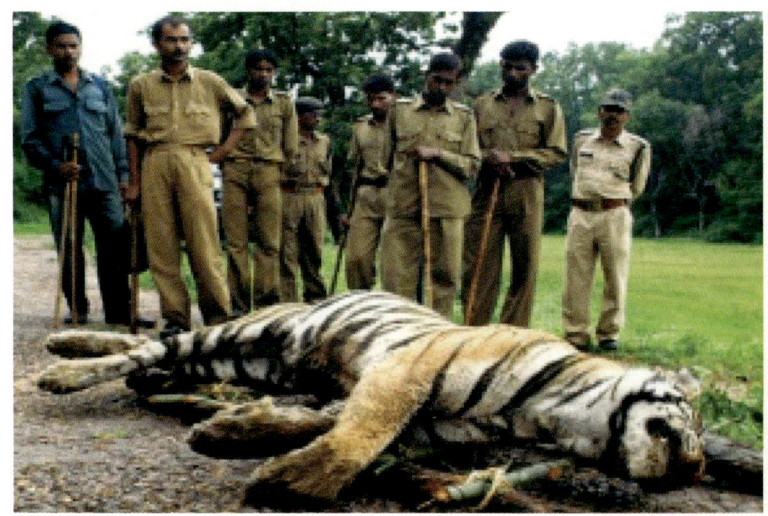

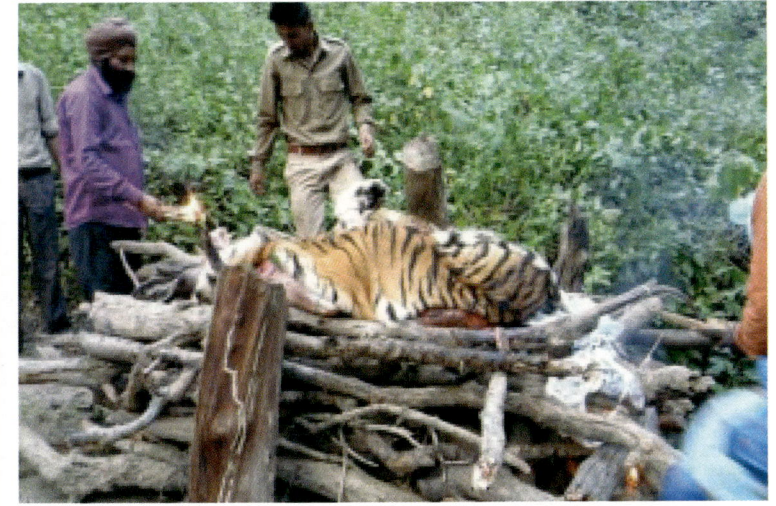

A tiger found dead in a steel-trap set near Deepnagar village Kheri district is being consigned to flames by foresters and locals. *(Photo credit : Sardar Kuldeep Singh)*

A leopard being chased by villagers *(Photo credit : Vidya Atraya, WCT)*

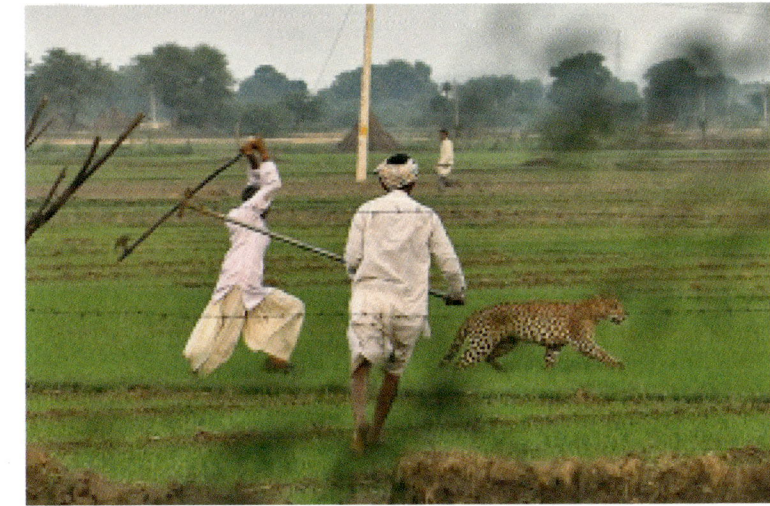

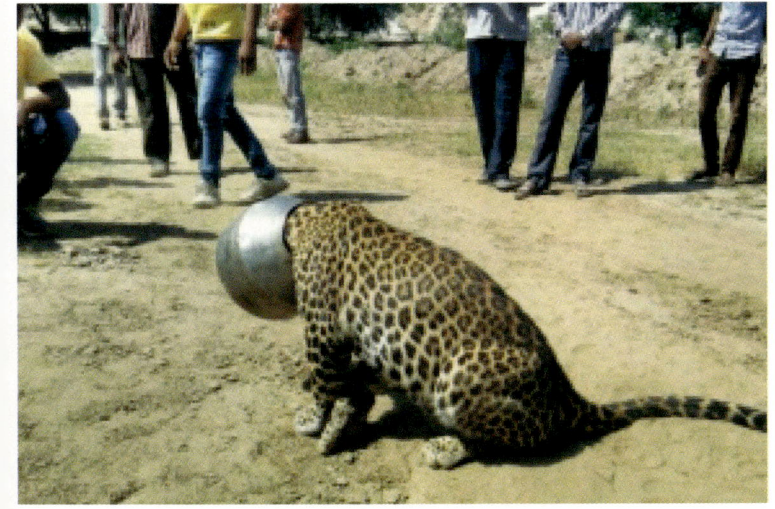

A thirsty leopard gets its head stuck in a vessel *(Photo credit : Sanjay Kumar)*

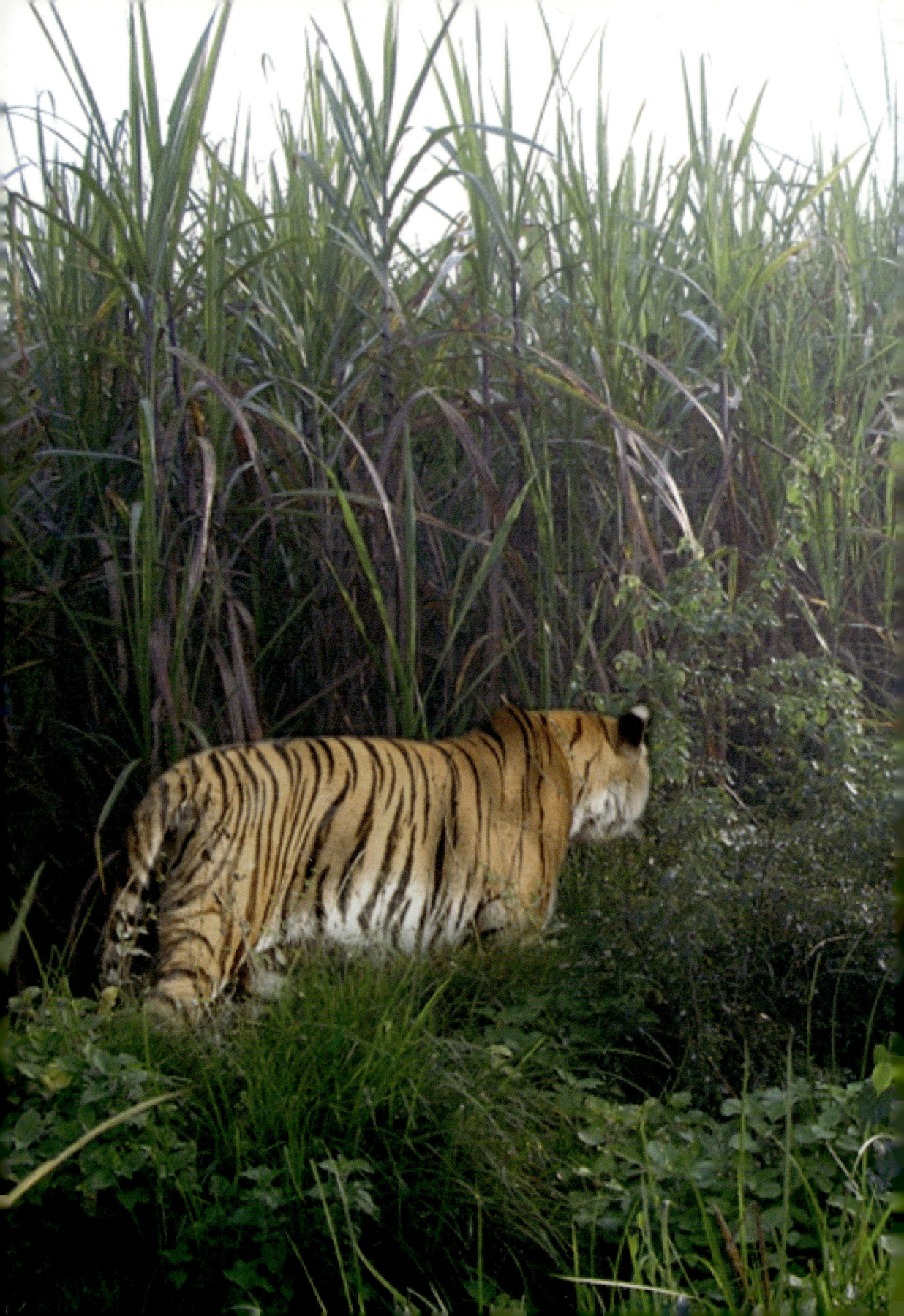

I decided to take a sporting chance. My men, too energetic in their quest for adventure, again lead the beat towards nets banging an assortment of pot, pans and empty tin-cans when there issued a savage grunt. The beast, now thoroughly disturbed, came out of hiding in a fast trot if not gallop. Then he lurched briefly, leaped into the air, and tossing his huge frame about crossed the *nala* entering a large patch of yellow sugar-grass.

By this time the natives had already mounted trees and some 200 onlookers crowded the escarpment to get a grandstand view of this unusually thrilling entertainment. I vouchsafe that it afforded me far less thrill than any of the fine share of might have-beens. In an attempt to flush the tiger again I certainly had no intention of endangering the life of beaters. The man-eater was now in an impregnable position, ready to exact vengeance if disturbed further and if things went wrong then we will have to shoot to kill as a last resort.

Fog and darkness had already clocked the land. Our luck had once again tricked us, providing us with two glaring examples of just how bad it can be at times. We called halt to the proceedings and while returning, we collected the nervy probationer, who had thus far not been able to muster enough courage to clamber down the tree.

People are often tempted to ask what a forest officer is worth if he has never been treed by a tiger or an elephant. This honour is reserved for few. When I told him that he had earned the distinguished honour, he said, "It is definitely better than having the tragic distinction of being eaten alive by a tiger."

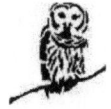

The Next Strike

"This tiger wants to drive us away from our homelands but we have no place to go"
- Prem Sagar, a resident of North Tanda

The exaggerated stories of tigers killing and eating humans had made the species suddenly unpopular and there was an insatiable hatred for the animal among villagers. However, one question has always bothered me — when a domestic animal goes wild, like a dog killing goats, it is called feral. But a wild tiger sits at the top of life pyramid, its menu biologically includes all live weight of his domain – including apes that the mankind is – and by nature's scheme they have preyed upon apes for incalculably hoary ages. Man-eating could thus well be within acceptable parameters of tigerine nature under nature's selection pressures. Then, how this history should be addressed as? Should it be by modern human rules or by natural rules in scientific terms?

The tiger has been a fellow wanderer on our evolutionary trail but paradoxically in last 20,000 years, mankind has changed a lot, but the tiger still remains the same as it was in Paleolithic times. If we need to protect these legendary predators to survive till breeding age with shrinking jungles and ever-exploding human population in their neighbourhood, then we need to inform ourselves thoroughly about them. In nature's law, creatures around a tiger keep him alive; hence we need to define whether this tigerine behavior of man-eating in present times is purposeful adaptation to a new order or reverting to old order? Either way it is no crime against the law of nature. Animal behavior is actually ordained by the law of nature. To repeat, it is the creature around a tiger that keeps him alive, no matter if it is man –the quintessential destroyer of nature. May be it is the law of nature in its purest form; a few humans must die so that many may live.

In any case, the tiger was connected to the world of human beings in a way no animal should ever be. The relationship between the tiger and man had indeed changed due to the animal's dietary changes. Never had so much of menace emanated from sugar fields in the memory of Kaanp Tanda villagers, and destiny had made me come there to rid the country of this awful infection.

Man-eating is as shocking as it is abhorrent and alien to human beings, but is not out of the ambit of a tiger's biological behavior. It falls within the fundamental rules of predatory beasts, and no human effort in particular can change these. When such most-focused land carnivores come to live in the neighborhood of man, preying on humans, crossing over into the realm from which there is no return, it is not at all uncharacteristic of their species. Terror grips the entire community. People realize how defenseless they are against a resolute tiger, which quickly develops a sweet-tooth for human flesh.

The villagers, meanwhile, were continuing their risky forays into the sugar country and overlooking my instructions. A village woman Ram Rati had paid with her life for her foolhardy conduct. Towards late afternoon we were having lunch when a forest patrol arrived with the news of the kill.

In less than ten minutes I was in jungle fatigues – high boots with leather breeches, buckle-strap cartridge belt and leather jacket with strips of thick linoleum attached to limit the claw wounds. I ventured to comb the perimeter of compartment 5 of Kishanpur sanctuary in search of victim's body. The rangers were armed with guns and high power nine shot pistols wearing thick overcoats. When you get all this paraphernalia hung about your person and you hold the gun you cannot stop yourself thinking about the killer stripes whose physical armaments are still more superior and dangerous from close range than your hell of the fire power and protection.

The jungle comprised elephant and tiger grass. My only hope of success rested upon taking up this task instantly, for here the tiger was last seen entering the thicket with the hapless women clutched in its mouth the way dog holds a juicy bone. The woman was heard screaming the frightening scream of the condemned. This alone might provide a reasonable chance to find the brute gorging upon the body.

Stroking my Jeffery .400 double HV –with which my senior generation had settled some half a dozen tigers in the past – and followed by Vijay Bahadur, warden of Kishanpur, S.N. Singh, SDO, and Om Prakash, ranger of Bhira and a few guards, I entered the heavy morass of vegetative growth that lines compartment number 5. Having killed the woman the tiger had taken it inside a grass patch and had probably devoured it there. Though the villagers had surrounded the patch but they were so panic-stricken that no one had dared to enter it yet. Some claimed to have heard the brief sounds of a struggle, which took place inside the grass. The poor woman had probably fought the tiger till the end of her life. We reached the place shortly before five-o clock. Several villagers were still standing there with axes and spears held in their hands. On their side sat a woman wailing and beating her chest, she was the mother of the victim.

It was easy to follow the route man-eater had taken as he had stopped several times to change grip on the prey. It seemed that the woman was alive and aggressively fighting every moment for life. I proceeded on the track, followed by my teammates all equipped with repeating .315 Indian Ordinance. Pools of blood marked the halting places. Further on the marks, seemingly of drag, went through a swamp land that still held two foot high water. Here apparently the woman had finally succumbed to her injuries or her head had sunk in the water and she had died of asphyxiation. We were waist deep in the wet grass. My shoes squelched in the muddy water and dripping stalks of reed grasses struck my face but we kept up a good pace.

The man-eater had finally entered a formidable cover and in this confinement of thickets further tracking was dangerous. At one point a hog deer gave a sharp alarm cry and dashed away. Then a terrifying and uncanny silence followed that seemed almost to vibrate with evil.

Our footsteps were slow and deliberate, rangers were better than good, they were even sweeping rifles in an arc with military precision searching for a target and our nerves were strung out. In case of man-eaters your sense of self-preservation becomes extremely acute if you know that your margin of safety is to be essentially maintained otherwise a slightest mistake on your part might become your own death sentence.

Naïve man-eaters don't tolerate being disturbed and shifted while they are eating. They are known to threaten intruders angrily and even attack them, going to the extent of making a second kill. In such cases, their range of attack is limited to the distance they can spring; rarely do they launch an attack from a distance. The greatest danger of their attack is from behind and to a lesser extent from either side. Such urgent situations are to be dealt with in a matter of split second and there is no time to align sights. Only a couple of lead balls with some 10,000 pounds of wallop are expected to stop 400 pounds of flesh and bone limp in its tracks.

Although we were seriously out on this task to destroy the man-eater this time, I could give no reason as why I felt so nervous. My skin began to crawl as if something deadly was in the offing.

We finally found the victim's body, a mile inside the jungle, of which nearly two-third was eaten by the tiger,. Fellow humans had never witnessed such a gruesome sight of a human being annihilated in this manner. The victim's severed head rested at the stump of a tree with long hair spread around, giving the impression as if she was buried in the earth, with only the head projected outside. The victim's family was collecting her remains when a barking deer began its nervous ventriloquist calls near fire-line. It was evident that the tiger was apparently hanging around. I directly walked in the direction the tiger had taken, insisting on complete silence.

I selected three of the best men to accompany me as I went ahead, while signaling others to follow at a distance behind. Old lessons of stalking came back to my mind – just as cycling or swimming is never forgotten in life. It is least a matter of watching your step; it is rather a matter of keeping your eyes at the place where you want to be and then every nerve becomes your eye and each muscle develops reflex action. You do not guide your body but you trust it to be silent and you walk confidently and soundlessly.

Slipping from tree to tree and walking much faster than my team, I covered some 100 yards when a giant owl let out a series of muffled hoots over a *Pakar* tree; and below it I got the first glimpse of the stealth of the solo hunter, its hindquarters more than half-hidden in a bush. It was the last hour of the day. The shades were lengthening and I was also a bit unsure of my aim for if things went awry the situation could become difficult. Moreover the spot was more concealing than the rest of the surrounding country. Vijay Bahadur caught hold of my shoulder and asked me to withdraw. For a long and anxious minute I was reluctant, holding my gun, afraid to open fire, in case I only wounded it and then gave up the chase. We both knew well that darkness was only a few minutes away and then even the most heavily armed man will be no match for a tiger's stealth at night.

Tired of an exhausting stalk – for it needs every bit of skill to move without a sound – we came out of the jungle. The sun was on the verge of setting and its slanting rays were sailing over the rise when to our surprise, the man-eater emerged out of the jungle and stood on a knoll looking at our retreating team. The fireball shone like a mighty spotlight across a cosmic stage and the gray-yellow tiger edged with brilliance seemed to have acquired a new mysterious glory. Like pure death in the evening light, he stood in the middle of the rise, etched against the sunlight, a vague figure literally throwing his long shadow over us.

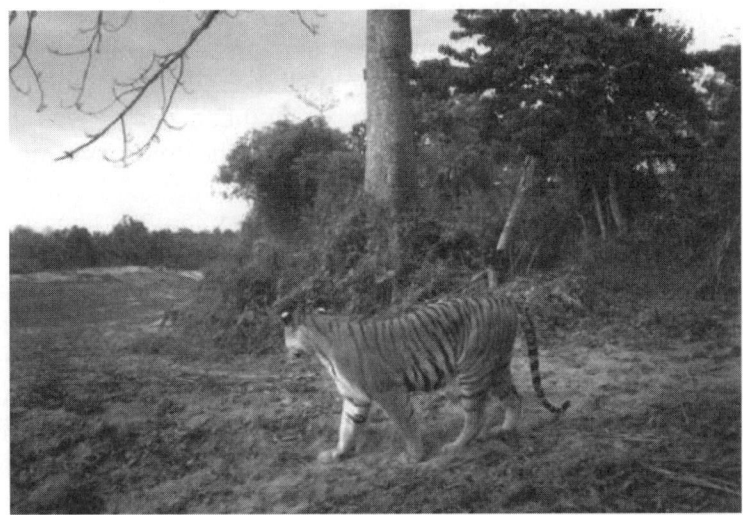

Even so called wilderness tigers are now confined to all those little fragments of isolated vegetation, separated from each other by vast open farmlands that they have developed the habit of residing in them.

He was some fifty yards away and in the evening silence the short admonishing sounds coming as vocal expression of his ire were clearly audible. Undoubtedly intensely curious as to where his food had disappeared so suddenly, he was induced to leave the shelter of the jungle and expose himself on the knoll, perhaps to check if we were the cause behind his missing meal.

I could see that the tiger's curiosity was pretty well unsatisfied and he was least willing to melt back into the thicket. So what was going on his mind? Was he considering someone amongst us as his prospective meal?

The members of the team looked confused, whether to bust him or not. There was no firm government sanction to kill the tiger yet some had gripped their rifles hurriedly for a snap-shot, feeling the metal; even I looked at him through the scope, my finger gently caressing the safety catch and my eyes probed the open space illuminated by the last rays of sun. The rising fog had slowly started covering the vista in a hazy effluvium, and the roosting calls of peacocks tampered with early yapping of jackals appeared straight out of an Alfred Hitchcock horror movie. Just then the wily animal perceived danger from guns and within no time, the sun and the tiger both went down the knoll.

The jungle had assumed the mantle of dusk. The afterglow of sunset was deepening when the wild trumpet of a red fowl echoed over the swamp and sugarcanes with strength, like the farewell note of the day as the twilight lowered itself quiet gently and sank below the earth. And the night fell like a dropped shutter.

❖

Arriving at the camp after dark I fished out a bottle of VAT-69 and poured a huge shot into a plastic cup. As I sat sipping it, my crew was already prepared for alcoholic abandon. The gory scene, the dark bloody earth, and the severed human head with its features set in a hideous grin of death, haunted me again and again. Even under the influence of alcohol, the morbid scene kept coming back to the mind's eye despite the horror and unease it caused. Amongst all these intense thoughts that fired my imagination, my repertoire of experience with these beasts was the only consoling factor that I could bank on. Still the terrifying incident gave me a new respect for the dangerous animal.

It was confirmed by the long intervals between human killings that the tiger was also living on other forms of prey. One of most difficult factors in tracking down this animal was that he behaved differently in different circumstances. Had he become a casual killer of humans because he could take for granted humans as easily procurable meal than any other prey? It is more a habit of man-eating leopards than tigers. Their depredations form no pattern because they usually take humans when opportunity arises. And in the meanwhile they carry on with their normal prey list. But once tigers become man-eaters, they consistently become stuck to human flesh and their victims take it with typical Indian fatalism: "What has to happen will happen."

That is why one wonders why Indian tigers in comparison to leopards made bigger scores of human killing than anywhere in the 13 tiger range countries. It is not easy to forget the scale on which Jim Corbett's man-eaters' operated. The Champawat tigress and the Panar man-eater, by far the worst, shared between them a record total of 836 human souls and probably many more that went unrecorded. The Rudraprayag man-eater lived both ways on normal prey and humans with equal efficiency; not particular whether his prey was beast or human.

I am a historian by profession and natural history tells that up to the middle of 19th century the tiger was considered a dangerous vermin because of being in direct spatial competition with man. Brander and Champion say that in certain parts of India like Sunderbans and Chhattisgarh, as well as in some pockets of Tarai, it was debatable whether man or the tiger would eventually survive.

Man-eating tigers have had almost an unbelievable influence on Indian subcontinent since first European explorers and developers begin to open up the jungles in earnest and their writings reflected the grim situations. Buchanan Hamilton tells as how tigers had turned bold in Gorakhpur and carried off people even in the middle of the town. R.G. Burton records a catastrophe in the famine year 1769, when most herbivorous animals had perished. "The tigers were famishing, and great numbers infested the town of Bhiwapur, where in very short time they killed 400 of the inhabitants; the survivors fled, and for some years the town was deserted." This incident tells that as in jungle a tiger's predation pressure shifts from species to species with seasonal changes, famine conditions bring the eminently adaptable predators to prey upon humans, with some of them developing a purely anthropophagous appetite.

To my mind their preference for the meat of *Homo sapiens* than any other is largely attributed to presence of extra salt in the human blood, which is horribly demonstrated in the case of almost all the potential man-eaters of the Tarai which were in full bloom of health with plenty of prey around. These were essentially different from Jim Corbett's man-eaters that belonged to disabled category of 'wounded and aged killers.' But now as norms have changed, despite human killings the preference is to capturing of animal rather than applying lethal control. Adrian Treves' studies prove that error rates in identifying problem animals are high and 71% of carnivores killed to prevent conflict showed no evidence of having been involved in recent conflicts. A report of United States Department of Agriculture Wildlife Service shows that from 1996 to 2001 federal agents killed some 13.7 million animals to control agricultural damages. "If error rates resemble those cited above," says Treves, "1.5-9.7 million animals were killed without cause." We can't afford to take such chances with *Panthera tigris* for after all it is a Schedule One species that is nearing extinction.

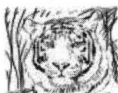

At close quarters with Tumbling Tiger

There is nothing freer than a wild tiger on the loose
- Charles McDougal

The dispensary was our temporary headquarter and its daily routine was regular as that of a well-ordered household. Our rifles generally rested against the vast trunk of weather beaten banyan tree that stood in the backyard of the building and our vehicles were parked on the ground around it. The distorted roots of the banyan stood up among the low trees like the ribs of a skeleton and were so twisted as to form one or two convenient armchairs, where we could sit in the shade and read or smoke.

The camp is daguerreotyped on my memory; a jackal, a civet or a pariah dog usually hung around eating the leftovers and towards night four pressure-fed storm lamps burned with 300 candlepower at the door of the camp. I have never ever known of even the most indomitable of man-eaters to venture into that dazzling blaze of light. My men knew this and were quite comfortable to remain in the dispensary with me. They were of course trained enough to awake at least once during the night and inject pressure in lamps when the level of kerosene dropped.

Two weeks passed. In this short duration our hunting had been very intensive and stressful. One evening as the afterglow of the sun lingered in the west, the rangers brought a pig to ensconce inside the bait cage. The idea was to slay the pig, throw a few fresh meat chunks around and deposit the rest of the body inside the cage. The pig was heavier than average; and the bigger they are the tougher they are, for their hide is as rough as the tanned boot leather. The pig was roped with its legs pulled apart and when a guard Ram Kumar butchered it, the swine screamed in an ear-splitting shrill. The squeals of agony, of course much prolonged, blended and magnified by the closed environment echoed in the ravines and were heard far and wide. Tigers are extremely sensitive to alarm calls and death cries of their prey animals, which carry far through the silence of the night and invariably draw them to investigate any commotion.

As if true to my hunch, the man-eater had already entered the village, slinking by the hutments for he knew somebody will certainly come out to empty his bladder and provide his evening meal. It was there that he heard the horrendous squeals and came running to investigate the cause. Without warning and seemingly from nowhere, a figure appeared above the mound and stood framed round a bend in a festoon of saplings. Suddenly we realized the man-eater was standing right above us.

The tiger had come straight from his 'buffet table' of the village - meaning thereby a possible human death had been averted that night. He was looking at us attentively from the escarpment about 20 yards away, his white chest exposed, neck raised and his huge paws soundlessly firm on the brown clay. Om Prakash and a forest guard were directly beneath him.

The rounded edge of the half-moon had emerged over the horizon. For a brief moment the tiger stood over the saddle of knoll gazing purposefully down the ravines, his preying eyes looking for the wild boar which had just screamed. There are a few things as breathtaking as a wild tiger in its natural setting; all magnificent and spectacular, commanding the aura ordinarily reserved for gods. What a sight, we gazed in fascination?

The tiger could surely smell the human odor mixed with the smoky scent of evening fires as well as the irresistible smell of pig's blood and urine that he had let out at being butchered. Several searchlights and hand torches instantly focused upon him as the great predator blinked his eyes in an overture of obfuscation, presenting a perfect target. In a reflex, the stock of my.400 was at my shoulder and within an infinitesimal moment, the highly-accurate and hard-hitting bullet could have gone blazing right across him. I found it impossible to resist shouting that "there won't be another opportunity like this", but hell, there weren't any orders to shoot this animal.

However, the tiger's immediate attention seemed to be on grabbing the boar's carcass that lay immediately underneath. He had only briefly halted; when suddenly a part of the knoll broke loose as his leg slipped and he fell down the embankment. In the middle of the fall he stumbled upon a log that lay spanning and took a complete somersault. Recovering instantly, the tiger came down sliding at a great speed and bumped into a guard who took on a defensive posture to protect his neck and head, and was knocked flat and then into the ranger Om Prakash.

The crowd was aghast. Their eyes and mouth wide open, they watched the tiger in dumb amazement. Then rifles begun to boom close to my head, followed by more booms as the guards started firing their weapons abruptly in haste while trackers scurried away like rabbits seeking a place to hide, when Neta in acute nervousness snatched the gun form my hands and two big feathers of flame erupted from .400 as he pressed the trigger, firing the twin shots abstractly.

The radical predator growled in defense and stood facing us with a threatening countenance, swinging his claws full out but missing the men by a narrow margin. A tiger at such a close quarter is a monster indeed. The two inch talons driving up to bone could

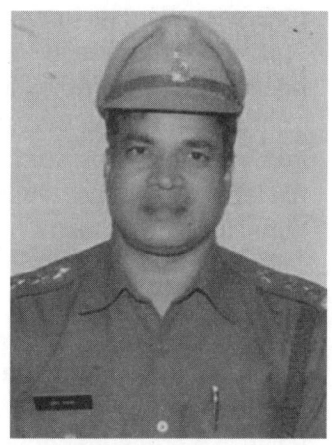

Om Prakash, the Ranger of Bheera; my untiring partner on Kaanp-Tanda man-eaters trail.

have held anyone like great fishhooks as his saliva erupting with growls splashed upon clothes of the people in the vicinity. Om Prakash swung his empty rifle, hitting the paw, while others just watched wide-eyed and awe-struck. The tiger wheeled about and made off for a short distance, but returned in confusion. Grabbing my gun back from Neta I automatically broke the action, dunked in two fresh rounds, but as more shots were being fired around, the animal took to his heels and dashed away; getting an extra burst of speed as the bullets whistled past him, throwing up spurts of leaves and dust.

The knoll ringed with the constant report of shots. Neta and I ducked behind the bole of a tree, more to save ourselves from bullets than the tiger as the animal rushed past us a few meters away. I could hear a vibrant thrust of breath through partially closed lips much similar to the noise made by horses when they clear their mouths and nostrils and his padded feet thumping like drumbeats in full gallop. Although the tiger is absolutely noiseless when stalking, he makes a surprising amount of noise when he runs.

Man-eater's escape was least of a charge but his route of escape, indeed fell only 4 meters away from my tree, where his fleeing showed all the outer elements of a charge. The awe-inspiring speed of tiger left a great impression on me. What I and Neta saw was an enormous head that seemed to be coming straight at us and at the same time rapidly increasing in size and the whole body seemed to be masked by the head only till it rushed-past.

The ranger miraculously survived without a single scratch to show for the encounter. The nerve shattering experience had shaken him to the heart because he was so powerless to do anything. The guard knocked flat by the rush of the tiger had played dead till the animal departed.

Greasy cordite fumes stinging our eyes hung in the evening air. The freshly-butchered carcass lay at its place. We counted the heads, in case the tiger had taken any one among the crew. We all were intact. In his hurry to flee a forest guard Ram Kumar had fallen in the slush and then quickly shut himself inside the iron cage that was set for the tiger. He came out of the cage dripping and jerking his legs, wiping the lumps of mud. He told the incident with gusto, as he laughed at himself as much as at his humour, his jokes going on with a lunatic hilarity.

Hearing their laughter, I wondered whether humor can be legitimate response to such horrific, near-death situations. Yes, to some this may be the gross violation of sensibilities but to some it is a necessary outlet towards exercising the demons of the hounding past no matter how terrible they are. What is often referred to as sick humor is believed to have psychologically therapeutic value. It acts like an escape valve in a pressure cooker. A tiger victim's jokes are a disgusted form of aggression; that are carried away far into an imaginary world but in this case the victims of aggression had gained their reward through jokes. This is the way with the light-hearted people; they replayed the death-dealing and lifesaving moments and turned them into a joke.

Yet, all that is real around them are the haunted forests of sugarcane, and the dreadful tiger which includes humans in his natural prey species.

❖

One may say that when the squad's armament consisted of over 20 rifles and shot guns, and it had been used so lavishly in the excitement, then why in such a poor show of marksmanship the tiger was missed at close range. But the answer is that the staff had been sensible enough to not to perforate the tiger. In a great show of awareness no one had pointed his barrel at it.

Though blood for blood has been Tarai's eternal rule of life but I am comforted to say that this operation was gentlemen's war against a hardened man-eater where none of mine or my teams' blood had ever got involved. Moreover when survival instincts come into play the race-memory of every species tells it to escape rather than confront the ordeal. The same had happened here.

Having had three hair-raising, gut-pulling encounters with this man-eater within a fortnight, I and my crew one day sat down mulling over things carefully and thought of going back to our respective business than doing this messy job. But tigers are alluring. There is something irresistibly spooky about them that places their pursuit – historically and morally – in a category of its own; a deliberate exposure of one's own life to real leeway of death, that 'icy clutch of danger' purely for the sake of adrenalin rush that drives people to skydive, speed cars or even feed killer sharks in the depths of the sea.

In the Grim Reeds of Sharda

"The silence sank
Like music on my heart"

Samuel Taylor Coleridge

The heavy going of the three previous days had so utterly fatigued me that I decided to spend next day in the camp to rest. Shortly after 9 am a runner arrived to inform that the tiger had killed a dog around the very village South Tanda, we had left the previous evening and some graziers had sighted him relaxing near the knoll. The people in the village had thought it best to leave the tiger undisturbed and wait for foresters to come and deal with it.

An hour later we were on the trail of the man-eater but when we arrived on the spot there was no sign of him. With the increasing light of the day he had left the knoll and gone inside a dense mass of green river reeds, which extended for nearly two miles down the river below. The reeds were some ten or more feet high and no ordinary fire would have burnt down that tangled mass. The threat of pushing out the 'lain-up' tiger therefore could not be put into operation till the reed was dry enough to burn, and that would be at least a month. However, it was essential to know about his whereabouts. I was sure that the man-eater was somewhere within a mile in the either direction of my map, so we entered the reeds.

Small packs of foraging mongooses chittered at us as we passed and then vaulted into the cover. Coots skittered away in the occasional pools that were left by the flood waters and red fowls wearing rufous winter pelts pecked the grit. Sharp-eyed and alert with our rifles ready we spent around three hours down on our hands and knees peering under the dense growth and into each tiny islet of bush for a glimpse of the striped hide. We hoped to hell that when we spotted the killer, it would not be bearing the countenance of an open mouth and bare teeth hurtling at us from close range. The problem is that a hunter crawling on all fours resembles a medium size deer and is more vulnerable to get eaten, especially when everything in the grass is in the tiger's favour.

At the moment the standard procedure for me was to keep intoning Lord Krishna's name as *Kavach* (spiritual protective armour), be slow and soundless and try to keep the rifle handy. Such a dangerous and hard hunting requires patience, endurance and courage. There are much greater chances of a slip after which the hunter could end up being chewed up easily. We spent the entire afternoon in the reeds, heard no alarm calls and save for a single hog deer that scurried in the manner of pig from which it derives its name, we didn't see much wildlife.

It was extremely cold with an almost frangible quality in the air. The sun was dropping and a glitch near the Sharda where the villagers dumped dead cattle had yet not been investigated. It was a favourite place for scavengers and in this incredibly dry winter when much meat tended to mummify than rot, this left almost no invitation of odor to blow around and draw meat eaters, as happened in acute summers. But we knew that the tiger knew the place and he regularly checked it, and so did the foresters.

Instead of following the trail of the man-eater industriously, we decided to proceed by the shortest route to the riverbanks. The night had plunged when using flashlights we reached the fringe of the belt towards river. An old Blue bull called at us with his nasal cry and bounced a few yards, stopping to stare at us again. Our movements alerted the game birds, roosting in small water puddles that litter the banks of Sharda. Disturbed by flashlights, hundreds of ducks, mostly bar headed geese, teals and garganey rose with a flutter from ponds that rang like drumbeats over the glitches. Amidst the honking of Siberian guests, resounding in the atmosphere and a flock of mallards circling over our team, we finally found the fresh signs of the wanted animal. Due to the loose sandy texture of the soil his pug marks were easily readable; we wearily registered the last location of tiger on geographical positioning system or GPS and informed the headquarters where the confirmed record of man-eaters' daily activities, through satellite imagery system was kept on scaled topographic maps, digitized at the home range analysis superimposed on the ground maps.

Again, as on the previous days, it was almost three hours after sunset when we got back to the camp deep in the blackness of night, utterly fatigued and fell on the cots with a sigh. We felt we all needed sleep more than food.

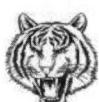

Tiger-Serenade

"Everyone needs a dog to adore him, and a tiger to bring him back to reality."
— *Unknown*

Far off across the Sharda, and settled on a huge mound, the village of Paraspur revealed itself in the flimsy sunlight. The great trail of North Kheri forests encircled it from three sides like a dark formation of clouds giving it a picture postcard setting. During the decade of the 1980s, when my research on sugarcane tigers was at its peak, this village and its people had been my constant companions and their association had held a special brand of thrill for me.

Next day passed without incident and we were all glad of the opportunity of a welcome rest. The following morning my team was still tired and sulky and I was in

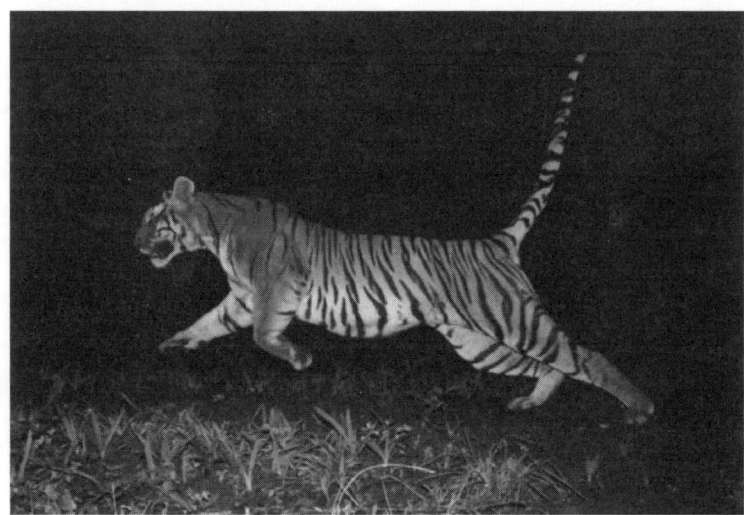

When tiger get ready to give demonstrations of their talents,people often fail to perceive the threat and stand mesmerized under their spell. *(Photo credit Wildlife Conservation Trust)*

a mood to spend the day in the camp and read something. Just then another messenger arrived with a report that the man-eater had been sighted near a village called Nairosa. Hurriedly we scrambled into a jeep and bounced away to the place. Again the day was spent in useless effort where in the ardour of the sport all personal comforts were forgotten. However, the day turned rewarding for while returning home we got an outstanding experience of tiger serenade; though not as much dodgy and threatening that I and Aftab had had with the Ghola man-eater a quarter of a century back.

After a daylong jaunt of miles, KK Singh and I were camp-bound. The sun was at the edge of the trees now and flashing copper crimson spears through the foliage. We were accompanied by local trackers, forest guards and a pack of six dogs that I preferred to use in field to avoid the accidental onslaught of man-eater. Within a few minutes the sun went down and a temporary period of uncertainty between light and darkness commenced. Grass bushes and undergrowth that had been so clear to the eyes in the brightness of the day now assumed the shape of some menacing beast as the light suddenly gave way to the stunning fears of the night.

The expanding evening became resonant with the enticing notes of peacocks. In the fading lights a pair of wild sows with a large family of sucklings crossed our path. A porcupine also emerged near a dead termite heap and was astonished upon seeing the dogs. She uttered a horrified grunt, spread out its quills to resemble a pin-cushion and bolted at top speed, seeking shelter in sugarcane. Dogs barked furiously but remained stationary as their reigns were in trackers hands, preventing them from chasing the animal.

The last tinge of twilight was dimming just then from across the Sharda a tigress rendered its mating calls. Taking its time, it initially issued moaning peripatetic vocalizations thrice, announcing that it was in season. Her calls were immediately answered by a male from our side of the river. It seemed loaded with the dominance required for a meaningful mating. Singh and I felt sure it was the young man-eater who was reciprocating the call. The veneer of the resident male had come upon him by default because he had come to occupy sugar fields to hunt humans, but in tiger protocol this was not his standard territory. The calls had come up from the reed beds and then suddenly it broke out like a strange concert of barnyard noises that lasted for a minute and then suddenly died away.

In the density of sugarcane, it is difficult to estimate the correct distance of the source of sound. The thick growth of fronds and high tangled grasses muffle the reverberations and echoes and the unstable air currents also make it difficult to mark the location of caller. Though the tigers were not in sight and it was certain that they were also not anywhere near us, yet the behavior of dogs turned acutely nervous, squealing in horrid noises, they tucked their tails, stood between our legs and freely urinated. Such is the power of fear that the alpha killer had exerted upon them.

The thickly sickle rim of moon had now risen over the vista. Its pale beams shed a diffused light over fog covered cane fields creating a ghostly atmosphere. Then another tiger, perhaps the real big one seemed to join his kens from Jhadi Tal compartment. Some three miles away an awe-inspiring thunder clap of sound boomed off from darkened cores of *sal* forest that electrified the whole atmosphere. The female wailed again and again as their calls succeeded each other, much like a rapid chuff-chuff of a locomotive.

Adrenalin pumped through my friends arteries. No typewriter is ever invented that can give a true impression of these sounds. The only way to appreciate their intensity is to hear them first-hand and feel the 'bomb-like' force of a heated god. When roars turn into a rising rumble they seem to come from everywhere at once and you don't know from which direction they actually emanate. I recall a Tharu once telling me, "The tiger roars settle as a vibration through listeners' body, disquietingly and scarily so that *langoors* fall off trees, dead with heart attack." No doubt this sensation is due to the fear which is more pronounced when one is alone at a place where danger lurks by night, and the sounds lend substance to the fear of supernatural.

The great matrimonial advertises, primordial and instinctive quickly swelled into thunderous *gurgle-warble-burble* and rumbled out across the expanse of cultivation and the village.

Fathoming what was happening we threw the torchlight around and saw a large monitor lizard making its way along the sandy patches. It looked as if it was sniffing something, much as a dog would do in trying to sniff the buried bones. Its incessantly flickering snake like tongue, was actually trying to know as to where bird or reptile eggs might be buried. The evening serenade had now begun to cast a spell on the landscape, making its denizens stay transfixed. A million heads must have lifted wonderingly at the ever triumphant sounds but the monitor was un-affected. It knew tigers were far off. It hung about, searching for eggs and then abruptly disappeared.

The worrying serenade continued intermittently. Like the very essence of Tarai, healing and lyrical, rhythmic and implacable, it had raised the level of adrenalin in our blood and the intense pleasure that all sportsmen feel, made out journey interesting. Some natives had drawn the hunting blade from the sheath of their belts while others were totting their savage spears, and even homemade .315 *Kattas*. It was all excitement so that the length of the road did not register much on our minds.

As the rim of moon rose further over the horizon, the calls finally ceased. Even after that the chilly night, a brilliantly clear sky studded with stars, remained electrified for long with their portentous energies. The shrieks of protest from the peacocks, from here and there, were noticeable whose slumbers had been disrupted by the explosions of the noise.

Well it is the world of super predators, the beasts of essential wilds who have changed little in thousands of years. Theirs is the ultimate world of violence and savagery, sheer power and fierceness where life means little. Therefore it is not easy to face such nerve-wrecking situations when two such lethal beasts are testing the strength of their lungs, strained to their uttermost and you know that one of them is man-eater. You need not be a coward to tremble with fear but in an unmitigated desperation of danger your tongue does feel parched like sand as at a close the range tiger roar is not as much a sound, as it is a full body experience. It so overwhelmingly scrambles one's neurology that even the stout-hearted can fall and faint. If you keep hearing it for enough time without seeing the noise makers -hidden in the night shadows expanding impenetrable around you--then definitely that hour can be terribly exhausting.

However to romanticize, there is nothing less tempestuous with assertive tigers. They need no embellishments for they are the best at their rawest and you know you are really alive when you move among them.

As I tumbled on the bed, the sleep overwhelmed the tired limbs but the deadly booms reverberated in my stomach as a sense of menace emanated from sugar fields.

"You can stay here and be eaten if you want but I will be off tomorrow," KK Singh rendered his good night compliment as he went to sleep.

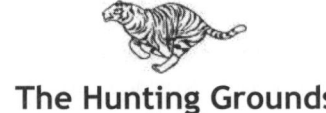

The Hunting Grounds

They are hyper-alert, hunt mainly by night, and live in a habitat of maximum concealment. There are far more people sightings by tigers than there are tiger sightings by people.
- Charles Mac Dougal

The Kaanp Tanda sugarfields wedged between Dudhwa National Park and Kishanpur Sanctuary is a favorite farmland habitat of tigers and is never known to be unoccupied. People usually sail well along them but if an aberrant animal arrives and generates an outburst of emotional anger, then suddenly the communities' psychology changes. The animal loses its respect as valued animal and is relentlessly chased.

Late Sir J.P. Hewett describes this area as full of immense grasses and rich rainfall that shielded a selective breeding and holding ground for tigers. I have the original copy of his book *Jungle Trails of Northern India*, wherein the hunter gives a vignette on a left page, showing the Sharda River and its rising mounds. It was a century ago and the land still looked surprisingly the same. As I moved amongst the beautiful scenery there, watching a pair of crocodiles raising their heads and then dipping away, I recollected my early ambitions and the picture in the book that gave a touch of romance to the scene.

Much of this landscape is under agricultural use and massive utilization of place by the human population has degraded the system to an irremediable travesty of its former richness. The grandeur of wildlife is much reduced but wooded plants continue to dominate farmed landscape and the elements of that old ecosystem that still mark the place are yet not fully altered. These were just as green as when Hewett had hunted here in the early years of the last century.

This area is like an old home, which has crumbled but its last few rooms still continue to house the residents. The fragmented pockets of savannah and swamps, supported by enough natural food like pig, hog deer and blue-bulls induce tigers to frequent this historical landscape. In winters this feature accentuates, as many guests arrive and sometimes create a temporary overcrowding in the area.

The extent of knowledge on requirements of tigers that use farmland areas as hunting grounds and the areas where natural vegetation patches prove most beneficial to them for staying purposes is poorly understood. Viewing Tarai farmlands under the lens of 'large predators as beneficial agency to agriculture' would easily cover and validate the tiger's presence because it would in fact include species like blue bull and feral cattle that damage the crops, and the tiger serves as pest controlling agent. Indeed this matrix, otherwise considered a blind spot, points to fundamental clues that show that big cat conservation is not inherently incompatible to sustainable agriculture.

Next day we again heard the tigress calling as she moved about the sandy banks of the river. She called intensely and her sounds appearing as preliminary invitation to love-making were enough to attract males. Indubitably the juvenile man-eater was affected by them and was often crossing the river. However, these calls did not seem to have the true element of unvanquished tiger calls that show overconfidence and fearlessness, they rather had frenzied impatience which broadcast the need and urgency for a mate.

Her itinerant communications again showed that despite her being in season, the male had not attained dominance over her, mandatory for profound mating either for lineal descent or his age. They perhaps stayed together for a day and then parted. Then the female vanished from the area and the tiger was seen loitering alone.

I later discovered that the range harbored a large resident male which we had heard calling from Jhadi Tal area. He had gone inside the jungles or temporarily vanished from the vista while on his territorial round, and the calling tigress was actually seeking his company. This occurrence gave rise to a note-worthy conjecture that the juvenile, which had till then avoided to venture in this trans-Sharda zone due to the fear of the large male, had sensed the absence of the male and immediately crossed over to meet the female. But often it happens that only the dominant male of the range is permitted to breed and it is simply the female that determines the eventuality as to whether it would submit to any other paramour in his absence or not. The courtship had thus not been consummated. In this case the tigress had rejected the juvenile. In such conditions the female only submits to another male if it can subdue her.

The juvenile, apparently stressed at the intolerance of 'ready to breed female' for she had abandoned his immediate company, remained in the same range for four days and then struck again near a village called Nairosa.

The story of what had happened was amazingly queer. A group of women was going about their daily routine in the morning, when they found a tiger feeding on a *langoor* monkey that it had just killed or perhaps found dead. They didn't know it was the man-eater, as they stopped and raised an alarm. To their surprise instead of running away the tiger looked up and took a few steps towards them and came up to an irrigation channel that flowed between them. It was not correct to disturb a predator on its meal, especially when he had started making demonstrations and advances towards them.

The intimidated women turned about and started moving away from the place when suddenly the tiger rushed through a mustard field and caught hold of a girl that had lagged behind. But the scene was witnessed by no less than a dozen cane strippers who raised a commotion and rushed out with spears in their hands, and the tiger was forced to abandon the girl.

This incident pronounced three important points. The man-eater was constantly crossing Sharda and alternating between Paraspur and Kaanp Tanda agricultural fields in an attempt to rationalize an existence which was increasingly interjected by constant chase. By confidence and persuasion, essentially a nocturnal animal had now begun to operate during daylight hours, and that, it had half way abandoned eating a *langoor* and grabbed a human. It is likely that the tiger considered humans just another form of monkey or ape that is part of their species' normally extended menu.

This is a point where cold analysis falters. It is difficult to label this act just as 'aggressive behavior'; perhaps it has something to do with the taste of human flesh. However, if tigers are not inveterate homicidal, then their natural instinct does not instruct them this kind of killing. I think unless the tiger is seriously hungry, injured or sick this aggressive behavior may have some interim survival value but leaving a meal half-eaten and going for a human kill does not ensure any survival value in evolutionary terms.

This was more like the behavior of a steady man-eater than just a novitiate in the game. Old timers believed that once a consistent killer becomes stuck on human flesh then it prefers only human meat than any other. I have even known confirmed man-eaters to charge through the herd of cattle to get at the herdsmen. Some tigers that accidentally discover human vulnerability are not averse to include the species into their prey list. These are vulnerable to take up to steady man-eating.

The tiger lingered briefly in the trans-Sharda area, successfully evading the fiery barrage of lead from engineers and then crossed back to his previous haunts.

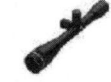

For Delectability of Human Flesh

The major problems in the world are the result of the difference between how nature works and the way people think.

- Gregory Bateson

Tigers attempt to capitalize on their chances of finding prey by focusing their search efforts in areas where their prey tends to concentrate in good numbers. The man-eater was never absent from Kaanp Taanda for long. It was an area intensively used by humans and almost every day somebody from us had always spotted it. People were even able to anticipate his movements for he entered the village towards evenings, circling its lanes and by-lanes without killing any cattle that were essentially tied at the door of every hutment.

Winters were intense and this had made the chase both protracted and wearisome. The fields lay covered with lifted fog that would reduce the temperature further by 2 to 3 degrees. The sun came far to the south, glowing palely beyond

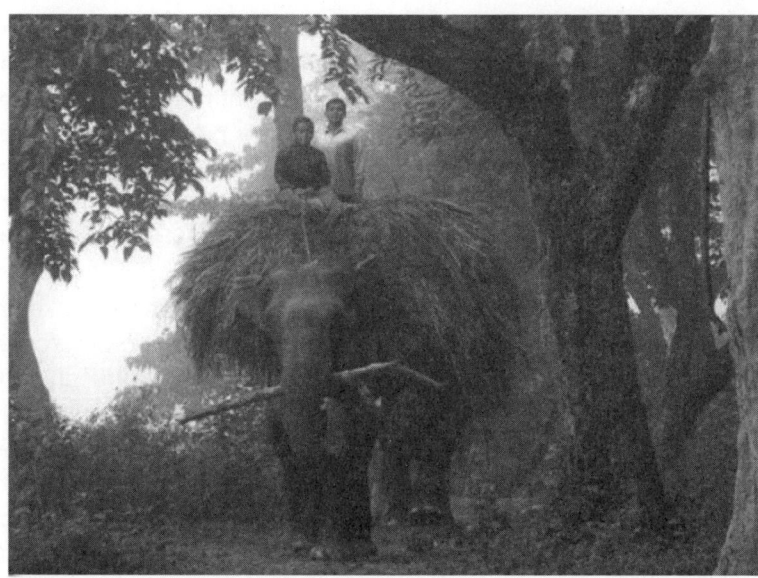

Elephants bringing their
fodder from the jungle

the mist, rising shadowlessly to the mid-sky and setting colourless and almost imperceptible, as if God was smoking to produce such a sunset.

On February 26, the sky was clear when around 4 pm we closed upon the village of Dakshin Tanda. We had approached it within a hundred yards when a guard signaled me to stop and showed me the spoors of the tiger leading towards the village. The village was all silent and certainly unaware that the people there were in real danger for the killer had decided to menace them tonight. We followed the spoor, approaching the village on the assumption that the man-eater was still there. All five of us readied our guns and entered the village in dead silence, taking advantage of every bit of cover we could find. Not a soul was seen moving about anywhere, not a sound indicated the existence of human beings. It looked a ghost village where every resident was wiped out by some deadly plague. Just a few wisps of blue smoke emerging through thatched rooftops indicated that the evening meal was being prepared where people had all ready locked themselves inside with doors tightly closed.

One safe bet in tiger tracks is to follow them for ample time and you will eventually arrive at the tiger unless the tiger arrives at you. We crossed the first line of hutments, when looking towards the far end of the village I suddenly became aware as if somebody was watching us and voila! He was there.

A leopard in a village may sound normal but a tiger's entrance in the village is not part of normal state of affairs. There can be nothing that so chills the blood with horror as the sight of a sinister brute deliberately seeking a human prey.

The tiger was standing near the grassy wall of a hutment, looking for a weak point to enter. He understood the relationship between humans and their hutments or perhaps he had always understood for he was a man-eater. He had become aware of our approach and seemed to smell the air as if it had picked up our scent. Encounters with tigers incite reflexive reaction and in a moment the gun freezes on the shoulder. My hand instinctively went on the trigger of my heavy caliber, while perhaps due to the experience of falling down the knoll and facing the barrage of fire, the animal instinctively recognized the guns. He faltered at my gesture and before I could properly train my sights, he was gone – like ectoplasm vanishing into space.

Night in the equatorial region doesn't fall, it positively plummets. Soon the darkness fell but we continued to search for the tiger inside the village with the aid of torches. The snorting ruminant gurgles of the cattle were very soothing sounds and the smell of their fresh dung was so overpowering, herby and natural in an odd way that I liked it. It reflected that the smell had not changed in the Tarai for centuries because no artificial fodder had been introduced to pollute its ancient ways.

The young juvenile was a true man-eater. It was obvious from his dangerous familiarity with humans that had impelled him to boldly enter the villages, like a cat loitering at the mouth of a mouse hole to claim its food on a grand, sinister scale knowing well that mice are bound to come out. Similarly for him the meaning of a human being had no bigger purpose beyond its potential as prey.

We started for the camp-site, carefully avoiding passing too close to the thickets of sugarcane and clumps of bush that might conceal the killer crouching in wait behind it. Man-eater hunting is a terrible job that continues to flutter in your stomach like so many bats; and to know the tigers' competences thoroughly is what makes you fear it thoroughly. Tigers can see and detect the movements of their prey under extremely low light levels; therefore in total darkness you never know when they come close to you. Tiger's soft padded feet allow it to feel the substrate and avoid crumpling leaves helping it walk unbelievably silently. His whiskers allow it to touch and feel objects close to its forequarters, giving it the ability to sense its way in darkness and absolute silence through dense cover. This exceptional perception of touch enables an animal of that size to get close to his quarry without a sound.

We were hunting the tiger and he being a man-eater, was just as certainly hunting us too. We had forethoughts and strategy and he had the tactics of surprise. It was a game in which neither could afford to make the slightest error, which would mean not only the end of the game but the end of the one that made it.

The cold silence pervaded all around the place and with fog having intensified; the distances had lost their perspective. It was horrifying to know that tigers also use fog as cover to stalk the game. Remembering the sophistication of man-eaters' thought process, the way he had come out to check our departure after we had collected Ram Rati's remains, I thought that though the killer had already proven that he had no natural fear of man, but it is this very fearlessness that gives the hunter an edge.

Next day, we learnt that the tiger had not gone out of the village. He had in fact entered a cattle enclosure and spent long nocturnal hours in it. I had a hard time believing it till I myself saw his defecation at two ends of large pen, following which he sat amongst one 150 head of herded cattle. Respecting the compact, excessive density of cattle, he never attempted to raid them nor did the cattle create any flutter. Both lounged peacefully at a reasonable distance without disturbing each other. I am sure the livestock that regularly goes inside the jungle to graze grows familiar with the carnivores' smells, which like many other smells, is a part of this landscape. And when cattle, by some good fate, don't acquire any experience of aggression from this agency, they turn complacent to a great degree against danger just as human beings do. Their instincts of self-defense dilute and a kind of recklessness and carelessness seems to grow on them, which makes them behave unworried. This also explains why people as well as cattle whose anti-predatory responses tend to be casual are so easily killed by carnivorous animals.

I cursed my stupidity for not checking the cattle pen though we had passed by it quite a few times and Kailash had dimly perceived a cow sitting aloof at the far end of the pen, which was in fact the tiger.

It is said that man-eaters are engineered by human delinquencies but my experience of Kaanp Tanda tells that unless it is possible to excise particular areas for wildlife and allow them to remain inviolate, association with humans and their domestic livestock creates an exceedingly subtle impact on tigers and is therefore more lethal in its final consummation. There are some logically delinquent tigers, who by the process of familiarization with human life style anomalously engineer human doom at first opportunity. The defecation indicated that tiger had staked the claim not only on the pen but to the entire village premises and all the live weight it contained.

The old treatise *Mragaya-Mayank* (The Hunter's Moon) of Balrampur Raj tells that "Man-eaters are shrewd learners through process of observation and they are in their own way quite analytical about events. They can assimilate much information, ascribe it to a source, absorb and remember relevant data about easy meal and learn from their experience, accidental or otherwise. If they produce successful results, fulfilling tiger's motives, they will seek to live through such situations repeatedly and never hesitate to add humans to their kitty."

The tiger had finally moved out towards morning, initiating a game of nerves. He was seemingly asserting that Tarai belonged to him and gladly letting us know that this was his home turf.

This was a particularly challenging hunt and there was no shortage of drama which shed a different light on every aspect of legendry predator. Tigers are capable of very perplexing behavior. Inherent and designing man-eaters are a class by itself. Behavior patterns of predators with man-eating urge are classified as aggressive, lusty, adventurous and eventually circumstantial. To my mind this tiger represented the adventurous category, which is an aberration of the highest kind. Every interaction with this radical animal gave us great formative experience on a different scale. For example his tracking style revealed not only his condescension towards human beings but also the immense power and confidence in which normal fear of the two-legged animal was overruled by contempt.

The tiger continued to base himself near the village for a couple of days. Since it was now entering the village, it was important to warn that nobody should be found outside his hut after dusk. I asked why the hell should people loiter outside when there was a known man-eater in the vicinity? I even announced that anybody found wandering in or around the village premises during the night would be shot as the man-eater, so better keep yourself and your children inside. But the answer of a man to my threat completely bowled me over. He said, "Sahib, it is hell of a time when you are sitting in the dark wondering what to do. Our imagination runs riot. It feels as if something big and dreadful is going to burst through the frail grass walls and grab you. And when this feeling grows stronger you feel like opening the door and bolting out even if danger lurks outside. Sahib, we will go out."

My curt sentences had a temporary effect on people. A grocer named Ram Dayal said he was mortally afraid of tigers and had shut himself into the hut for over a month except for going to the loo. It is certainly spooky how some people seem to get singled out for attacks by killers as this time the slain man was none other than Ram Dayal. The man was passing through a path flanked by canes when without a warning the killer swarmed over his upper body. Wedging a point blank charge in his normal stride and with a crush of fangs into his neck and shoulder, he quickly dragged him off. Unlike the claws of wolf or bear that are predominantly designed for digging and traction, tiger's anchors are like fine surgical tools that become slashing blades when pressed into flesh of victim that is not so much sliced as is shredded like a tattered cloth. Within matter of seconds Ram Dayal was dead meat as the scissor-shaped incisors sheared away the body and the man-eater ate huge chunks of meat from buttocks and thighs, chewing with the side of his muzzle until his face and chest were covered with the dark gore.

On hearing the news I went out with rangers to collect the remains. The pool of dried blood on the crusted blanket where the man had received his fatal hit was very saddening. My sympathies went out to those unfortunate people being killed owing to our ineptitude when every valid reason was there to shoot the culprit. Ram Dayal's torn body lay covered with mud, with eyes wide open, lip cut and teeth bare with a grinning expression of unendurable agony. I doubt if men killed thus by tigers can ever appear sleeping peacefully. Most of the corpses I have recovered from killers' dens in sugar-fields look hideously traumatized.

The expression of intense predatory fear that I witnessed in the eyes of Ram Dayal was so authentic and so unfeigned that it filled me with primal fear. I felt a sudden overpowering aversion to tigers that was peculiarly eccentric. I had never

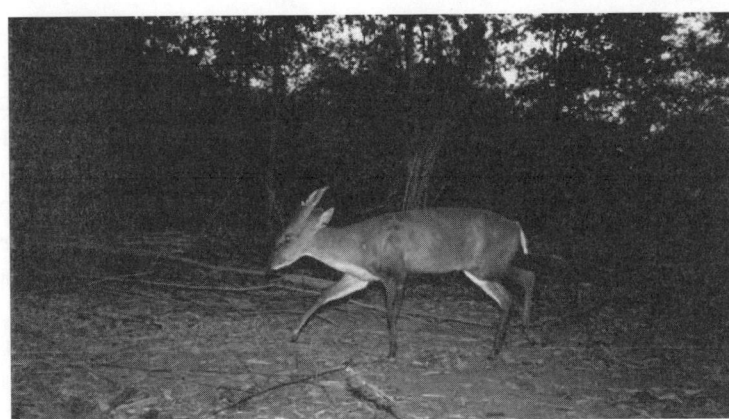

The barking deer also called Muntjac keep to more or less thick vegetation and come out to graze in the outskirts and open clearings fairly didiurnalay

previously experienced such a strange numbness of mind, despite the fact that I had recovered quite a few human corpses, half and almost fully eaten by tigers and the dread of the grieving villagers huddled in their huts, with the piercing and lonesome cry of women weeping for their dead, on cold nights. Ram Rati or Ram Dayal's fate could easily be our own, had our strong social network that exoskeleton of technology called 'firearm' had not been there to safeguard ourselves. I patted my gun and felt overtly contented that its twin barrels contained nearly 10, 000 pounds of wallop. I am not the squeamish type but you do think this way when you have just finished collecting a man remains in a plastic sack. I wondered if the authors who had first coined the phrases 'as cruel as a tiger' or 'as bloodthirsty as a tiger', which brought them into universal circulation, had witnessed similar occurrences.

The sky had turned grey. The funeral pyre of tiger victim burnt far away with the leaping flames casting gloomy shades all around. The dark lumbering shapes of park elephants and mourners silhouetted against it. They were seemingly concerned with nothing but the scourge and curse of the land where people yield life but others stay on bolstered by the fact that they have nowhere else to go. The singular thought in our mind was that if anything went wrong and the man-eater strikes again then anyone from us might be reduced to a simple corpse, mortified and debased like the one that was being burnt.

The very night a terrific rainstorm raged over the vista, lightning cracked incessantly in all directions and along with it we heard nothing but great rain-lashed wind which beat upon our shelter like sea waves, making straight for the open slits of our windows and freezing us in the bed. Earth, air, fire and water, the four cardinal elements seemed to have gone mad in the nature's fury, especially that stirring experience of blinding flash, followed by a first rate exhibition of fireworks exploding in the sky. How comfortably we take them for granted in our moderate urban homes but how brutally they can assert their despotic power in this land of Tarai.

A couple of days later when the water had dried and the roads became motorable, I was passing through a less travelled road that was known to be used frequently by the man-eater. The shades of evening were longer and the crickets chirping, when I suddenly saw a tiger sitting calmly in the sugarcane. I stopped the vehicle. I had no doubt that we had been in his full view and he was hearing through our noisy discussion. I picked up the rifle, and peeping through the telescopic sight studied the fellow closely for some trace of irritability but it went on gazing at us calmly. Behind me, were half a dozen villagers, sitting expectantly, eagerly awaiting the act of vengeance what they obviously regarded as a score to be settled.

Ishwar Chand was garrulous. "Shooting him is the right way out. They won't shoot it until it has eaten ten people," he mumbled. "Yes," the natives responded. "It will not be called a man-eater until it has scored that number." They asked me – rather, dared me – whether I would bust him or not, for buying time now could mean further loss of human lives.

The sun was sinking just above the tiger and none of us were sure about the identity of the beast. I examined the animal carefully through Nikon Buckmaster 3x9x40 camo rifle scope casually aiming at where I thought the animal's heart would be, but gently held the fire. The tiger, a male with massive forequarters was facing me placidly and his apparent harmlessness was disconcerting. With flies buzzing incessantly around him and many scars and wounds slashed across his muzzle, he never showed the slightest sign of unbecoming behavior.

The natives were grumbling. "Who will be responsible for further deaths? The foresters must feed their wives and children to this tiger to achieve the score! Some of us could as well turn crazy and catch them, beating the hell out of them. Crap..." Their angst was palpable at my reluctance to give in.

Though my tiger time in the Tarai has made me accustomed to the anger and snide remarks of the crowd, but at that moment pressed by their will, I must have aligned the gun quite a few times, rationalizing that hunting man-eaters is hunting in its purest form. With the memory of Ram Rati and Ram Dayal's grotesque remains hovering in my mind, I was confused with rising adrenaline and enhanced alcohol-driven energy. Alcoholism, incidentally, is a cultural norm of the Tarai and I had dabbled in it that day. It had made me imagine that my reputation was at stake, and so was the credibility of my gun and telescope. This nasty predicament lasted for some time in my mind but then suddenly I felt a jolt as I returned to myself – and to sanity.

It is not that the old sport killing is still deeply entrenched in my psyche, in fact a hunter has to be highly selective, because eliminating a member of extinction-threatened species (although justifiable in extenuating circumstances like self-protection) is a crime. Wild tigers are chattels and diddling with them means landing in a whale of soup with the government where no benefit of doubt works to your advantage. It is a legal problem that may cost you your job if it does not remove the cause of resentment amongst tiger traumatized citizenry of the area. However, the tiger was giving us the thrills and something was telling me inside that it is not the genuine man-eater.

For the next ten minutes the scene remained unchanged then I lowered my rifle and handed it to Neta. The great predator also thought that mutual inspection was finally over and he lethargically rolled on to his back and with paws in the air, giving a dime to us.

Ishwar Chand was naturally disappointed doubting if the peaceful tiger was not the murderer that I had allowed to live. It is not easy to leave people who place implicit faith in you against the ravages of an aberrant predator. Nevertheless they accepted my view point, that man-eaters being relentlessly pursued do not behave this imprudent way. You can't out-tiger a man-eater this way on his own terrain.

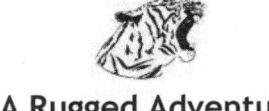

A Rugged Adventure

"A tigress is most likely to demonstrate but is easily turned away and if a tiger once demonstrats he is more likely to charge and charge home than tigress"

-A.A Dunbar Brander

Darkness works as a stimulant for predatory animals. Once the evening set in, the man-eating tiger was almost a different animal and I am sure he had a reason for it. In the darkness large predators believe themselves to be invisible. They feel safe because of the difficulty anybody would have in spotting them and their reflexes sharpen. It is a time which offers the greatest danger from the felines. In the advantage of night, the soft-padded man-eater can walk through fields noiselessly, enter into human settlements and come upon their quarry unexpectedly.

It was late winter now and the tiger was still operating in the vicinity. As the dusk fell, a hush fell in the village. The entire village community that lived in fragile hutments was gripped by terror as they realized how defenseless they were before a stubborn tiger which intentionally sought human prey. The village vigilance committees were on alert. They had the knowledge that the tiger had been without meal for quite a few days and it would certainly strike again at the first opportunity presented.

In the chill of that foggy evening I was lying in my tent. Nearby a campfire burnt brightly. Tea was boiling, and Neta was in great vein, giving the events of previous days a through going over when the cultivation fields to my north resounded with the frightened cries of alarm. A spotted deer hind, munching on wheat crops screamed the preliminary warning, *Aiow! Aiow! Aiow!!* in her sharp and whistle like sound. It was taken up by a peacock roosting somewhere on a bough. It squawked in the unique two-toned siren. The farmland was alarmed and alert. Where there is menace of a man-eating tiger, the carefree blithe feeling gives way to intense awareness. You may call it a 'premonition of death' for the tiger was out on hunting: going to kill someone.

This alerted Mohan, a member of the protection team. He moved his torch all around and from under a mango tree besides the barn, a pair of lambent eyes reflected the glare. His friends immediately set fire to the pile of grass to take a better view of the animal. It was none else than the man-eater which had arrived to take its toll.

Conventional wisdom says that tigers nurture a fear complex against man, which has been passed down over timeless generations of inter-relations between two species. But here the tiger was in direct spatial competition with man. Instead of getting disturbed by the shock operation, it came out boldly in the open within sight of five other men who were sitting on a cot next to their hutments. The men raised alarm as several others came out of their homes for assistance, ensuing lusty and frenzied commotion that drove the tiger away.

Then an uncanny silence followed that seemed almost to vibrate with evil. Although I could give no reason why it should feel so, except that I suspected that the tiger was approaching. I am not of nervous nature and I was seriously out to deal with the man-eater and this was no reason. But darkness definitely makes me weak as I have already said a certain percentage of my boldness disappears with daylight.

At the same time, a quarter of mile away from my camp a woman named Anita and her niece covered with a quilt had gone behind their thatched hutment to relieve themselves. Why they had committed such a reckless act is not explicable, as everyone was aware that the man-eater was in the habit of systematically proceeding from dwelling to dwelling and any person stepping outside would be ringing a dinner bell for him. The women kept the oil lamp on the ground, when suddenly the tiger appeared from the darkness and seized Anita with the quilt, grabbing her by the shoulder. The cat sank its fangs through the meat and bone and started pulling her on the ground.

The girl screaming in alarm ran towards the village while the victim's cry rose in crescendo into the most blood-curdling shriek of pure terror: *Bachao, bachao, baghwa pakris* (Help help; the tiger has caught me), echoing hollowly through the stygian darkness. The lusty cry was caught up from house to house and not long before pandemonium reigned everywhere. The protection team instantly ran for her rescue.

The women's husband immediately started his tractor and began to chase the tiger going a few meters behind it. The women was screaming and fighting hard. Clamped in the jaws of her attacker she scratched and ripped its face with her nails, pulled his ears and continued her battle soaked in her own blood. She hurled abuses and cried for help. She was alive by the fact that her upper body was still covered with the quilt and the quilt was dragging along.

The big cat covered a furlong then feeling troubled with the tractor roaring behind him and also from its victim's continuous resistance, tried to shift the grip from shoulder to neck. He kept the women on the ground, and hooking his claw in to her belly, leaned upon her to grab her throat when she threw the quilt upon the cat's face and tried to blind it. She was doomed if she did this and damned if she did not. The big cat caught her arm through the quilt and pulled her inside a dense sugarcane plot.

Within minutes another salvaging party arrived with three more tractors on the spot. One was driven by the owner of the sugarcane crop where the tiger had hauled the woman. The man did not hesitate to flatten his standing crop with a leveling plank attached to his tractor and open up a few lanes for a better visibility. Soon the tiger was located and from all the sides the headlights focused on him; it was now pulling on the woman by feet. The drivers screaming very unprintable phrases quickly brought their machines near the animal and almost sandwiched him in between.

The sounds of commotion reaching our camp could only mean that an attack by the tiger was in progress. I could hear the men and women shouting lustily. Grabbing my eight-cell flashlight and bandolier of ammunition, I stuck a pair of soft points in my .400 HV Jeffery's Express double barrel rifle, flipped up the ivory night-bead sight and running a quarter of mile, lateral Arabesques ,when on gaining the spot, I found my gun about as much use as a tennis racket in my hands, for its night bead colliding with some hard object had tilted to one side and a chance shot with the weapon in such odd circumstances may have wounded the tiger and thus aggravated the trouble. Though the gun was dunked with hyper-lethal bullets and shot in every sense of word would have been a positive 'sitter' but it was quite difficult to sight the rifle in the dark, when the half-circle of people stood in the backdrop of man-eater. With a broken night bead, the fear of endangering people's life was imminent in case I miss the target.

The tiger was now bold and not ready to relinquish its quarry. His gaze was still and resolute. A threatening rumble emanating for his chest caverns kept the crowed shuffling 10 to 15 feet backwards. In that particularly dark night, his wicked blood-shot eyes peering over foot high undergrowth positively scintillated with devilment. When challenged, it kept holding the victim in its jaws but yet gave a terrific demonstration of snarling to the rescue party which raised an explosive din at the top of its voice. Luckily a spear thrown at the beast hit it in the back and the tiger turning to bite it, dropped the lady from its mouth. Her husband instantly parked the tractor over her, bringing her between the wheels that provided her a protective covering.

The animal hovered around with purpose looking for the chance to grab her once again. Blood was dripping down its foreleg as it moved issuing very impressive A-R-R-O-U-N-G-H followed by a number of angry snarls AR-R, AR-R, AR-R that could freeze the plasma in one's vain. His behaviour was fitful; he was even awkwardly licking his right foreleg and knee. First we thought that some thorns was embedded but soon we realized that it was the blood on his body that was not his but was of the lady that he was licking. By this time over a hundred men had gathered in a fever of excitement and their morale was high. With their hackles raised like a fighting cock more tractors pushed ahead when tiger sensed danger and disappeared in the dark.

The entire right shoulder of the unfortunate woman had been smashed, there were lacerations on the neck as well as a small throat wound but the windpipe was intact. She had suffered a good deal from the shock and loss of blood. She sat on the ground in the puddle of her own blood but refused to accept that she could have really died in the fang-hold of the tiger.

Still shaking from the effects of 700 yard wind sprint I had made, and realizing that there was no time to lose, Kailash and I followed the beast in the dread of the night. The fog was getting dense and it was bitterly cold. Several armed guards joined the search with intensified longing to get this tiger as soon as possible. It was bush country with plenty of reed all around that was too wet to be set on fire so we stalked the tiger from one clump to another.

Every tiger has its heavy acrid odour and this one exuded a rank and musky smell that we felt with changed winds. Now and then we caught the glimpse of his golden yellow hide in flashlights and his flashing eyes floating through the wreaths of fog as he slipped behind the trees and undergrowth. We crept forward soundlessly and almost imperceptibly. The distance separating us could not have been much more than 30 yards but it made for an almost fearsome atmosphere in the tight confines of the night where squeezing the trigger seemed a futile gesture. Unfortunately the reeds became longer as we proceeded and prevented over vision. Finally we were compelled to abandon the chase. A few peacocks calling in a scolding retort indicated the tiger's passageway through the *narkul* grass. For long time afterwards nothing more was heard.

In the meanwhile Om Prakash took the lady to Bhira government dispensary, where after immediate first aid attention and penicillin injection against likely infection from putrefied meat found under tiger's claw and teeth, she was carried 200 km to King George's Medical College in Lucknow. The doctors saved her life with four bottles of blood and many more million units of intravenous penicillin. Her recovery was remarkably rapid. She is definitely one of very few, incredibly lucky people who have come out alive from the grip of a super predator. When I asked her in the hospital how she felt in the jaws of tiger she claimed to have sensed no pain. It is quite likely that people or animals caught by predators are drugged in a state of

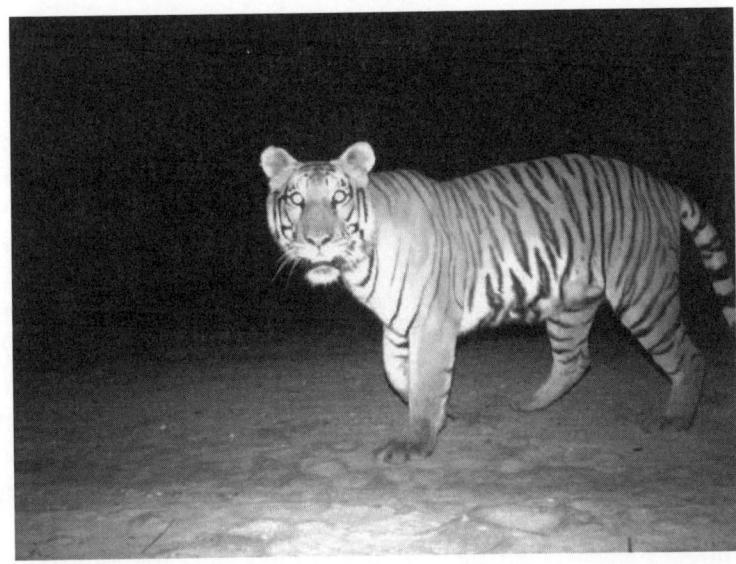

Tigers cut a magnificent picture in the night. Its worth a sight to see at least once in life. (*Photo credit : NTCA*)

terror-induced anesthetization and they never show an indication of pain. Even wild dog victims that are literally eaten alive as live slabs of flesh are ripped out of their body don't feel pain and the death is normally mercifully quick.

The woman's health has deteriorated. She claims to feel feverish all the time, with her normal body temperature scaling over 99. She feels heat, rage and growls sometimes as if temporarily affected by some mysterious rabies. Perhaps all this is a psychological disorder the result of a terrible memory she carries in her mind.

To be caught by a tiger is a singularly malicious way to have your overdose of the Tarai.

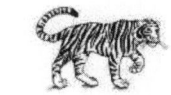

The End of the Affair

"I never heard of a successful programme where an established man-eater has been relocated and rehabilitated in the jungles. I credit such attempts as being too risky in terms of human lives as they generate public outcry and hatred towards tiger, pitting native communities against the ethics of conservation. Of course different from the Nazi terminology, the imprisonment of tiger is the only 'Final Solution'.

- Author on Kaanp-Tanda Man-eater, in a conservationists meeting at Dudhwa National Park Headquarters.

By this time the first huge beautiful tigress no 5 that had crossed Lucknow and Barabanki was shot dead at Faizabad district. It was disastrous that the simpler and irresponsible solution of destruction was adopted for her without meeting the requirements of "stating the reasons thereof."

The capture of a tiger involves skillful persuasion and patience and when you fail to remedy the situation you shoot. And when the operative decision lies solely with CWLW as final authority only bad managers play the last card as first option over priorities of conservation. Instead of issuing orders for a scoring man-eater of Kaanp Tanda, he had got a young healthy tigress killed. It also tells that poor managers use their powers as authorized dispatcher to pronounce the death sentence for a Schedule One animal because they lack official commitment and sympathy for the cause of endangered species.

My campaign to 'Save Men from Tigers' had helped me visualize that such decisions are made through default or inertia while the cultivation of 'Conservation Will' results in increased levels of forbearance towards carnivores by local people and promotes a viable path towards coexistence. Unfortunately instead of addressing this line of approach, news bulletins were flooded with the reports about the tyranny of tiger and any reaction on the part of people could bring death to other tigers that were sharing the safer heaven of sugarcane in the area.

Panic was at its height in the anti-tiger campaign and the actual fulcrum of my intervention to capture this wild cat safely was repeatedly failing. The word had gone out that I was conniving with foresters by sparing the tiger's life each time. The village chief along with a number of villagers held me personally responsible for Anita's episode and so was Ram Rati's husband who was having a mental breakdown as a result of her wife's death. He knew for years as Honorary Warden of the Sanctuary so he constantly blamed me and my team for his tragic loss. The situation was no longer a safety issue for tiger or men, even the Forest Department's credibility was at stake. I feared that this confusion might result in setting a death trap for the tiger or the poisoning of some meat bait, as the priority was to let the humans live in peace. I had great apprehensions that if something was not done quickly this tiger was going to die the same evil way in which the Dhaurarah leopard had been done away in October 2008.

❖

Having spent a long tiger time in Tarai, I have not only witnessed the misery of people, living aside predators but also travelled through a time warp, visiting remote pockets with danger at my elbow, where a lot more of Tarai got into my blood stream than its malaria. I understand its pulse and when there is no way for people to leverage out of such situations they strike with vengeance. History records that during 80s and 90s, their rebellion against government's moratorium on hunting had put a more daunting array of predators to rest in peace by poisoning, trapping and even with their ungodly guns, the muzzle loaders.

This particular beast had injured 6 women, killed four men, three children and preyed upon fifty cattle in Dhaurarah sugar-fields, namely in Pundit Purva, Bela Haar and Sisaiya villages. The case-hardened offender seemed to have realized that humans were unable to defend their cattle and they could be picked right from

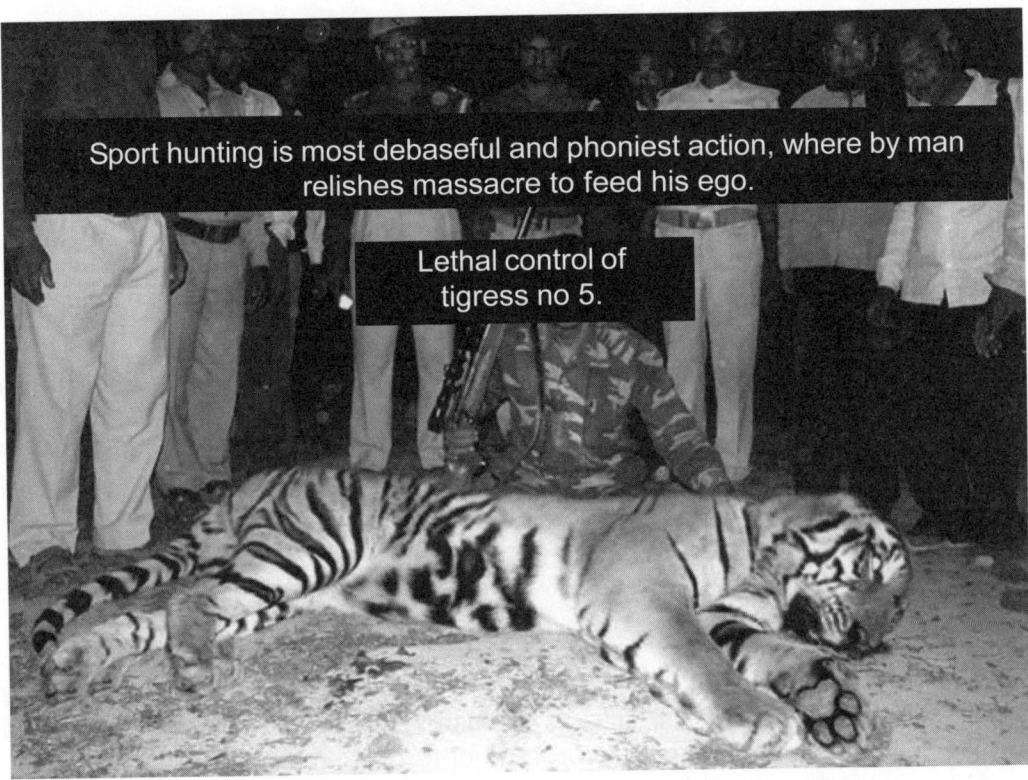

Sport hunting is most debaseful and phoniest action, where by man relishes massacre to feed his ego.

Lethal control of tigress no 5.

their doorstep. Day after day he snatched pets and injured people, when on the call of Chief Wildlife Warden, M. Ahssan, I went to assist the team to track and capture the animal.

The very evening, I was holding a council of villagers, orienting them as how to deal with predators within farmlands when a forester came running to me with the news that the leopard had just killed a girl but was brought to bay by a pack of five trained dogs, which belonged to a local landlord.

The place was just half a mile from the village. I picked up my magnum and rushed to the spot. We were midway when we saw two injured dogs coming towards village with their lacerated and bleeding faces. They took us back to the mangled bodies of the other three lying dead. It may look odd but one must perforce admire the thoroughness of an irritated leopard, for all the three dogs had been disemboweled so badly, limb by limb that all of them croaked within a short time while the jungle ninja had escaped.

Only next day it attacked a labourer duo, pulled out the intestines of the senior and tore open the scalp of another so that both had to get over a hundred surgical stitches. A leopard often allows people to pass close by him if he thinks people have not spotted him but the instant they stop or look towards the bush he is hiding, he dashes away or comes like lightning. A leopard can easily rip a man literally to ribbons, in a very few seconds. The labourers had committed the same mistake of stopping by him. The damage has to be seen to be properly estimated and believed.

(Such kind of aggression in which the leopard rushes out of concealment without warning, and mauls some unfortunate victim and then decamps without making a meal of it is certainly complicated. I have no explanation for this bizarre conduct; it is something unique unless it is some kind of infection like rabies. But I am not qualified to discuss that because I never heard of mauled victims developing the disease.)

Stealing of a predator's kill leads to increased natural predation rates and makes it more troublesome. A week after this incident I was going to Pundit Purva where a trap cage had been set, I crossed a small patch of grass and tree forest where I happened to discover the withered remains of a black buck. A pile of neck hair with half-chewed innards and crushed bone fragments of ribs indicated it to be a leopard's kill. The antelope was ambushed in the night, party eaten on the ground and moved away. I glanced around for a suitable tree into which the leopard might have stashed the buck to place it out of the reach of jackals and other competitors and there it was, on a Dhak (Butea-monosperma) tree. The natives taking advantage of an easy meal held upon a tree wanted to grab it for their pots but seeing the rangers eyeing them sternly, they lost courage and came along. However, appropriation of predator kills, if it is a wild animal and the killer is incautious enough to leave it in the open is a normal practice of natives.

While returning the same way at evening I crossed the tree again. The tree looked strangely empty; the buck had gone. I examined the ground and discovered that it was the work of natives. Surreptitiously our guides had informed the location of kill on mobile phones and the miscreants had collected the carcass.

Three days later the spots, still going hungry was seen entering a barn. Local antagonism had already created serious management problems, hence no one informed the foresters and villagers quickly surrounded the barn and set it on fire. The trapped beast was charred to death in the leaping flames.

❖

Luckily by March the park elephants came back from Lucknow and were immediately employed in man-eater operation. Ashok Kumar, the vice chairman of Wildlife Trust of India (WTI), New Delhi had sent Anjan Majumdar, a qualified expert of darting to deal with the problem.

On the day of reckoning the tiger was spotted near the river and was immediately surrounded by four elephants. The *howdah* elephants must be staunch and steady and must be ready to stand the threat of an angry tiger but at the growl of the tiger these turned unsteady and clustered closely, their bodies shivering with excitement. There was a danger of their bolting or dropping to that fast shuffling stride that elephants use when frightened, just over their first panic. They can walk at the

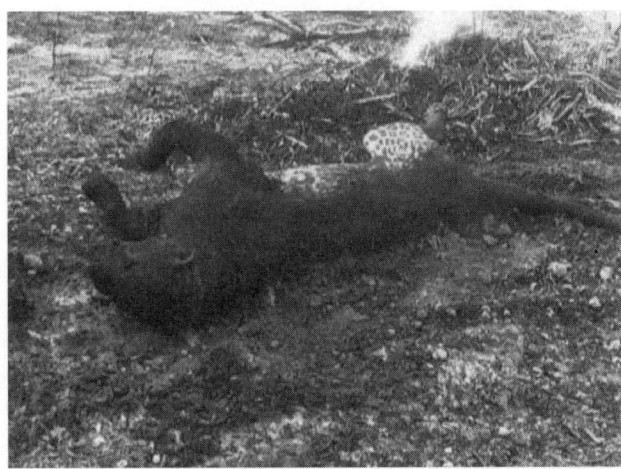

The charred carcass of marauding leopard. *(Photo credit : Abhishek Verma)*

approximate rate of six miles an hour but length of their stride is so extraordinary that in acute nervousness they can go about 20 miles in an hour.

The difficulty of finding staunch elephants is no doubt greater in present times than in the hunting era gone-by, when they were trained over the bodies of dead tigers to make them overcome their fear. Campbell, the old forest ranger, describes that elephants were later fed with the balls of sugar dipped in the blood of the tiger. This gave them an attraction to trample the predator under their foot and taste its blood.

However, the mahouts didn't let the pachyderms bolt. They were solely concerned with delivering the maximum number of stimulating blows to the stern of the beast upon whose back the vets were precariously perched. This kind of driving is not always unattended with risk for then the elephants huddled still closer and started rubbing their huge bodies with each other, this dangerous maneuver of the nervous beasts presents a threat to riders' safety. The foresters were busier in saving their legs and feet from getting chafed in between the grinding monstrous bodies than rounding the tiger.

The mahouts were putting hearts and brown into their job. Seeing the tense situation this exercise was justifiable, because in nervousness, the propensity to charge is the elephant's worst fault for it upsets the darter's aim. And if the elephant opposing the tiger kneels, as he may do in fear of mortification at the moment of determined rush attack, he may throw the occupants out of the *howdah* including the mahout who perches on the elephants neck.

The giants had their trunks risen in unison, issuing loud trumpeting, and all their nervous fidgeting presented a picturesque feature of the old days of sport – the splendid system of tiger hunting with elephants and shooting it in its midday retreat. However, amidst this chaos Anjan managed to fire a dart shot from a temporarily attained convenient commanding position, which took the target in the rumps. The tiger bolted inside the reed bed and fell some hundred yards away.

The anachronistic animal was in the bloom of good health and carrying on human genocide in an area where excellent populations of prey base was around.

Darwinian neurobiology links healthy man-eating carnivores to homicidal maniacs among men for indeed they just eat humans for the hell of it. A South African game ranger, Peter Turnbull-Kemp's table of man-eating lions tells that age and condition of 91 percent of man-eaters were fair or good when disposed of, 13.3 percent were aged but uninjured and only 4.4 percent were aged and injured.

Similarly Kaanp Tanda was a healthy man-eater, sleek and more than fit to pursue his normal food whose trail of violence and destruction had now come to an end. Needless to say trying to save a tiger is a formidable task, before the tranquillizer effect is diluted and the animal injures itself in its struggle to escape, its immediate deportation arrangements were made for Lucknow zoo. The news of capture had spread far and wide, a strong crowd of no less than 10,000 people poured out of various villages and farms to take a look at their tormentor. Most of them had never seen a tiger from so close, people patted it, spat on it, kicked its cage and abused it, while anesthetized by drug he simply stared impassively through the bars. It seemed like a fair for photographers and tourists from Dudhwa who had joined the melee.

Ram Rati and Ram Dayal's mother rendered a deep cry when they saw the tiger. They wanted to have it killed. Their cries touched my heart very deeply, making me feel sorry for their children.

Despite the calumny of the ferocious and blood-thirsty monster, with which the species is still burdened today, these hard-pressed animals are most fundamental expression of life on earth. They are worthwhile of conserving and making a cause for the life, worthwhile to battle for their existence, to cherish and raising funds; for their very awe-inspiring presence electrifies the atmosphere. I touched his unsheathed claws sharp as razorblade and even his fangs, yellowed but absolute sabers, curved with single cutting edge. It made my skin crawl and I liked it. The wrought physical vigor with which I had so doggedly pursued this mighty predator, I had actually drawn from it; and perhaps in some intriguing measure, I also partly belong to their world as a well-wisher.

The sky was turning from amber to deepest bronze with gathering darkness – when the truck carrying the outlaw left for Lucknow zoo. As my Gypsy King followed the vehicle, I couldn't help thinking that this magnificent creature of untamed wilderness and sugar Savannah had met this fate simply by the fact that unlike other tigers who were simultaneously sharing his own ground, he was disoriented with the nuances of living in agrarian area and had been wrongly thrust into the proximity of mankind. Instead of fulfilling natural survival functions and giving wide latitude to man it had yielded priority to making them his meal.

I knew that besides this man-eater, there were two other tigers inhabiting the same terrain but these seemed experienced fellows, the self-oriented ones; they never created any problem and continued to live genuinely in the safe sanctuary of farmlands.

MAN-EATERS CALLING

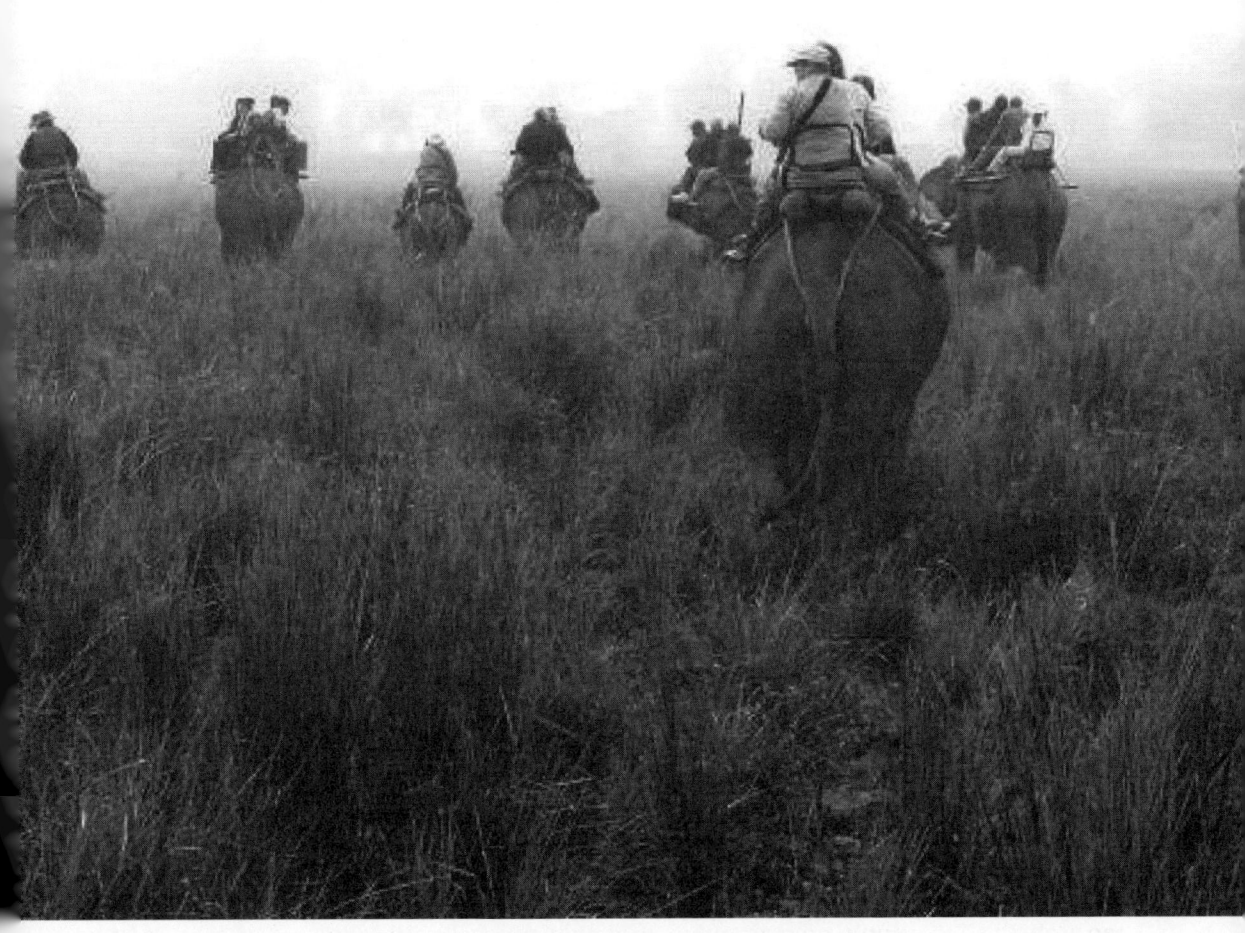

CHAPTER 8
THE MAN-EATING TIGRESS OF MORADABAD

Chapter 8

The Man-Eating Tigress of Moradabad

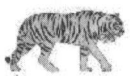

Because of much greater concern for human welfare that exists in all societies, usually wildlife gets eliminated if the conflict goes unresolved. For example, over last few centuries, most conflict-prone wildlife species in India have suffered range constrictions of over 90%.
- Ullas Karanth

SHE WAS DEFINITELY HIGH ON TESTOSTERONE BUT SHE WAS NOT LOOKING for a male to tantalize, tease and mate. She was rather deeply anguished, showing an angered hurry that she did not bat an eyelid before tearing six people into shreds and making mincemeat of them in a short span of 16 days. And then she vanished like ectoplasm, as suddenly as she had emerged, leaving behind not just a long trail of blood and gore but also a trail of half a-dozen enlisted sportsmen, all heavily armed, frantically following her pugmarks and also an army of angry people out to get her at any cost. In the end, her body unperforated by bullets, her limbs unmauled by traps and her whiskers intact, the marauding tigress of Moradabad had the last laugh.

This particular tigress made her appearance towards late December 2013 in the vast thickly populated region around the borders of the states of Uttar Pradesh and Uttarakhand. The single-minded vehemence with which this raging dynamo of energy went about her killing spree, pushing further and further into human zone, not only shook the national media but triggered the biggest ever operation by forest authorities in recent memory to nab a destructive killer.

The operation was a miserable failure but that is not the point. Rather, partially hidden in this narrative are some important questions which beg for an answer, and which I suspect do hold some crucial lessons for the entire wildlife fraternity that hopes to protect this lethal yet endangered species. My old associate Aftab Wali and his team members were continuously tracking the tigress for over 10 days and therefore I was privileged to have first-hand information about every twist and turn in the dramatic chase which ultimately turned futile but brought a great determinative experience.

But first, the facts. On December 26, 2013 the partly-eaten body of an unidentified man was found near Hasanpur village in Moradabad district. The village is about 200 km away from the Corbett Tiger Reserve's southward belt, the Jhima-Kalagarh division in Uttarakhand, and therefore nobody at the time thought of a possible connection between the carcass and a tiger. It was taken as a body thrown by a murderer that was later feasted upon by hyenas and jackals.

The second death took place three days later in Mithapur Muja village of Moradabad district. It was 28-year-old Vijay Singh on the outskirts of the village and tell-tale pugmarks of a tiger were found near the body. It sparked off a widespread alarm in the region.

Till then, the impression conveyed to the people was not necessarily the true realization of the actual danger involved but this discovery plunged the entire Moradabad district into inevitable panic within hours and also confounded the Forest Department of Uttar Pradesh. Dramatic encounters, life and death situations and the tiger's potent deadly charges became the talk of the city. Nobody in living memory had ever heard of a tiger roaming in the region. And here no ordinary tiger but a man-eater was moving, making people realize that they were nothing more than plain and simple food for her.

Without wasting any time the Divisional Forest officer Bonik Brahma assembled a team of foresters. He was not the man to sit idle when the house was on fire. Cages with live baits were strategically put up in the area and elephants and tiger experts with tranquilizing guns were brought from Dudhwa and Pilibhit forest ranges. The team deputed to deal with her comprised Aftab Wali Khan, Imtiyaz Siddiqui, a police officer from Sitapur, Wazir Hassan, Deputy Ranger, Jaipal, Pushpendra and a verternarian Dr Bharat Singh. vet

Apart from hyenas and pariah dogs no other animal ever approached the baits at night and all the traps remained empty. However, the tigress – for this is what the killer turned out to be eventually – was still giving them a wide berth. She had plans of her own. On January 5, 2014 she stuck at Changeri village again in Moradabad. Incidentally, this was her most audacious attack so far. The victim, 30-year-old Rajiv, was working on the edge of sugarcane fields with his father when the tigress pounced upon him from behind. The terrified father could do nothing to save his son, and by the time a large group of villagers arrived to claim the body, it had been dragged 300 meters inside the sugarcane fields and partially devoured. The killer had stripped the body of clothes and then eaten, showing more intelligence than the cannibals of Central Africa who cooked Christian Missionaries in their boots thinking that they grew on their feet.

When the rescue party reached the grim spot a flock of red fowls was clucking around the body as they racked their curved claws through the blood damp soil searching for meat scraps. They had not yet touched the body though the tigress was nowhere to be seen.

That night, in order to keep the spirits of the villagers high, the foresters tied a few baits at strategic points and stayed in Mithapur Muja village. Far away in the solitude of sugar fields the jackals let forth their weird howls. With a couple of shooting stars in the sky announcing bad luck, their hideous ululation told on people's nerves. In such an atmosphere the tigress called twice, a sort of monosyllabic *aoom* that wailed in the open air like the single note of a pipe organ forcing the jackals to fall silent. "We lit torches and walked down at the outskirts of the village, but she was in sugarcane cover that none of us could dare to comb. The tigress did not touch the baits that night and moved away," remembers Aftab.

The third killing was important for many reasons. While it did not establish the method in the killing madness of the tigress, it pointed out clearly the trajectory she was taking. She was now going back towards Uttarakhand border, from where she had presumably come. But why did she take the trouble of walking 200 km away from her home range to make the first human killing – a typically eerie behavior – and what prompted her sudden retreat? The answer to these questions would naturally come out with the unfolding of the story but first let's take a close look at macabre drama which had by now clutched the entire region in its grip.

By January 6, the tigress had become the talk of several towns in the district of Moradabad and adjoining Bijnore. A sense of menace emanated from the sugarcane fields, where people had stopped going. A sort of paralysis had set upon the area. It was as if the clock had turned back to some two centuries back where man and dangerous animals had lived this way only. Farmers stopped venturing into sugarcane fields and by sunset all houses were tightly shut from the inside. At night not a soul dared to venture out in the open. For the next seven days, the killer tigress occupied the front page of all newspapers of the area with other national and international news pushed inside.

At around the same time, the Forest Department pressed the panic button. Fear in the region had turned to anger and at several places villagers armed with guns and spears had started scouting the area in vigilante moves. Efforts to wean such animal from habits contrary to normal mode of existence are the matter of policy of the State Government. The Forest Department did not lose time in issuing a death warrant for the tigress, allowing teams of 6 hunters to move in and finish her off – if they could. It was this phase when on the invitation of District Magistrate Sanjay Kumar I reached Moradabad, finding it worthwhile to wear a pair of hunting boots for a short stint.

Sanjay is a passionate photographer while his wife Aparna, an IPS officer, is an ace mountaineer. She has recently hosted the Indian Tricolor and the UP Police Flag on Mount Everest, the world's tallest peak.

In the mean time, sporadic news of tiger movements poured in from various places. Wildly fanciful rumors also flew in the air. It was said that she was checking doors in the night and was found seeking entry through the windows in a farmhouse. Amidst these came news that an unknown man was seized and devoured among the cane breaks. Only a few blood stained rags were found in the morning and the tracks revealed that the tigress had been the culprit.

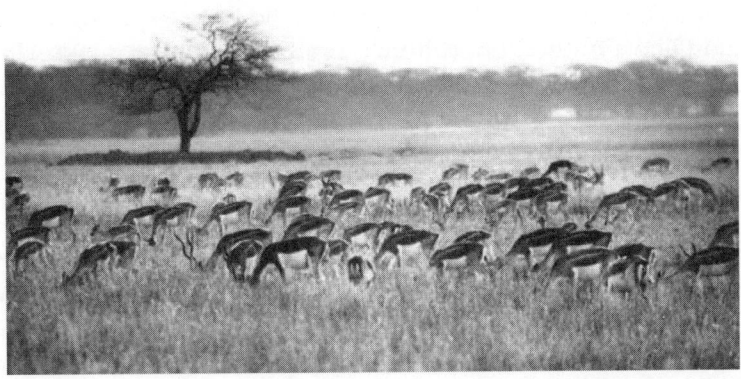

Black Bucks heard were plentiful in Moradabad during 1980s until a forest officer very fond of antelope kebab got posted there. By the time he left, black buck heards were almost eradicated under his patronage.

There was no record of her leaving any person in mauled condition. All the victims had died and were left half-eaten. She was rumored to roar and rush at the intruder, always charging with intent to kill, not merely to terrify or to prevent interference.

The tigress was permanently ill-tempered. She was eating humans and living on other prey too but in priority she seemed to stick to the diet of human flesh. Many thought that she was afflicted with some wound but this was doubtful as no grounds had been stated for the supposition and her footprints seemed normal. Thereafter, the tigress made two new headlines in quick succession. On January 7, she killed a six-year old girl, Shobha, near the sugarcane fields at Mallivala village and two days later, a woman Dulari was killed at Dariyapur village. Both had been half devoured.

Dulari was a 35-year-old fair and good-looking woman. Her features, eyes, her admirable young breasts required no artificial aids. Even so terrible a death could not blemish her beauty. The man-eater, in her usual habit, having eaten her haunches and thighs had left the upper body intact.

For years, humans have paid the price of doing business on tiger's terrain but now here was a tiger doing business on human terrain. This had awakened primal fears and made people conscious of the possibilities of being eaten by dangerous man-eating beast. Evolutionists call this "awareness of being meat", which is acknowledged among the earliest forms of human self awareness. This fear humbles us, make us aware of our mortality and that is why the human reaction against big predators is more direct and sharp than anything else.

The villagers were so paralyzed with fear that they refused to build a platform on the tree where the hunters wished to watch for her return. By now the tigress had turned for her home and was now inching closer to Uttarakhand. Each human death was causing a profound impact on people. I remember experiencing a creepy feeling when for the first time I saw her tracks at a pool where she had quenched her thirst. She was certainly the deadliest, the most determined and mightiest of man-eaters I had ever chased.

The situation was chaotic, communications were chaotic and it was no longer simply a security issue. The Forest Department's credibility was at stake. The villages in Uttar Pradesh situated close to Uttarakhand border now clearly fell in the danger zone. A newspaper report appeared with a nasty headline, "Man-eater scores while the foresters wrangle" and suggested that more people were destined to be killed. The word was getting around that Dulari was not the last.

Making peace with a killer tigress seemed a maddening idea and at the same time there was no way to forestall further human casualties. It is not possible to fix a period during which an uninjured, irate tiger, in a series of fits – that often make a domestic cat race round and round the room – can be considered fully dangerous, that is liable to charge at the sight of man. Though cats, if the series of fits continues, finally die dashing around the walls like those stunt motorcyclists riding the 'Wall of Death' but activists lack similar experience about tigers. Hence she seemed destined to be shot. It was most urgent to report the villagers to take precaution against her and avoid confronting her.

Reaching Moradabad I primarily took care to implement my programme of 'Saving men from Tigers'. Thousands of pamphlets were distributed in over 50 villages. The people were given firecrackers by the Forest Department and advised to not to venture alone after dusk for they scarcely knew about the predatory ways of attacks in closed environments that the sugarcane crops provided. The pamphlets also counseled people that the killer was heading towards Uttarakhand and they must stay clear of her path and avoid the welter of tall crops otherwise they would be a gift for the man-eater.

Incredible it may seem, nobody let alone any hunter or photographer who was alive, barring the third victim's father, had even seen the killer tigress, Her pugmarks on a blood splattered trail was all that the villagers, forest officials and the hunters had to contend with.

The next killing on January 10 took place barely 12 km from the jungles of Corbett Reserve. The victim 22-year-old Shiv Kumar of Mania-vali Garhi village could not prevent himself from becoming the sixth meal of the man-eating tigress. Like other victims, he too was working in a sugarcane field when the ravenous and ferocious tigress jumped at him with ruthless violence and feasted upon her ghoulish meal. Having done this, she abandoned the kill and moved out towards the *nala* side where during the midday she took a siesta in the sunlight and kept herself warm.

That late afternoon, a colorless sun was at the edge of the trees and fog had started to simmer over the landscape when Aftab and I reached the tract, daring what is commonly known as "tiger hunting on foot". Ram Dev, the then Director General of Police ATC Moradabad had provided me with sufficient police force carrying AK-47 and SLR's, and two private vehicles to assist in hunt. Shiv Kumar's body had been recovered, most of his buttocks and part of his side had been eaten away and a lot of dark blood had coagulated on the fallen leaves of cold and wet sugarcane.

An hour's search in sugar grass yielded nothing of tigress' whereabouts and then the sun set and the sky became flecked with bulbous clouds. A slight drizzle also started, making the conditions for shooting critically adverse.

Unaware that the tigress was resting in a thicket, we had reached extra close to her hide-out, when suddenly the air seemed dark and heavy with feline excrement. On sudden intuition, Aftab stopped and retreated quickly at a point (later we found at that time he was only eight yards from the tigress.) She produced a deep short *whoof* and rushed horizontally through the canes into another plot, continuing the loud *whoof, whoof, whoof.* The sugar crops shook swiftly by her gliding body. The cops took it to be the grunting of a wild pig while I and Aftab knew it without doubt that it was the tigress. The *whoof* usually constitutes a form of warning telling an intruder to keep his distance or face the consequences.

We at once halted in our tracks. Motioning back the men, we retreated to consider the situation as the contour of the terrain influences all hunting of dangerous animals. The visibility was less than ten yards and the possibility of an average shot was only fifteen yards in case one is lucky to determine which part of the animal's shadow-dappled hide makes him vulnerable. This short range is enough to rattle the nerves of hard-bolled professionals. It was impossible to overestimate the degree of danger my team was subjected to. I checked the loads in my gun and as a marginal precaution against the stabbing tooth of predator, wrapped the woolen pullover round my neck and knotted it.

Meanwhile, 50 yards away three policemen, combing the crop saw a streak of movement as something flitted between two thick sugar plots followed by incredibly sinister gurgling and sounds of thumping paws. When a disturbed tiger suddenly retreats it often gives this call. When trying to break a line of surrounding human beings they roar, but this they do when they are pushed by the beaters. This noise is quite different from the cough they make when intending to attack.

The police picket was considerably scattered and any one moving singly was vulnerable. In the advantage of darkness, the possibility of the soft-padded animal, noiselessly sauntering up to them and ambushing unexpectedly could not be ruled out. Moreover all man-eaters, whatever their type, will essentially take the inevitable straggler —separated from the group, entered a bush to urinate or just lagged behind to tie a shoelace. It behooved me to be on high alert. I quartered the ground slightly in advance of combers and warned loudly, "beware, the killer is around."

Those who have dealt with aberrant tigers would understand what I mean to say. Despite a life-long acquaintance with super cats I am still no less afraid of them than I was in the beginning. My heart slammed in my ears as adrenalin pumped through my system, reminding me of an old jungle adage that man is a soft cucumber and tigers don't need any strategic modus to kill them. The tigress had naturally left the cover, whoofing, a fairly clear indication of her bad temper and if there is a long pause you must not assume that she is gone; the fact is often contrary, she may be coming.

The species of *Panthera tigris* is *numero uno* at killing you if you give them just a little bit of chance. And in times of such attacks, their movements are nothing but a blur, a very unnerving fact at a time when one is probably scared witless. Their typical charge from 40 feet (which is their ambit of attack) takes the blink of an eye. It comes like a streak of death, a muscular javelin, knocking the victim down. However, I was deeply impressed to witness that the well-trained policemen had dropped on their knees on my alarm call so as to get a level shot in case the man-eater breaks cover.

Finally not fancying the possible results of following a stressed man-eater into the dark, who seemingly too was not liking the idea of tackling so many people at a time, I withdrew at once; though I was a bit distraught at having missed the opportunity of exactly locating before attempting to kill her.

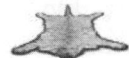

Bane of Human Delinquency

"There is no off switch on an enraged tiger."
– An adage of Big game hunter's

That evening it rained torrentially and continued all the night. Next day towards morning the sky cleared and the foresters again started on the trail while I, with my leave over, started back for Lucknow.

After January 10 no fresh killing was reported. Calm returned to the troubled zone but her behavior left many questions that still needed to be answered. The circumstantial evidence established by tigress' route and pugmarks proved beyond a shadow of doubt that she had come from the Corbett Reserve, covering a more than 200 kilometers and returned after 16 days, but why had she done it in the first place?

Crime investigators believe that no crime is committed without a motive but what could be the motive of this apparently healthy tigress, plaguing the area with a sudden killing spree and then halting the killing as suddenly? I am sure if India's beloved Briton Jim Corbett had been alive he too would have been bewildered by the cat's ostensibly abnormal behaviour. But then, had her behavior been really abnormal?

I attempted to fit in a few missing bits in this jigsaw puzzle through information which Arvind Chaturvadi and Aftab provided me.

On December 16, 2013 there was this widely circulated news of the arrest of 12 alleged poachers near Amangarh forest range situated on the border of Corbett's Kalagarh range. Skins of two freshly killed tigers were seized by Special Task Force (STF) from poachers named Rahees and Saeed. Both the dead tigers were sub-adults, merely a year old, implying there was a mother tigress too somewhere and

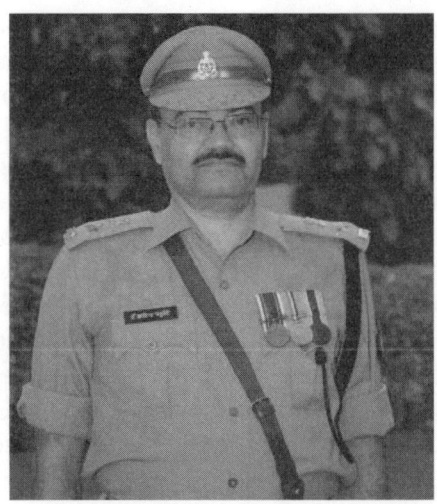

Dr. ArvindChaturvadi, Superintendent Police, S.T.F, U.P at National Police Academy Hyderabad; Decorated with the President's award for gallantry, he has confiscated over 100 leopard and 10 tiger skins.

in all probability, siblings were accompanying the mother. All the carnivores, birds as well as animals have strong maternal instincts, they keep their young around until they are mature enough to take care of themselves, and train them for hunting. The parents are known to go to any length to defend them in the time of crisis.

The Superintendent of Police STF Arvind Chaturvedi who caught these poachers corroborated these facts, saying, "Tigresses ensure that their cubs don't stray for longer times and if they do they are desperately searched out. It is difficult to imagine such a transformation in the attitude of a wild animal within a fortnight unless her pathetic circumstances are fully understood."

Yes, no tiger ever becomes a man-eater by choice. In the officer's words lay the key to the riddle, with sufficient *raison d'etre* to connect things together. The reckless molestation of motherly sentiments and the psychological injury to her own self had made the tigress extraordinarily belligerent. It was yet another example of how mindlessly a man can work. First he upsets the balance of nature then its serious repercussions overtake him and he eventually pays the price when nature strikes back. It also proves the horrendous conception that man-eaters are not born, they are created by man. The same applied to this tigress.

In this book I have already cited the story of a man-eating tigress, shot by my maternal grandfather Kunwar Sahib that was known to go about with a male during mating season, which claimed and ate no human flesh, meaning that man-eating is a deviation. Every time it is the pressure of circumstances that forces a tiger to seek an alien diet. In this case the familiarized predator never deliberately sought human flesh but she rather learnt that humans are easiest to kill and are most prolific prey species. In academic lingo her depredations formed no pattern because she usually took men when the opportunity arose along with hunting her natural prey. I think the main reason for the man-eating predisposition was undoubtedly the pressure of human population upon her as the cane harvesting season was on full throttle.

Let us fast forward to January 12, 2014, the day the last pugmarks of killer tigress were seen at the very spot on the outskirts of Amangarh brick kiln from where the skins of two tigers were seized. I am sure many of my readers will lap up the deduction – for there is none other to negate it that the killing tigress is none other than the mother of the two dead sub-adult tigers. In my decades of tiger time I have found that normally a tigress leaves her territory only when it is driven out by another stronger female. However, going strictly by the circumstantial evidence it was not the case with this particular killer, which proves the old apothegm that man-eaters are generally created by reactionary human activities.

Aberrant tigers that attack human beings because of hunger, inexperience or injuries or in defense of cubs have always existed. But such occasional killings do not necessarily lead to persistent man-eating behaviour, giving way to such a terrific manslaughter as she energetically accomplished. But it is also true that some tigers who discover human defenselessness don't hesitate to include the species into their list of prey and later become steady man-eaters. The difficulty experienced by a tigress with cubs in obtaining food, sometime becomes a motivation for killing humans.

Eventually, I tried reconstructing the case history what must have happened. Distraught at the disappearance of her cubs the tigress came out of the forest cover and started moving towards human settlement. Supercats share a special rhythm with their cubs and when separated by distance or their abrupt disappearance, they feel an imbalance and turn nasty but when they rediscover them or get closer to their lost progeny the imbalance begins to stabilize. The search for the cubs took her all the way to Moradabad district but her emotions did not stabilize, till she realized its futility and turned back. Failing to locate the cub the tigress took out her anger out on six unlucky humans who came in her way. This proves how a normal tiger can be easily diverted into unnatural ways by human delinquency.

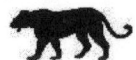

The Bottle-Neck Factor; Emotional Explosions

"A trademark of something that works well, the cat body has hardly changed since its inception. Like with today's cats, their digestive systems could handle only flesh. The lesson of the cat is that if you are to become a full-fledged carnivore, you have to commit everything to it".
- Craig Childs, Uncommon Encounters in the Wild

Cubs are a key factor in making a normal tigress so incredibly dangerous and a vast majority of human deaths come from cub-bearing tigresses. That is why more tigresses are recorded as man-eaters than males. Disturbed cats searching for cubs are prone to travel to long distances. An offhand case, quoted by Williamson in *Oriental Field Sports*, tells that his men brought him two cubs found in the jungle; he shut them up in a stable, where they were very noisy. Two or three nights later the mother came to the place (some 30 miles away) and was so fierce and

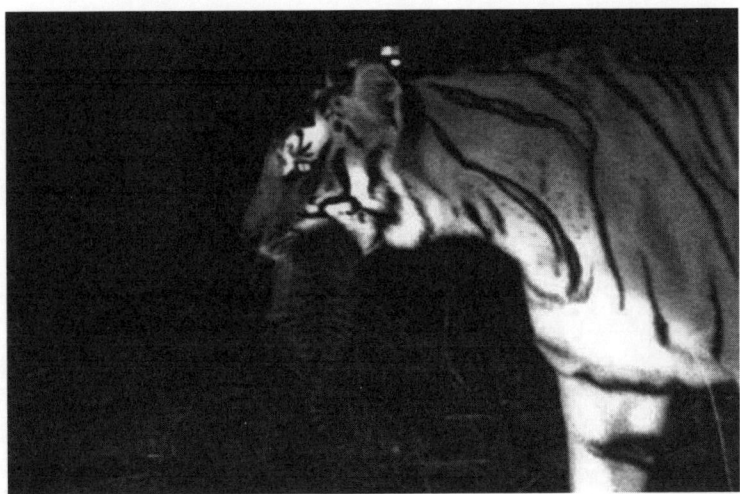

Maneating is more frequent in females than in males because the difficulty of finding food for cubs and the pressure of rearing, keeps a mother constantly on tenterhooks. *(Photo credit : NTCA)*

aggressive, roaring and trying to break in that the men in charge of the cubs threw them out of the window; she picked them up and carried them off.

Corbett comments in *Talla Des Tigress*, "Under stress of circumstances any animal, and a human being also, will eat food that under normal conditions, they are averse to eating. From the fact that during the whole of her man-eating career the tigress had only killed 150 human beings –fewer than 20 a year – I am inclined to think that she only resorted to this easily procured form of food when she had cubs and when owing to her injury, she was unable to get the requisite amount of natural food needed to support herself and her family."

Time does not deface the events graven deep on memory tablets and invokes many keen memories. Back in 1979 while tracking Barauchha Nala man-eating tigerss at Gola Gokaran Nath that I had earlier observed at the banks of Katna river at Larti in 1977, (*See author's Tiger! Chapter 8; The Katna Tigress.)* I had recovered the kill of a man named Ram Das. The tigress had overpowered him and dragged him for over a kilometer into dense sugarcane to feed her two generations of cubs, (one male about a year and a-half old, and the other two were around four months old) who dined on the corpse's both legs and genitals. The mother was famished and naturally pressurized in adverse habitat conditions where she had been previously driven away by natives from many normal kills she had made to sustain her cubs. She had really gone on rampage killing thirteen people before she was shot on the very victim's half-devoured body that was used as bait.

The case of Moradabad tigress, besides being an extremely horrifying instance of a mother's revenge is also an interesting case of journeying in the course of PSI trailings, a perfect example set by a man-eating cat to return to her in situ position. For she was recorded to have passed once again only 30 yards away from the very depression near brick kiln in Bijnore, where the skins of her two cubs were seized by STF.

I had chased exactly six man-eating cats in sugar farms before this experience and all these individual animals stand out in my mind as being nightmarish. But this consistently nasty feline stands as particularly challenging, where Aftab and I had inadvertently come close enough, theoretically, to become a statistic on this occasion. She was a killer, no doubt and her peculiarly aberrant behavior, technically called temperamental or explosive man-eating, was the window to her pathetic soul that was moaning due to the loss of cubs. Modern scientists prove that while the female is pregnant, she develops a new psychic quarter of brain called baby brain compartment whereas males are devoid of it. This helps her to understand her progenies uncommunicative needs as well as her progenies to understand her. Predators naturally possess a developed baby brain because their cubs are born blind and helpless. Therefore if the essential dignity and way of the life of a large predator is ignored and family is violated then such biologically gruesome conflicts are liable to happen.

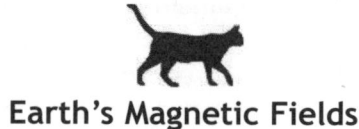

Earth's Magnetic Fields

"When the world's human population crossed the six hundred crore marks with more than half of humanity living in Asia….. Paradoxically it was not ecological or biological data but the social, population and economic statistics that reinforced understanding of what truly were the key challenges to tiger conservation".
- Hemanta Mishra, J Paul Getty Wildlife Conservation Awarde, Nepal

Straying is an abnormal behavior, however PSI (pressure per square inch) trailings, a term that Dr Joseph Rhine of Duke University has coined to refer to the animal's psychic capacity of homing in, attempts to explain a cat's ability to travel a long distance to return to their home again. It suggests that felines have an internal compass that is sensitive to the earth's magnetic fields and if a cat is lost for a short distance it can usually find its way back home. But its chances of finding home become smaller as the distance grows (more than 10 miles). Something called the homing instinct is an ability to detect direction using something other than the normal five senses a cat uses. If a pet is fitted with magnets, he loses his ability to find his way back. This appears possible with pet cats and feral cats but it applies on wild cats too when the place of their original home is concerned.

In time and space continuum they use the earth's gravity to determine their place in the world or in better terms, their *in situ* position against their *ex situ* wanderings.

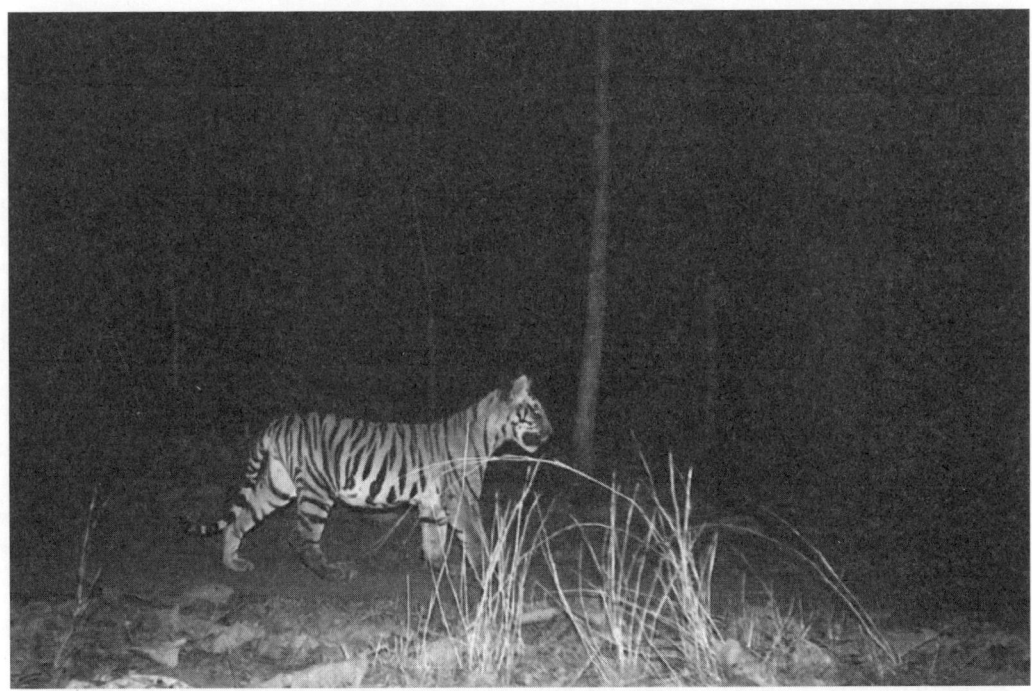

Tigers are bound to lose in man tiger conflict. We need to consider that man eating is the last ditch activity of a desperate beast rather than its standard behavior. (*Photograph credit : Wildlife Conservation Trust*)

This new vocabulary once again acquires added value here as I wonder idly about tigers because something that is *in situ* can most certainly be subjected to control and the tigress entering jungle, by definition means coming under controlled conditions, the defined boundaries of the forests.

Finally after this long journey of more than 500 kilometers, both ways going and coming, her pug marks were found up the jungles of Jhima-Kalagarh belt in Uttarakhand, entering her original range where she was initially established. When it's certain the other five senses could not have been used by her to find the way back home, PSI trailing may explain the causes of her incredible journey towards home over a long distance, through places and territory she has never seen or been to. It is the homing instinct of cats on a different scale that had brought her home. To repeat modern ethology's principals that animals are not instinct-driven automata (as perceived by old authors), but are complex beings that need not stick to a limited set of prototypes.

After this the man-eating cases abruptly ceased, the canard of old hunters that once a man-eater is always a man-eater meets doom in this case. Man-eating is an unnatural function for big cats and it is only in the extreme cases of maddening compulsion that they hunt a human or develop anthropophagous appetite. I am unable to vouch for delectability of human flesh, though monkey is priority prey for tigers, which is the nearest available alternative creature to a human.

A central guideline issued along the aegis of the National Tiger Conservation Authority (NTCA), responsible for policy on governing this specialist subject, states categorically that a man-eater will only be declared a man-eater designated to be eliminated, if it has devoured more than one person. So this man-eater, by the text-book definitions as well as by circumstances and being consistently nasty, was *de facto* not a man-eater by choice compulsively seeking human flesh. She luckily eluded hunters and proved that tiger's natural disinclination to seek sustenance on human flesh is strong.

The tigress is reported to have returned to normal conditions and goes for more acceptable prey animals available. Wung Longwa, Project Director of reserve forest in Uttarakhand, told me that "the tigress behaves impeccably. Her scars are healed by nature as she has now raised another family."

The journey of this tigress is a unique benchmark case of PSI trailings that qualifies all the four stipulations created by Rhine that have to be met to decide if the trailing is successful. Reliable witnesses, a positive identification of the cat, consistent and credible details and lastly, other witnesses who could give additional evidence. This is also one of its kind and rare case of nature that contingent, secondary man-eating began abruptly and ceased equally abruptly. What is more significant, it suggested that by no means do all such encounters and temperamental man-eating cases lead automatically to human predation. Hence, many cases require no further management intervention than compensating the victim's relatives.

Do I need to add that in all I have the private satisfaction of seeing her restored to normal existence?

Book 5

THE NOMADS OF FARMLANDS

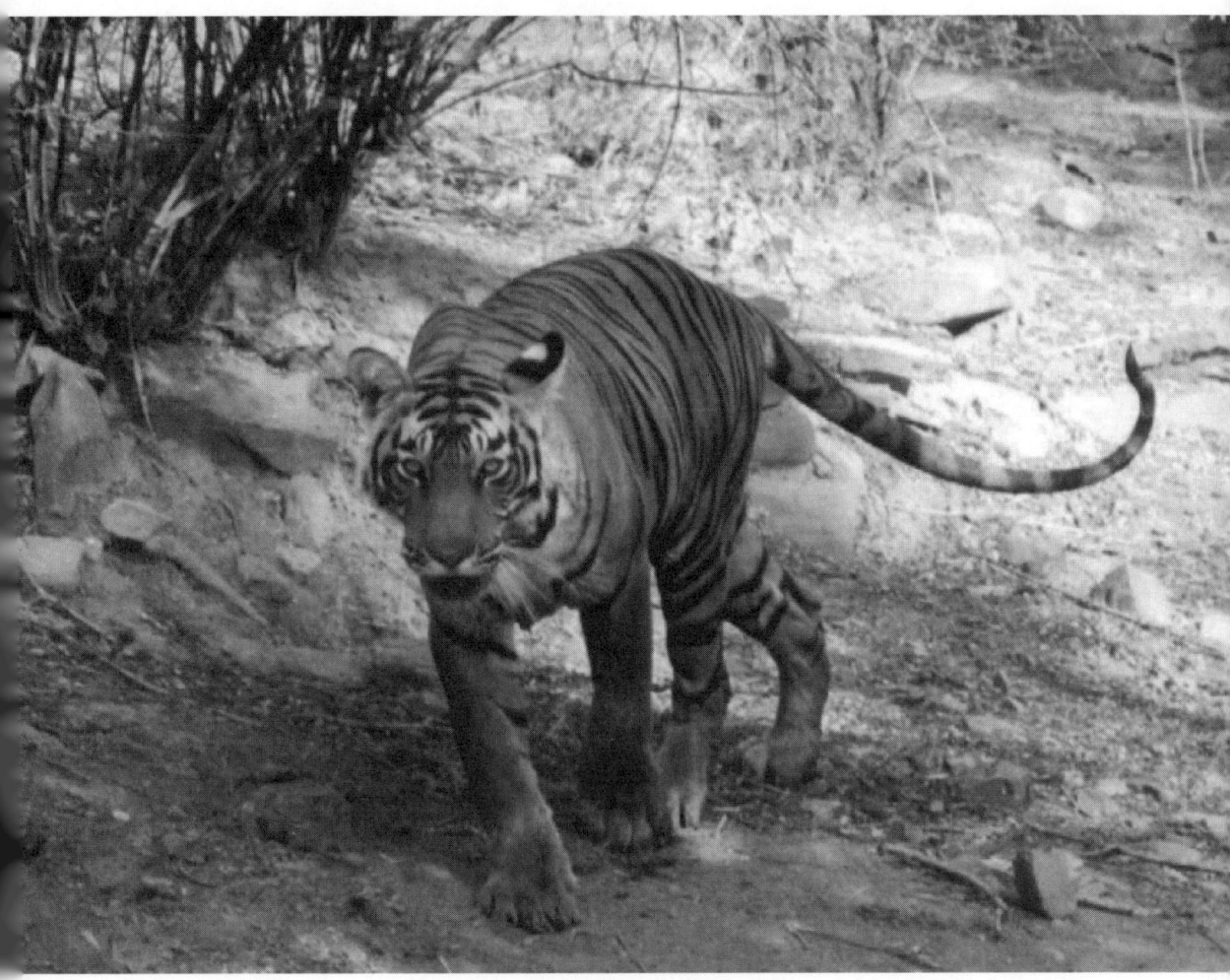

CHAPTER 9
LIFE-STYLE OF A CONVIVIAL
BACHELOR

Chapter 9

Life-style of a Convivial Bachelor

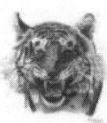

What makes a species survive? It is not the strongest of the species that survives or the most intelligent that survives. It is the one that is most adaptable to change.

- Charls Darvin

ON THE MORNING OF THE DAY THE YEAR 2012 BEGAN, FOG AND MIST covered the land and a biting cold wave swept across the landscape. I was returning from Delhi where I had gone to attend a seminar at Jawahar Lal Nehru University. I was driving my newly-acquired vehicle, a 4-wheel drive Toyota Qualis, and moved cautiously, hoping that the swirling fog would thin out as the sun rose. My daughters Shrivriddhi and Samriddhi, who had come from USA and Germany to spend the winter vacations, were happily sleeping on the backseat.

Chanting *Hanuman-Chaleesa* to keep myself awake from the fatigue of night drive, I drove slowly as morning was breaking and Lucknow was nearing. Suddenly, a yellow stripped form emerged in front of me, standing broadside on the road, looking at my vehicle with its glowering eyeballs obfuscated in the headlights. The brakes screeched as I halted the car abruptly. I was totally unprepared for what I saw, jumping out of my skin as the driving wheel slipped out of my hands. It was a real beaut tiger, well over eight feet, standing in front of the vehicle. No matter how many times I blinked my eyes, but there he was, staring at us. My wife too was gawking wide-eyed when all of a sudden, like a flash of lightning the noble predator lurched and melted in the swirling mist.

Anita and I exchanged glances, both of us whispering under our breath that it was indeed a tiger that we just saw. I got down from the vehicle and feeling imbued by sheer magnificence, and mystery of what I had seen, I spent some time on the spot looking for his signs. The paws of solo hunter were clearly imprinted on the ashes of grass, which had been burnt only a few days back.

"Don't disfigure the tiger trail Papa, walk next to it," Shrivridhi said observing the smoothly made tracks, that looked like gorgeous art of nature, while I tried to determine the gender of the animal.

An hour later having arrived at Lucknow I called the Chief Wildlife Warden and broke the news of the newcomer. He discussed the matter at length with promise to

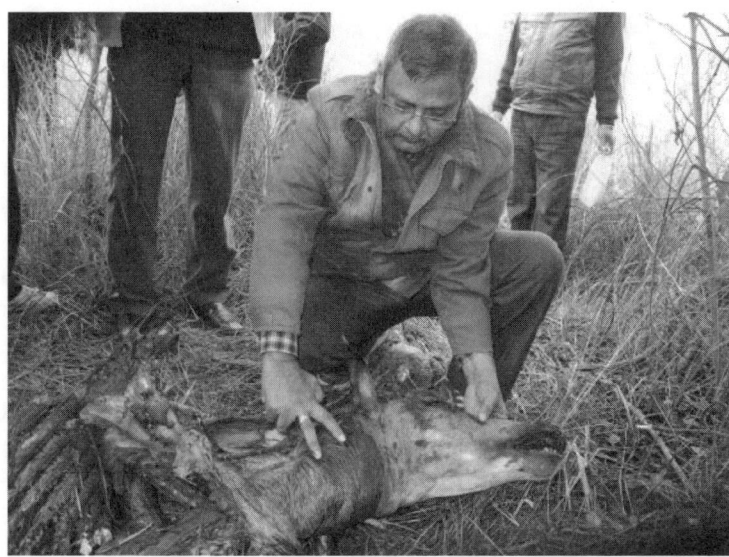

Author examining a half-eaten Nilgai; the first recorded kill of the Convivial Bachelor inside the premises of Mango Institute.

investigate immediately. "Nothing to investigate, the chap is awesome," I insisted, "a tiger is there and you better be up and ready to face the music."

"And anyway Sir, try to keep its name clear of the infamy which was heaped upon the earlier tigers that visited Lucknow. I don't want you to give it same reception you accorded to its predecessor. Its mere appearance should not become the reason for its destruction," I added.

The spot was some 20 kilometers to the south-west of the city. I then called Neha Shukla, a correspondent with the Lucknow edition of the newspaper *The Times of India* and gave her the information.

"The Forest Department has yet not confirmed the identity of the animal. Are you sure it is a tiger?" she asked.

"Yes, it is a tiger," I said and hung up.

In the next one hour my telephone and mobile was busy as I got calls from correspondents of *Dainik Jagaran*, *Indian Express*, *Amar Ujala* and a few others. Next day the newspapers were full of news about a tiger having lost its way in Lucknow district.

Like the previous visitors to the city, this animal too was a likely affiliate of sugarcane component of the tiger population, rather than a direct immigrant out of the forested regions. In the case of internecine, con-specific confrontations or anthropogenic pressures, temporary random emigrations of tigers do take place in farmlands. Young tigers, that come under transit parameterization are much prone to leaving their area at the first whiff of tension. They typically follow the contours of local rivers that often make them turn towards villages and townships and further towards cities. Once a tiger ventures far enough, its esoteric telecommunication system and territorial organization breaks down and then it gets lost. There is then little scope for it to retrace its steps back to the original holding ground.

This homeless male, later dubbed as Badshah by media had embarked on this unusual voyage after monsoons. In absence of sightings and kills on its journey to the city, the beast remained unreported. It moved through cover and never made itself visible yet he fed properly on regular kills.

Covering some 250-odd kilometers, it finally halted in the vast 300-acre campus of the Central Institute of Sub-tropical Horticulture (CISH) a Central government establishment in Rahman Khera, engaged in research on mango and other fruit species. Comparatively a small area, it was but certainly a special piece of forest where the conditions easily provided the tiger with a safe hide-out. It made its home in a grassed landscape not far from the main office building of the institute and continued to remain around it for good five months.

Establishing a Routine – The Daily Chores

I'm learning that human pressure on wildlife is becoming increasingly dangerous. You've got to be more alert because more animals have been pushed around, wounded, subjected to human harassment, ambushed, all kinds of stress. When they attack, it's totally predictable.
- Peter Beard

Emotion is a useful motivator and tigers inspire powerful emotions. Therefore all the conservation enterprises in the fight to save the tiger are emotionally laden. Four days had passed when I went out to check as how the new immigrant was faring on his new-found terrain. The countryside around the institute held a substantial number of wood and grassland patches. These sporadic forests, extending from 5 acres to 200 acres in land area are composed of sub-optimal tiger habitat that fall under jurisdiction of the state Forest Department. The bigger struggle for these patches is to survive ever-expanding human settlements that for multiple uses depend heavily upon them.

There were no less than 11 species of carnivores in the agricultural expanses surrounding CISH campus, using temporal and spatial aspects of their environments in accordance with their nature. According to a professional theorist's Rule Book it was an adverse habitat for animals to live where a certain minimal wild prey population could barely exist but in reality it was different. It was indeed an ideal habitat for wildlife.

There were tree-cavity and burrow dwellers, jackals, hyenas, foxes, cats, rattlers, ant-eaters, mongoose, hawks and owls, monitor lizards and small mammals, grassland birds, game birds, and songbirds that nested and collect seeds and insects in the fields. The stock of large antelopes like *nilgai* was satisfactory to

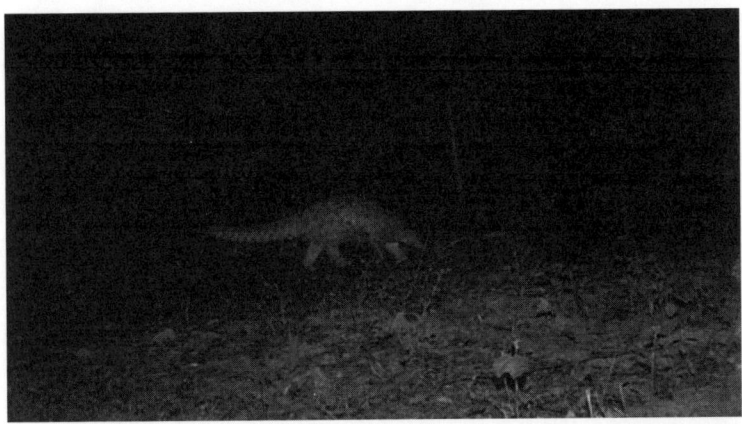

Indian pangolin is commoner than is generally believed. It usually moves about only in night and is seldom seen.

good. Feral cattle and pigs in duos with their snuffling piglets ran around water ponds competing with each other. Multitude of *Langoor* and rhesus monkeys, rodents, porcupines, pangolins, amphibians and reptiles used the place as breeding grounds and relied on close-by flooded rice-fields and wheat for winter food. There was enough "requiem" of snakes to delight a herpetologist, including Russel's vipers and saw-scaled viper, cobras, regiments of krait and pit vipers, and not to mention rat snakes that are active during the day time.

Hawks, owls, hyenas and jackals lived in the campus of the institute and used it as their hunting grounds, and small mammals, grassland birds, game birds and songbirds nested and collected seeds and insects in the fields. During winter journeys migrating birds were often found resting in the gram and rice fields before and after the breeding season.

There were so many sympatric competitive species with in predator guilds and there was so much of protein pack of prey just about 20 kilometers away from my city home that I was not prepared to believe it, and now a tiger had come to put up in middle of them.

Completive interactions among predators generate selective pressures upon land terrains. Only time would tell whether the land could take the pressure of a tiger or the tiger could take the pressure of the land without coming in conflict.

By January 20, the tiger had made four natural kills in the campus – two blue bull females, one male peacock and two dogs. For the time being the availability of natural food, needed to support a large carnivore seemed to have biologically naturalized him in the area. The fortunate situation for the managers was that the institute campus was so well stocked with legitimate prey where the tiger had completely free choice in the matter of prey selection. It seemed that after months of long run and no respite, the mighty predator had not stayed here in vain, he himself had approved the place as ideal; staying put for three weeks, refusing to move out.

My past experience had convinced me that it is increasingly difficult for a travelling tiger to find a suitable habitat amidst human landscape and when the strayers chance upon any home of selective occupancy they naturally come to a halt and try to settle down at their best. This is a sigh of relief, where they feel stress-free and are favourably contented. The institute site seemed to have all the mandatory components of cover, water and prey to hold up this wanderer. The fine network of irrigation channels, supporting the agriculture cycle in the precincts had generated artificial patches of wetlands that provided an additional area for wildlife to use.

Throughout the tigers stay much was written about it in the newspapers. Not to recall those headlines and sensational stories, I would rather contend myself with relating some episodes which throw more light on tiger's mentality and his reactions in certain situations.

Towards the end of January the Forest Department finally took up the cudgels and arrived with all paraphernalia in the campus. Elephants were marched down from Dudhwa, steel cages were brought, a team of WTI darters was hired and the operation 'capture tiger' started in full swing. However, the mandarins' attitude was unprofessional. At no stage scientists, tiger specialists and conservationists were involved in the endeavour to discuss seriousness of the problem. The requests of volunteers, experienced hunters and NGOs like Tiger Terrain to assist the operation were turned down. The foresters thought that the war was made of guns, elephants, nets and courage and they had brought them all. It was their duty so where was the need for outsiders to poke their nose into this?

Iron cages were placed with goats tied inside. Given a favorable wind, it's a delectable invitation. The more strong the wind, the wider it would broadcast the presence of food.

One cage was kept with buffalo offals inside it. The effort ended in catching a couple of pariah dogs. As the trapped dogs barked and quarreled over the meat, the tiger was naturally attracted by their sounds. It visited the spot, hung around the cage all night eyeing the dogs, circumvented the cage but inexplicably, scrupulously avoided nearing it and then went back towards morning.

Amidst the Foresters exercise, I was on errand of my own; using this opportunity to test my thesis on the template of rural environs' ability to provide ecological needs of a large carnivore including its long-term potential of food base. It was not for the first time that I was following a big cat's trail near my city. I had earlier done it in three winters of distant years, but alas, all those great wanderers were officially murdered within a fortnight of their arrival. Though the line between survival and elimination of this animal was precariously thin, as there is much criminal element in stylish cities like Lucknow, I sincerely hoped that it would not meet the same fate of its ancestors and become an important study animal.

Tiger is a conservation-based species and will only survive if people want him to. Thus, my field work also had one more purpose that was to 'balance people with tiger' and orient countryside population with nuances to exist with tiger. At first my arguments were against the predatory animal and its evident dangers but towards the end a more realistic picture changed the situation and people agreed with environmental approach. The way tribals live with wildlife in jungles – as Tharus' in Dudhwa– indicates that humans are a part of the same ecosystem as much the tigers. Both happily survive without problems.

I believe an impartial view needs to be taken on this issue. There is an alarming surplus of every kind of feral stock in India from cows down the line, which are eating out all the vegetation and turning green belts into desert as many parts of Middle East and North Africa have become. In this situation, there is nothing wrong if an animal as precious as tiger lives on feral cattle that are redundant for humans.

There is nothing to feel sorry about, as this is the law of nature, the rule of predator and prey, and as long as the tiger goes for quadrupeds and not those who walk on two legs it is a no-problem tiger.

Now, a fresh affiliate ordained by God to subsist on flesh had come to live around Lucknow, the enlightened notion of co-existence was that he was a part of harmonious animal kingdom in which human beings were the only dangerous predators.

The farmland tigers with their inter-specific aggressions, including strayers, it seemed were least organized to receive a bit of a nudge from jungle world again. Perhaps Mother Nature just wanted to remind its so-called trustees to not to take too long over deliberations, to decide on critical issue of their protection in farmlands, and aid their management by identifying long term solutions.

My daughters Shrivridhi and Samridhi got involved in my endeavour and distributed the pamphlets of 'Saving Men from Tigers,' telling the simple tricks to people to save themselves and be careful – much the same way traffic rules are explained to city-dwellers. Points of this campaign suggesting a readjustment of human attitude towards animals and its proactive conflict prevention actions over reactive conflict reduction actions have already been highlighted in this book. Wild tigers are government properties; any interference with them makes you run afoul of laws. Even tracking them is illegal. But it was initial matter of saving human lives -a part of my individual tiger management policy in farmlands where enforced coexistence is sometimes unavoidable due to multiple compulsions'. So without worrying over legal ends I was never away from the place.

I followed the tiger along the courses of river and nalas with local people and from time to time assisted them in devising better livestock protection measures. As I searched the area with enough food for predators and enough food for their prey, I came upon multitude of paws and hooves, and encountered the tiger on six different occasions. Interestingly the incidents of natural history that marked the highlight of these rounds, made it possible for me to write this story on a different scale.

On one Saturday we had followed the tiger tracks for whole of the day without any success, when towards evening clouds covered the sky and lightning began to dance. We quickly abandoned the round and hurried back home. An almost inky black blanket had rolled over the fields when from near a water pond, I happened to hear a desperate honking of a bird followed by a flutter of wings. I shifted the torchlight, and found a fishing cat sitting on its haunches at the border of the pond. A whistling teal duck lay pressed under its body weight while the cat was plucking its feathers. A dark cloud hovered overhead, hanging much lower than normal as its outlines were sharply delineated by incessant lighting. Lights did not disturb the cat and she persistently ate the dinner in our presence. We stood there for over ten minutes and watched her engrossed in feast. She munched the whole bird including her legs and then vanished in the rippling wheat crops.

The presence of a fishing cat in Mango Institute was a rare proposition, no less significant than the arrival of the tiger. I excitedly reported the case to media but not much cognizance was taken because lesser lights of life are always shadowed by the bigger cats.

Meanwhile, on January 26 a milkman from Janwapur village brought his two buffalos to give them a bath in the stream. It was afternoon when the tiger charged out of the undergrowth without any warning. The cattle panicked and fled high up the banks. He wrenched one and pushed it down the embankment and as if in a confusion went into a hiding. The cattle fell in the water gasping and howling frantically, while the other one going in a blind flight bumped into a tree with full force and collapsed on the ground. Seeing this the tiger again came out of its hiding, ran up to the fallen buffalo and instead of strangulating it to death, he stood by it like a hunting dog that is trained to guard the trophy. Meanwhile the first victim, not lethally injured, got up in the water and ran away. At the same moment a group of vegetable sellers, approaching on bicycles was on their way home from market. On seeing the tiger they began to shout and wielded staves, which forced the tiger to move away into a dense lantana thicket. But he kept growling from there. However, the threat remained an elemental bluff and he never charged in earnest.

The incident created panic in the area; incredible it may sound, contempt-bred familiarity is a factor that often makes a tiger kill human beings. But as the days passed by no more deliberate attacks were recorded, though pariah dogs kept disappearing everywhere.

As the tiger was recorded to pass through a given area periodically, a steel cage was shifted to the particular place. The goat placed inside was next day found badly injured. On examination it was found it to be the work of a hyena. Its prints over those of the cat indicated that at the dead of the night both had separately visited the place, none had entered the cage but the hyena had made attempts on the goat, clawing portions of the unfortunate bait from the outside. The goat was

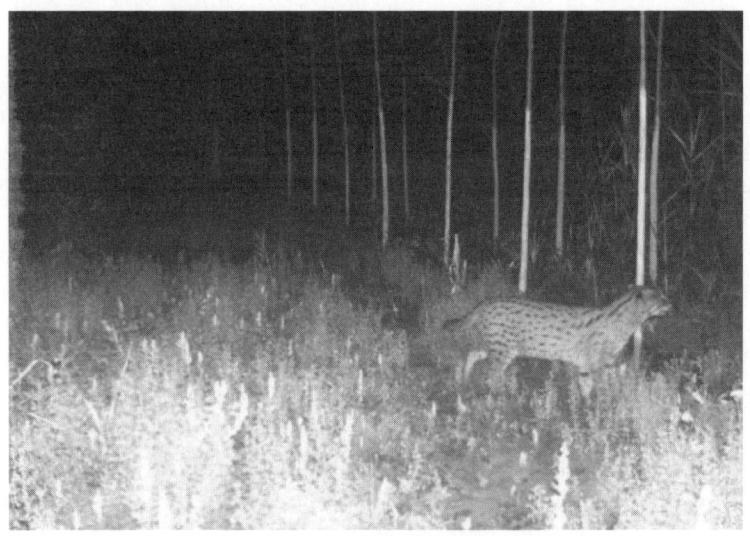

The rusty spotted fishing cat preys upon small birds and animals. It is noctournal in habit, seldom seem and hallows in trees are its favorite shelter *(Photo credit : Mudit Gupta, WWF)*

bleeding from rump injuries. The attacker had even plucked out a part of its tail, as its tooth-scarred back showed. While trying to avoid its tormentor the jumping, bounding goat had injured itself further.

However, there were no physical barriers to this super predator's freedom. He left the sanctuary after sunset, took rounds of some ten to fifteen kilometers and came back before the dawn broke. During these perambulations, confirmed by his pawmarks, he went up to borders of several villages even entered the villages in the dread of cold nights and crossed them directly searching for the prey.

One night the tiger entered a milkmen's settlement, claiming a buffalo and her calf. Yet, the cattle-owner Lakshman wanted this animal to survive. He told me on meeting: "It is true that we fear this tiger, but we had never felt the excitement and nervousness which this animal has given us. It is a feeling of acute thrill since he has come to live here", apparently it no malignant fate that held their minds in thrall but was a pleasant feeling of rare nature. His elder brother, a guard in the institute, said: "I have come across this animal many times. My fear tells me that an empty-handed man is helpless to challenge it but I don't understand the need to stand against such a mighty predator even with my gun."

I told them they will have to pick up the ways to reduce danger to live with it, just as we take precautions when we cross the road. You know cars are deadly and people get knocked down, suffer serious injuries, and even get killed by them yet we all settle with this danger in a way that allows us to live agreeably with motorcars and other vehicles like that. The guard valued the point and was happy to distribute my pamphlets among his friends.

Like Lakshman there were many villagers who had managed to retain their humanity. By a little stretch of imagination people knew that a superficially wounded tiger, inclined to blame his wounds on somebody is a nasty thing. But they also knew that you get along better with hornets if you don't stir them up with a stick.

During day times, the loner lay idle or slept. In few tight months, this juvenile had faced serious anthropogenic pressure and met much more human beings at hand than any jungle tiger might see from a distance in its entire life, and was consequently getting used to them. He even changed locations repeatedly, shifty and self-protective when labourers moved about mango orchards. It remained silent at the sight of people, never disregarded the chatter of their voices and started retreating for the cover as soon people crossed its personally defined safe 'line of control' at about 30 meters.

He was no competitor to man, showing gross disinclination to challenge human authority. In the milieu of its co-existence with humans, his cautious behavior had steered to a strange co-existence that did not require much intelligence but it spoke for certain flexibility on the part of both. And when hundreds of labourers, scientists, foresters, fruit pickers, grass cutters and vagabond villagers roamed the vista, passing through his resting places and all came back home alive, unmolested, this was enough to prove that combinations of tiger's own sound sense and a change of heart on the part of humans had helped both to survive.

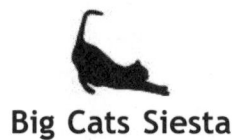

Big Cats Siesta

The tiger is confident, calm , collected animal that rarely loses its control , even in sudden, unexpected encounters with humans.

- Charls Mac Dougal

On February 2, I was in the campus of the institute when excited by the alarm call of a Langoor monkey, Dr BK Panday, a Principal Scientist and I went out to track the tiger. We soon came upon a drag and discovered the remains of a small feral pig which had been devoured the very morning. The kill lay in a secluded grass clump inside a ravine where the intermittently cackling jackal was still hanging around. It ran away when it saw us coming. A deep ominous silence seemed to reign over the place, when a burr of sound reached my ears, meaning thereby the tiger was sleeping.

He had chosen the best spot available to spend his day time. It was an isolated and impossible spot. Big cats are the sleepiest of all mammals and when they sleep they really sleep well from 10 to 14 hours of the day, because they have nothing to fear in their environment. In my younger days at Larti, I had twice walked up to within lethal distance of sleeping tigers. Except from muscular ripples up and

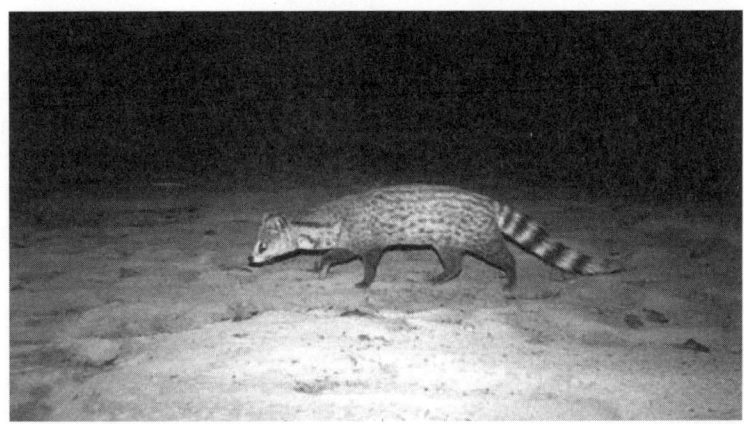

Small Indian Civet is a common creature living out of the forest in Tarai farmlands. Many live near villages and some struggle into crowded towns finding refuge in drains and outhouses. *(Photo credit : Wildlife Trust of India)*

down their flanks owing to heavy breathing they never budged and kept sleeping. But in farmlands, the situation is contrary. Human avocations dominate and natural fear of man does count, hence they prefer short sleeps and half-sleeps that the dictionary defines as cat-napping.

Suddenly the snorting burr ceased and seconds later, I heard a twig crack below me in the gulley, some 20 feet away.

The tiger was cat-napping along a flat bit of ground, when hearing our arrival he got up and left the cover. Like sport-rifles have their own peculiar loading sounds and the closing of a shot gun breech makes a metallic drainpipe *tonk*, sounds relating to tiger are also typical. Years of free lancing and wild scouting has made me so used to these sounds and I have a particular affinity for them. The languorous creature of long grasses and jungle pools had left the place and had gone towards the cultivation fields of Surriyapur, a village at the outskirts of the institute. We advanced some half a mile, carefully through stunted trees and shaded bushes and finally found him sitting in the water of Behata Nala. We left him undisturbed and retraced our steps.

Even in his changed location the tiger was not more than 200 meters away from the mixed fields of mustard, rice and wheat and yet none of the labourers working there were aware of his presence. Forced by circumstances to live in sub-optimal habitat and facing all manner of threats, the solo hunter had quickly developed the ability to live among high densities of people –though inadequately poor – yet selective occupancies. His cautious behavior was nature's way of enabling him to avoid aggressive encounters with humans.

Although tigers habitually return to the kill, which they have fed upon but they will hardly come back to a dead animal which they leave uneaten on their own accord. This tiger also never returned to his kill and the scanty relics of pig lay there as an open feast for the scavengers. Locke says, "It is hard to account for these apparently small kills when the tiger goes to a great deal of trouble to secure them, but the fact remains that such instances do occur. There is no apparent reason why the kill is left. I have taken great pains to ensure that cows killed in this way have not been disturbed and have checked by absence of footprints afterwards that no one went near them, but the tiger seemed to have lost all interest in them… It is only when the tiger has a completely free choice in the matter and elects to leave his kill uneaten that he can be depended upon never to return to it. I have known other tigers to be attracted to such kills, however."

Where the tiger lay was a sunny point to spend a good winter day, an isolated mustard field flanked tightly by wall-like circle of sugar crops. I later corroborated that he used the place as his regular day-time lair. The villagers could only discover this fact when they often saw him crossing the Behata Nala towards the evening.

A press reporter confirmed he had visited a garbage dump where pigs from a local piggery and multitude of stray dogs were gathered. Soon the dogs and pigs ran away as the tiger arrived and stayed there, hunting for edibles in the waste such as chicken and mutton leftover thrown away by butchers. The animal had not to come to the place in empty lurking. He knew that with the abundance of butchers rubbish and such prey as stray dogs, would help him earn his sustenance lawfully without troubling his human neighbours. Such as Tiega tigers do when they descend on Vladivostok peninsula in hard winters, living on dogs and thrown offal's.

The behaviour of an animal is controlled by the endocrine gland and nervous system that is deeply affected by the environment the animal inhabits. It is quite obvious that the behaviour of a large carnivore in such landscape will differ from that of an animal in its natural environment, as unstable environments usually restrict animals from performing some species-specific behaviour, which can manifest in abnormal responses usually termed as aberrations.

A day after this incident he killed a stray cow near a course of Behata Nala, but left it uneaten. Perhaps he feared that he had done something wrong and he may also be chased from this kill so before anything happened he abandoned the kill. It was discovered by a fire wood collector in the morning.

The uneaten 'kill' lay half a mile ahead, near a watercourse. Dr Panday, I and four of his assistant researchers walked upstream, keeping close to its sharp turns and hairpin bends till we reached a spot where we could see crows sitting on the trees. The presence of carrions indicated that the 'kill' could not be very far away.

The crows were still on trees meaning thereby the tiger was guarding the kill and was scowling at the alighting birds. Walking noiselessly in the jungles had become second nature with me. I negotiated the first turn in the watercourse and approached the second, across which the crows were sitting on the trees, kvetching raucously, while some of them swirled and flickered for a distance and then came back.

Life of field researchers that enters a predators den is never short of potential close calls. Similarly I never look for thrills but these come to me without seeking.

I walked up the last of the bend, which brought me on the high embankment of

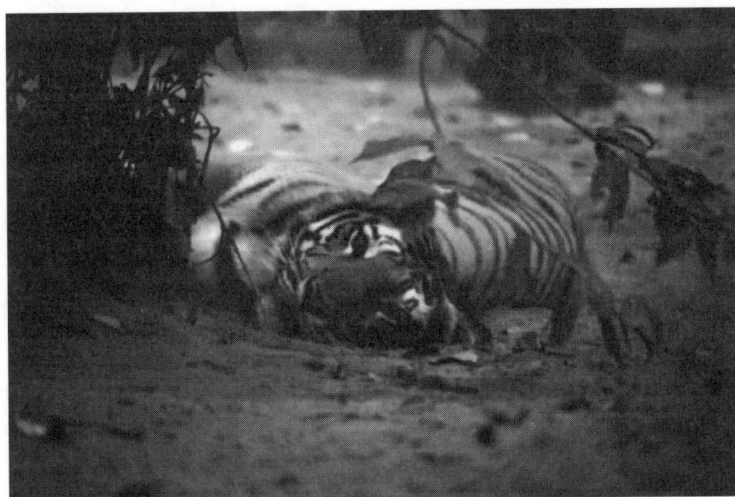

Cats are the sleepiest of all mammals. They spend 16 hours of each day sleeping. With that in mind, a seven year old cat has only been awake for two years of its life! *(Photo credit : Sanjay Singh, Director, Dudhwa National Park)*

Behata Nala, where I stood on the slopes hoping to see the kill. I was so involved in things that I had failed to notice a small depression in front of me. As I stepped forward, I slithered down the slippery incline and fell into a peat bog, 20 feet below. My stick also fell into the water and while I tried to pick it up quickly, I heard a soft whoof of surprise and saw the tiger sitting like a stripped sphinx, not more than 30 yards away. It would be wrong to say that only I was jolted, indeed it was a mutual feeling as the tiger and I saw each other simultaneously, but it lay rooted to the ground, staring back at me, without any air of tension. It merely twitched its ears to flap flies. Its emerald eyes seemed concerned, his mouth agape and the conglomeration of stripes, extravagantly marked aglow in the lambent sunrays that filtered from the tree leaves.

He neither lowered his head nor flattened his ears. He even did not hiss out any warning to me to move away. Yet feeling mortified, I kept sitting where I was. The animal contemplated me with a kind of quiet premeditation -like a chump-headed man fondling with an unaccustomed thought. I could hear the thumps, like distant muffled drums, which was in fact my own pulse swelling in my ears yet I remained confident. They say that when a person is in a mortal predicament, his whole life rushes through his mind but nothing of that sort happened with me. Instead my instincts told me to avoid looking at the tiger. While remembering the rules that one remembers, I got up on to my feet and cleaning my hands of mud, slowly climbed up the steep.

The tiger never meant any serious business. It was easy to figure out that he knew human habits well. He knew that they go snooping about every place, even impassable points, to look for something. He did not react at my slithering with fright or aggression. He gazed at me innocently for half a minute and then looked away yawning as if I did not exist, peering rather at some unfocused point. Then abruptly from there, a jet-black snake, locally called *ghora-pachhar* (meaning faster than a sprinting horse) speedily crossed towards the tiger scurrying into the grass. The grass was tallish and I did not see more than a flash of it. This shocked the tiger, and next moment the handsome yellow beast went bounding through in great leaps. My friends on the rise saw his glimpse like a mass of colors. They had already heard his whoof and sensing danger had walked on some 20 paces on the escarpment to investigate my whereabouts when they happened to disturb the snake in a bush that recoiled towards tiger.

"Don't worry Rahul," said Panday, extending his hand to pull me up, "this tiger is used to humans. He won't offend."

Possibility to emerge unscathed from practically all such nearly disastrous incidents can be attributed to sheer good luck and the fact that Dame Fortune has constantly been with me. There may appear quite a few narrow escapes from disaster in this account, it is merely because they occurred at widely spaced intervals of time and are in the nature of highlights in a longish pursuit of natural history observations and partly also to having learnt basic elements of hunters drill in early days; such as running, climbing, dodging, maintaining calm, quick loading and of course never loosing nerve. These escapes may be called 'The Cat's Cream'.

I ought to add that the tiger had been watching us ever since we had appeared on the escarpment and was keeping us in view therefore my fall did not come to him as a surprise. However, to see the tiger slink away from the group of people made me realize the man's impact as top predator. A combination of instinct and learning had taught him to fear man like no other animal.

As regards swiftness of the snake, I doubt that many people confronting *ghora-pachhar* in the wilds would have the inclination to check their speed with stop-watches but an estimate (probably exaggerated) puts it at 20 miles per hour, which could be vastly exaggerated. A herpetologist told me that *ghora-pachhar* is in fact a large rat snake with body length of nearly two and a half meters. They growl throatily and stand to impressive heights when nervous; their actual speed is 8 to 10 miles per hour over a short distance.

The Extraordinarily Versatile Predator

Many individual carnivores pose no threat to crops, domastic animals, or humans, despite having access to them for years.

- Jorgensen et al

The day of February 18 was fading as the sun transformed from incandescent white to crimson to carmine and slipped soundlessly behind mango orchards. Twilight was scarcely more than twenty minutes long as the day closed abruptly. We were on a Jeep that was moving on a mud path and its every occupant, including Vijay Kumar, then inspector General Police Agra zone, scanned the surroundings. Night jars and owls ghosted as many bush rabbits caught in the headlights ran before the vehicle. Their eccentric behaviour of zigzag locomotion is often ascribed to their indecisiveness, but actually this way the long-eared creature is easily able to dodge its predator for the trick gives him an extra edge in survival.

Within a short time the Jeep reached over the 20 feet high escarpment of Behta Nala. We put the vehicle on the dirt track running along the extended embankments, where deciduous leaf litter lay thick on slopes. We were negotiating a turn, just then the bright beams of light cut the darkness and there was an instantaneous vision of the tiger positioned in search of a prey. He sat in a depression looking like a heraldic ghost framed in thick shadows. Confused and obsfuscated, he gestured like a dazzled owl that shuts his eyes against the sharp lights. He then got up and ran towards stream. The cartilage of his great pads expanding with shifted weight thumped distinctly on the ground as he took an enormous bound and leapt across the watercourse. For a flash of moment he was visible airborne, and then abruptly he vanished in the sunset air as if swallowed by the skeletal line of waning light.

"Arey Nala phaand gaya" somcone said. The Jeep was immediately stopped. We got down and looked for him with the aid of torches. But the silent darkness brooded around. The tiger had gone, accomplishing a gargantuan feat in just little over two seconds with utmost elegance and ease.

The western bank of Behata Nala had a sandy surface and what had happened just now had got deeply imprinted on it. Next morning I came back hoping to record the distance the tiger had so casually covered. A careful measurement showed that he had leapt 37 feet and 10 inches despite the fact that he had taken a very short start. I wondered the way he had survived the impact of landing and how his strong forelimb bones and ligaments in the feet had helped him absorb the shock of his body weight.

The athletic sinewy movement in which he had crossed the *nala* was something to be seen to be appreciated. I think even thoroughbred stallion horses, which are trained for long jumps and hurdle clearing, cannot equal this sensational feat from a 20 feet high escarpment. Being hoofed animals they would not be able to bear the force of landing from high altitudes; their legs would shatter and break down.

The evidence left me in an acute admiration for the beast that is the biggest and the most spectacular machine of energy. Its elastic muscles produce nearly unbelievable strength at the time of need as their long hind legs enable them to leap forward and their small collar bone enables the length of their strides. This show stands as one of my most memorable recollections of a tiger's irrepressible vigour. Perhaps this is the reason why big predators fascinate us, their seemingly inexhaustible power fulfills our needs for instant gratification, beyond morbid titillations.

Cats have phenomenal strength. Many facts and figures pass before my eyes when I touch this subject. During my early years at Larti jungles, *(See author's Leopards in the Backyard)* I had witnessed Spotty, a 50-kg female leopard, carrying a more than 60-kg *chital* on a tree. Domestic cats are relied upon constantly by animal scientists around the world as a substitute for all the large felids and by all accounts are a thoroughly reliable model. A college colleague of mine named Denzil Godin, recorded that his domestic cat, weighing about five kg, carried a chunk of raw meat weighing 9 kg over a six-foot boundary wall, gorged upon it and then left. Such evidence may appear quaint but in fact is worthy of respect. Similarly I have also known a prime tiger weighing nearly 200 kilograms and measuring three meters from his pink nose to the tip of his tail jumping a six foot high fence with a large cow in its mouth.

During February 1998, I was camping at Maharajnagar near Kishanpur Sanctuary when rangers arrived with news that the previous night a tiger had raided a hamlet called Motiya Dhakka and in a frenzied attack slaughtered six adult cattle in a pen. This phenomenon amongst predators, politely termed as surplus killing, is practiced by all large and small cats besides mongoose and birds of prey. It may appear quite unnecessary and vindictive but nature never created a predator that would disturb the food chain and topple its balance, which will naturally go against its own survival in the long run. Yet, why they do it is an unanswered question.

Accompanied by ranger Shyam Kishore and Om Beer, my old associate from Paraspur, I reached the spot to investigate firsthand and settle the compensation. The scene was a reminder of Stevenson Hamilton's descriptions about a massacre of baboons by lions and the Russian records of Amur tigers engaging in the slaughter of wolves; a high energy murderous lust of youngsters, which manifests in a kind of spontaneous attacks. The tiger after having killed the cows had finally selected a 100 kilogram cow for a meal and tried to carry it away from the pen. He first tried to skip the barbed wires from below but unable to do so, finally threw the cattle on its shoulders and then in an explosive use of power, not to call a lithe spring, made a standing leap and landed across the wiring line. The tiger cleared the six feet high fence but the cow fell on the wire half way and a desperate pull from the tiger resulted in uprooting of nearly half of the fence that collapsed on the ground. Small chunks of flesh adhered to the barbed wire were axiomatic signs that the tiger had definitely jumped the fence with the cow clutched in his jaws.

The blood trail, of course of the cow, not the tiger, went towards the jungle, and we followed it. As we neared a dry *nala*, we were greeted by two woodcutters sitting on high branch of a tree. They told us that they were passing through the place early in the morning when a full grown male tiger suddenly materialized before them, and he was carrying a cattle carcass on his back. He exuded the confidence inspired by his enormous size and strength and did not seem affected by the weight of the carcass. The wood cutters had spent their life in the jungles but never heard of any such a queer thing in life and were now witnessing the horrifying spectacle as if it was something from other world. The predator was coming towards them, covering space in enormous strides, his chest and front legs were blood besmeared, dripping out of hideous wounds in the cow's neck. Ill-equipped to face the advance of a tiger, the men's confidence deserted them and, dropping their axes on the ground, they quickly climbed the tree.

We heard the woodcutters' story with skepticism. I was aghast at the unbelievable description of a cow slung on a tiger's back but they endorsed it repeatedly with wide-eyes as large as poached eggs. "Yes, the cow was on his back like a sack on a man's shoulder. Only its rear feet were sagged on the ground." No one amongst us could believe what we had heard, probably because we had just followed the blood trail over grass and not the tiger's spoors, but I was strongly aware of the fact that the cattle was not carried through a drag, for grass on the way was never trampled. My curiosity was aroused, "what happened then?" I asked.

The men continued. "Having climbed the tree we waited for the tiger to clear off. He came up to the *nala*, dumped the kill at its edge and inspected the terrain. We thought he will haul the cow in the dark shades of *nala* and eat it there but no he decided to act the other way."

Now what they saw next was simply mind-boggling. Remember it is not me who is making this statement; I am rather narrating the incident which the woodcutters claimed they had actually witnessed. The tiger did go down the *nala* as expected; he came back to the kill, caught it again by décolletage, swung his neck right and left quite a few times, as if trying to pluck out the animal's neck from the rest of the body. Then he abruptly tossed it in the air with a great jerk of strength. The lobbed body went flying across the 10 ft broad *nala* and landed there with a thud. The tiger then smoothly sprang across the *nala* and took away the cattle; this time dragging it along his side effortlessly in normal speed.

Having heard the account, I sighed in absolute disbelief. "It was a wonderful story and might well be true," said Om Beer, "Even if it is not true, still it is the sort of thing that could happen when it pertains to tiger." We examined the clear pad marks on the dust around *nala* and to our genuine surprise their story was correct. Tigers have elastic muscles that produce nearly unbelievable strength at the time of need. This particular case demonstrated rather exceptional power of a fat cat's neck that threw a 100 kg cow some ten feet away. I gasped in amazement as I saluted the singular strength of the super cat that has no match in the predatory kingdom. Perhaps for this singular reason even wild elephants and rhinos keep a respectful distance from them.

Incidentally, Valdimir Troinin, a Russian expert of Taiga mentions of a tiger that jumped one meter and a half into the air with a 50-kg animal caught in its teeth. The Russian had seen a birch tree 15 cm in diameter broken down by a tiger, and a dog – a fat one weighing about 30 kg – fly five meters away from the blow of a tiger's paw. He ends by saying that "Try to throw a 15-kg rock that distance with both your hands." However, my personal experience about the tiger's capacity to lift heavy weights tells that tigers are far more superior in strength than what Troinin records about them.

Thomas Pennant, a Missionary registers about strength of Sunderbans tigers, "The Pietists... often fall victims to these terrible animals; they have such power as to carry off a man with utmost facility; they will even go full speed with a buffalo, which they will seize out in the field." Big cats have wonderful control over their bodies and due to the quality of their protein-rich diet, perform incredibly brutish feats when pressed hard for survival; feats that draw gasps of admiration from onlookers.

I have personally experienced several episodes and accumulated a number of stories like this. All come to the same conclusion that big cats are extraordinary beings. This is the reason why I love to watch tigers. Indeed the radical animals never cease to surprise me. Their raw power, their fluid grace and suppleness with regal bearing never fails to stir my imagination and the more I know them the more I respect them -Godlike.

The halo that surrounds an adult tiger, so evident and alluring to a human observer – is not a pure invention of an admirer's brain but based on crude physical facts. Perhaps for this reason, in the Hindu Pantheon the tiger is the celebrated steed of Mother Goddess, and their dominance and superiority over their realm is absolute. This truth has given the world's most precious cat an incredible corona of reverence that captures our attention and finally a status for adulation as a super-deity in the animistic cultures of the Tarai.

To sum up in words of Troinin, "Nature was generous when it created them."

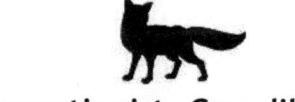

Conservationist- Grandiloquence

The solemnity reflected by this beast is not unreasonable. You can trust a normal tiger to be exactly like this one – it not an unnatural behavior as it is a trait of the species and never anything else.

- The author at a press conference of Tiger & Terrain in Lucknow

---

By March the extensive baiting had localized the tiger and even made it an object of curious attraction for city-dwellers. The mango season was in offing. Buds had come up on the trees, but preliminary crop management was in jeopardy. The resident tiger inside the campus had brought all outdoor activities to a halt. Mango trees were not being taken care of, pesticides had not yet been sprinkled as scientists and workers alike were too fearful to move around. The worried director

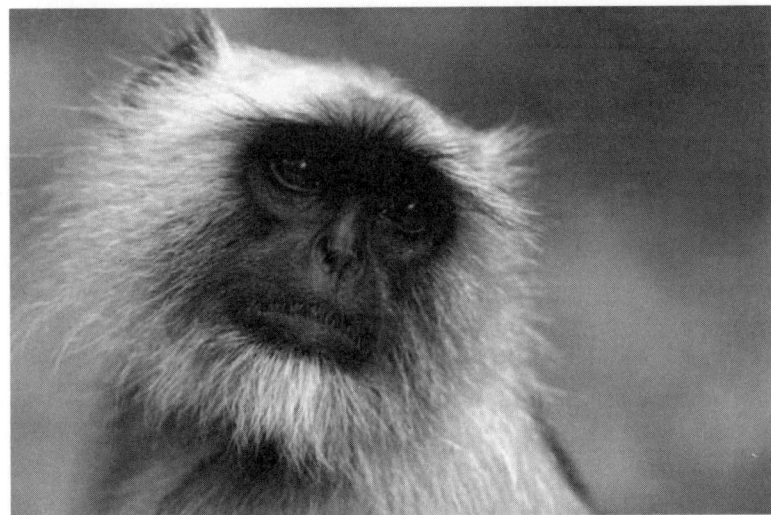

Langoor monkey are
common throughout
*Tarai (Photo credit :
Sanjay Narayan)*

ran from office to office, pleading to top Forest Department officials to sanction more equipment and redeem him of the problem. The Chief Wildlife Warden made it clear that things will move according to law and no outside agency would be entertained in this operation because the Wildlife Protection Act of India places total control of wildlife conservation in the hands of forest authorities and it is they who will perform the operation, no matter what time it takes.

Former field director of Dudhwa National Park G.C Mishra, then the Chairman of a city-based NGO Tiger & Terrain arranged an interactive session on the truant tiger in a hotel where wildlife connoisseurs and old game-hunting circles were invited. The forum examined the paradoxical situation which saw attempts to keep competent people outside the game rather than to bring them in to conclude the task at the earliest. An acrimonious argument started between the audience and pro-foresters. Newspaper representatives lambasted the department for behaving irresponsibly and for their poor understanding of problem, which seemed deeply rooted in a legal and elitist approach which could not benefit wildlife any way. It seemed that lines were already drawn on the ground and the mandarins thought they knew better than anyone as how to deal with this tiger. Never was there a truer example of an unworkable approach towards problem.

The meeting concluded with a specific pronouncement for the government that if bonafide sportsmen were not available to tackle the tiger, then the notorious poacher Sansar Chand currently languishing in jail should be brought out on parole and be immediately employed for this task. The man is true tiger catcher, whose expertise is known to have accounted for over 100 full-grown tigers, weighing nearly two hundred kilograms, besides many cubs and hundreds of leopards.

Against all odds of the ecological crisis, it was no doubt an important study animal for me, having provided access to the clinical knowledge which tigers are known to follow to survive during stressful existence in complex areas. I may add that scientists are more concerned with canopied forest and the study of its wildlife while those who enter the farmland have largely been away from their gaze – even off-limits of their radar. No one even picked up the scats of the tiger to analyze as what he had been naturally eating, their priority was on capturing it.

The drawback is that there is no wildlife research wing within the state's Forest Department where researchers can foster dialogue and interaction with wildlife managers. They are rather treated as unwelcome outsiders. The truth is that both researchers and forest officials can learn from each other's experiences. Knowledge production systems – both state sponsored and independent – seem to be under attack from the bureaucrats. A disturbing trend of marginalizing independent researchers and even making them subservient to the needs of the Government is clearly visible. The Forest Department has its own fix set of blanket rules with no capacity within its mandarins to judge the activists and their research output; hence farmland wildlife work was not of much use to them.

I am constrained to say that all through my tiger time in Tarai, I have not known any scientist or a conservationist ever being called by Forest Department to explain the applicability of his research for the management of wildlife problems. People like Ragu Chandavat and herpetologists like Romulous Whitaker, whose international reputation in contribution to reptile conservation in India is unmatched, were denied to carry out research inside the forest on the basis of unproven allegations. Even Billy Arjan Singh was ousted from Dudhwa many times and despite being a Padma awardee, his freedom to enter the park was hampered.

There are countless NGOs, activists, scientists and wildlife buffs whose role in conservation has been striking but they never get a chance to show their expertise in times of crisis. It seems that government policies are often just policies – nothing more or nothing less. The ridiculous manipulation once again brought out the limitation and failing of so-called departmental tiger experts. The linkage between conservation knowledge vacuum and bureaucratic approach often results in a combination of absurdities and foolishness.

One evening a live goat provided inside the cage bleated constantly throughout the night and attracted the animal. The tiger came, circled round the cage, watching the goat that fell silent at his sight, partly entered the cage but got suspicious and came out. After this incident, despite being hungry, it never attempted to step into the baited cage. A forester told me that it had rather made an effort to claw the animal from outside just as the hyena had done earlier.

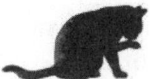

Solitary Tiger - Pattern of Survival

"Even when tigers are continuously baited and allowed to drag their kills into cover of their own choosing, where there is everything the tiger needs- adequate shelter, water and freedom from disturbance-this steady supply of food offered under ideal conditions does not succeed in localizing these big cats other than for temporary periods. Soon the tiger gets its priorities straight again. It moves on".

- Charls Mac Dougal

Three months had passed and the master predator was continuing elusively in the area, visiting a series of places at regular intervals. His nightly rounds covered as far west as Chandrika Devi temple along the course of the *nala*, and beyond the railway line in the south. It was roughly a linear beat of about 20 miles. The territorial animals by choice occupy only that much of area that is necessary to satisfy their few basic needs. He moved through river grass, crossed farmlands with humans in residence, killed smaller animals, chomped them then and there but never forgot his safe sanctuary. He never strayed in long perambulations. Even if a half-eaten kill was left in midway, he would delay his return to the Institutes campus until nightfall the next day.

The institute's sprawling estate was like his permanent home. It was kind of mega-enclosure, hundred times the size of a football field, where its perimeters might have lacked fencing and metal bars but the penalty of leaving it for long could be otherwise troublesome. The animal would be vulnerable to punishment for transgressing the boundary just as severe as it is for the tiger that slips through the gate of the zoo amongst people. If it behaved itself it would be captured and placed back within his boundaries. If it did otherwise, it would be shot dead.

The repeated return of the tiger proved that abandoning a sheltering area spontaneously is not part of the tiger's natural behaviour. Moreover, when a tiger's habitat is of selective occupancy the animal shows strong disinclination to move out of it and remains in residence as long as possible. This is a parameter on which the categorization of a resident and a transient is done by scientists and this becomes subjective when based on stable home range and detection histories.

Great excitement was caused one particular week when a large number of blue bulls gathered around the Chandrika Devi temple township. The priest at the temple of Mother Goddess explained "Blue bulls seem to have gone crazy at this time of the year. Their vagaries cannot be otherwise explained unless it is the fear of the tiger." The priest was dead-on, the predator pressure on this species had gone excessive.

One morning while based near Chandrika Devi temple I got the news that the tiger had just killed a blue bull a mile away. I quickly reached the place and found a massive antelope had been shot by poachers. It had run as much it could, and then fallen clearly unable to rise, but was still alive when I got there. It was amazing to see the tenacity of this animal. A .315 bullet had entered its lung and severed the main artery, entering further into the body and cutting the entrails. A huge quantity of blood had pumped out of the bullet hole, the rill of blood had trickled down across the road. A passing cyclist had seen this rill and had run away in panic, spreading the word that the tiger had made a kill. Incredibly, blood had spurted out of a hole of nearly half-inch diameter, and the red rill had dripped down to some twenty feet away from the fallen animal. Though the blue bull lay exhausted and still, its heart was still pumping out the blood with strong pressure. Like an invincible immortal he was continuing to breathe.

It was a phase of intense cold. Days dawned grey and gloomy and the sun as though tired of lingering with fog never burst forth with strength. The antelope lay there for good four days, providing a substantial feast to hyenas and jackals. I and my old photographer friend Yogesh Kumar, then Principal Secretory Institutional Finance also made a vigil till mid night, sitting on a tree with spotlights and a camera, but no tiger turned up and we were left watching the scavengers raid the meat-bait. Although it is extremely annoying sometimes but it does provide worthwhile observations. The 800 pound venison was devoured by jackals, hyenas, eagles and crows within four days. A week later when I passed through the place a lanky geriatric hyena was hovering at the site searching for scraps. All that remained of the grand antelope was a bare skull and some vertebrae.

I reported the poaching case to Special Task Force (STF) of the State Government; and after a week's tracking, STF officer Arvind Chaturvedi caught a gang of locals that hunted blue bulls and sold their meat. Their vehicle and three licensed rifles were confiscated and substantial hard cash, accumulated from large deals, was recovered.

Arvind is an old associate of mine and his work in controlling poaching and recovering contrabands is substantial. Some days later he made a presentation for Forest Department officials explaining variants in poaching. These included market-driven hunting that removes selected species, and local hunting, which is a more universal threat that targets a wider variety of wildlife. Since it is practiced by larger number of people than those that indulge in market hunting, it is biologically more tragic than selected hunting. This may be an academic matter as what fosters hunting and sustains it in farmlands including profit-centered options, but the warning siren is already honking, needing serious attention on the part of law enforcement officials.

Drawing on my years of tiger observations as well as several encounters, both friendly and aggressive, I can say that a tiger in its normal surroundings is a modest

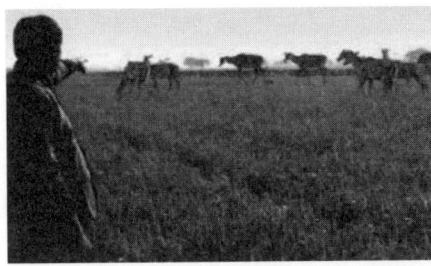

Blue bull gathered around Chandrika Devi at the outskirts of   Lucknow

animal by nature than most other felines. The exotic mega fauna is a symbol of unbridled and elemental power and equally of gentleness. Yet, in the popular mind, the tiger is the personification of ferocity, ruthless savagery and upraising cruelty, which is not correct. Perhaps the picture has emerged out of its mysterious and predatory nature. The fear of a normal tiger is more imaginary than real. It could be because they are such impossibly magnetic creatures.

Three and a half months had gone by and the beast was unblemished. His bashfulness was well realised by herdsmen who almost daily came across him. Jungle folk living within hearing range of a tiger's roar are habituated to witnessing occasional incident of cattle lifting and despite knowing the strength of the jungle monarch are never afraid of a wanton attack by a normal tiger.

So was this wanderer, a dangerous and powerful hunter, but unquestionably a conventional beast. Despite its adversarial contact with man and seemingly adapted to anthropogenic pressure, confined to small place and in competition with too many scavengers, he reflected no trace of aberration. It is said that isolated instances of human killings occur in chance encounters with tigers as they suddenly come into conflict with human interests but during my investigations, I had disturbed this tiger accidentally twice on its natural kill and so had many other people. But he had left all and sundry safe. Likewise one night, the tiger killed a buffalo and its calf at a village called Metheypur but when at the dying sounds of his cattle the farmer Ram Deen got up and raised an alarm. The tiger ran away and never returned.

Such behavior of tigers stimulates surprise and interrogation and what is not known about them outweighs what is known about them by many orders of magnitude.

Animals learn in human association. Domestication makes dogs more intelligent as civilization did to humans; similarly cats are quick learners in human environment. After quite a few unprecedented confrontations with humans this tiger instinctively learnt to respect human livestock protection measures, while simultaneously accepting potential food base around him in form of feral dogs that existed on garbage and feral cattle that damaged the crops. He learnt that domestic cattle avoid mixing up with feral cattle hence are easily identifiable and were a permanent source of food supply. All these factors reinforced by my personal experience of tigers convinced me that this animal had confirmed advantages of survival in this landscape where burgeoning human population was in demographic dominance.

This tiger exemplified little beyond itself, contributing little knowledge in terms of general principles that a normal predator instinctively follows when it comes to live by humans. This case establishes rigorous baselines, not just for tiger conservation in farmlands near principal jungles but equally for a change in wider set of norms in tiger study parameters.

I say this all on the basic knowledge of prey base in farmlands. There is a relative abundance of wildlife, especially blue bull herds which are considered a relative of cow and hence held as sacred by the populace. Then there are feral cattle that supplement domestic cattle as tiger's primary prey base. If this initial prey base collapses then all my bets for farmland tigers are off. It is only when we appreciate how they live without creating problem for people, whose work naturally brings them within the killing reach of these predators and yet they invariably fair well, that we can really understand their unusualness.

A tiger will truly fight for what he has and what he needs and is ever more courageous than most. But he is contemptuous of cowards, wary of his equals and never afraid. The master predator inevitably heard human communities passing by his hideout every day, collecting fuel wood from around his resting place but he never committed the mistake of growling at them, which would advertise his position.

Between February and April he had witnessed sugarcane, wheat and barley being harvested and his habitat of strong cover being reduced day by day. Fragmentation disrupts demographic functioning of wildlife populations and directly affects ecology and behavior of all animals. Once the composition of local wildlife changes it affects the predator too but he compromised with this human activity and developed skills to negotiate within diminishing cover spaces. He didn't leave the area in search of better quality habitat patches; he rather adjusted downwards in response to this human induced depression of vegetation, spending a disproportionate amount of time in last surviving hideouts along Nala. I am sure he even knew that humans squatted in these patches and behind trees to relieve themselves so he never ever sprang on them in confusion of their being quadrupeds.

While studying tigers, I got ample opportunity to review man-tiger conflict in Tarai farmlands that ascertained that many tiger attacks were not deliberate. The reconstruction of the exact circumstances of attacks, in some 50 cases, revealed that this particular position of humans squatting whether relieving or cutting grass was the main cause getting attacked. Believing men to be a quadruped tigers notched them, but later confused by the puzzling carcass, they left it uneaten.

Fortunately such ecological disaster never happened in Rahman Khera area, where unlike the forest, human density was 300- plus per sq km and man had every business to go alone. Mankind may not afford to give living space to a predator on their landscape but the predator, whose species is marching towards extinction,

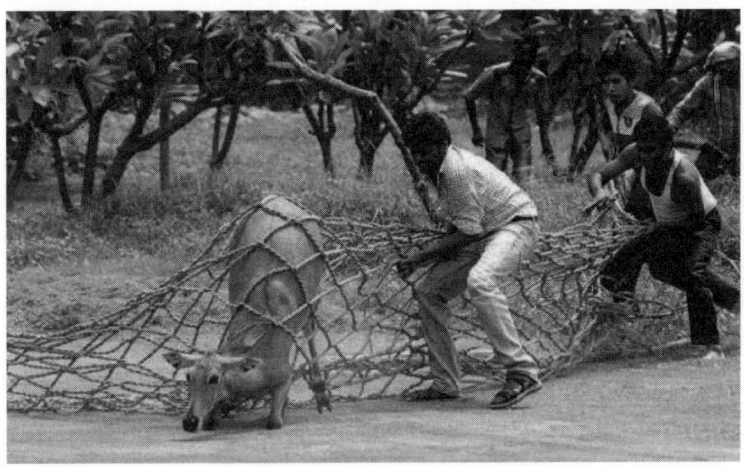

Trapping in nets is a clandestine operation which produces no gun shot sounds and culminates silently. *(Photo credit : WCT)*

still has the ability to create a safe place by their side and live on friendly terms. Vladimir Troinin says "tigers who lived for centuries with thrift, long ago adapted to human mismanagement." It is truly astonishing that in a short time a species can fundamentally remake its biologically meaningful relationship with the systems that keep it alive.

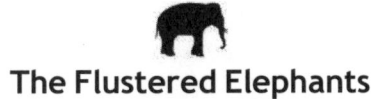

The Flustered Elephants

"Where tigers are strictly nocturnal, they have become so to minimize contact with man".
- Charls Mac Dougal

The DFO accountable for the operation operated from a quasi-heroic pedestal and claimed such a ponderous knowledge about tigers that it would have submerged many a lesser man like me. He had a great collection of *shikaar* material with him and might have gone down like a swimmer in a sea struggling with tiger books under each arm.

One morning he and a team of veterinarians from the zoo were combing the central area of the institute, a dense tree zone, when suddenly at the approach of domestic elephants, the concealed tiger exploded out of the grass, hurling himself upon his tormentors with an angry outburst of roars. The sudden upsurge of roars panicked the badly trained elephants that spun on their heels and bolted with their tails up in the air. One elephant was chased by the tiger for some 20 meters. The strange sounding roar of the enraged tiger and the thunderous blare of terror-stricken fleeing elephants shook the elephant riders. Equipments flew everywhere in wild confusion as the foresters had difficulty in saving their heads from overhanging boughs. They gripped the ropes or whatever they could in their bid to hold on to their seat despite the elephants' mad sprint.

For a few moments pandemonium reigned supreme as *mahouts* somehow managed to control the headlong dash of the pachyderms. In confusion two darts were hastily fired which failed to hit the tiger. However, good sense seemed to prevail on the tiger and he quit the chase. The DFO later said that the tiger had sprung on to the rump of the elephant upon which he was sitting, but was kicked off and thrown. The apparently hungry beast dropped flat and went back into cover, glaring and snarling (I don't think that elephants can kick like a donkey. They can of course trample but not bobble their hind quarters.) This particular elephant continued her flight, screaming and trumpeting and did not stop until she attained the camp.

I and Dr. Panday reached the spot four hours after the incident. The afternoon field was completely empty but for a hare family foraging in the open. At that precise moment an eagle swooped down and grabbing a baby rabbit in its talons, settled upon a nearby tree. The prey bird was immediately attacked by a flock of crows. The scavengers constantly poked their beaks on her head till it was forced to abandon the baby. The injured baby dropped down the tree but surprisingly, recovered and dashed to a shelter leaving the crows thoroughly disappointed.

While we were getting back to the institute building, a fox chattered in alarm at a tube well site, indicating that the tiger was making its way to the kill point. Apparently the tiger was disturbed and there seemed no point in following it further. In wildlife ventures the greatest risk to a naturalist comes from the unpredictable behavior of dangerous animals. A tiger on a given day would turn his tail at the first whiff of human scent, but the same tiger the next day may present a bluff-threat demonstration and for no obvious reason. And if it is a male with a female, or a mother with her cubs, then it can even carry through the intended charge. It is therefore not only death-defying but fatally perilous to regard tiger actions as elemental bluffs that some arm-chair experts may want you to believe. I would estimate that roughly 20 percent of all charges, including apparent bluff-threat demonstrations by uninjured healthy tigers, if generated under harassed conditions are genuine and in case of a wounded tiger the charge is always fully qualified. However, I would still maintain that distance is a critical factor in judging the seriousness of predatory charges.

Indeed all the methods invented by hunters to shoot tigers have now become strong tools in the hands of conservationists to save the species. Forest officials had initially resented my idea of sprinkling urine of a zoo tigress but when they read about this idea in a book, it was immediately applied and the very night, the predator was attracted to the spot and its first photograph, smelling a scent soaked brick was clicked. The picture became very popular with city newspapers.

The urine was continuously sprinkled around the cages for a week and the tiger took to prowling around them. He would make typical gestures and often call impatiently. He often lay down over the spot, saturated with the female's smell, his

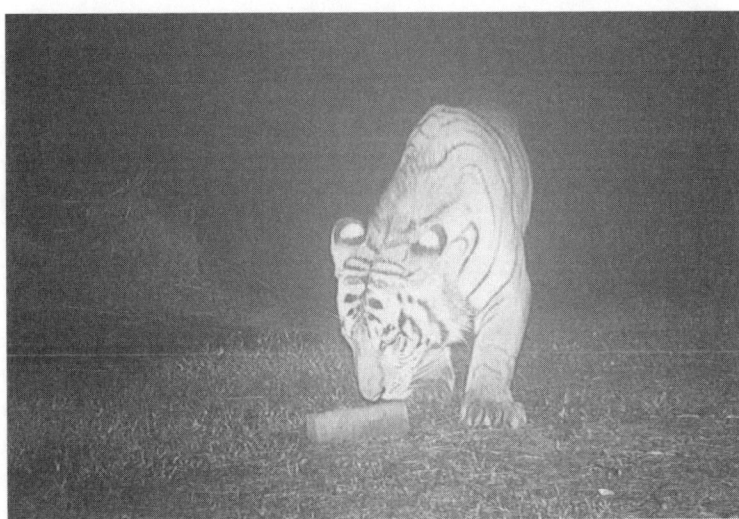

Bachelor smelling the brick
wet with zoo tigresses
urine

head resting on the ground and eyes closed, he seemed to absorb the seductive aroma of the tigress, much like sunshine through every bit of his body. Then he would rise slowly and move down the path where the scents lead and where the cage was kept. Towards evening, a cadence of its moaning calls floated across the immensity of space, meaning the male was on the ball by the smell of urine and was searching for the female. It is a patent vocalization of tigers, that is often much difficult to pin-point whether it is of male or female that tells the other partner is ready to mate. He would often call and circle the premises, searching for the elusive female.

Curious as ever, I observed his naïve style of functioning where the application of knowledge based solutions was completely missing. As a ludicrous charade a honeytrap was arranged. A stuffed tigress from the museum was planted into the cage with fresh urine of a zoo tigress sprinkled around it. Thriving in the solitude with no mate around, this bid to cage the tiger was appreciable but nobody noted the smell of insecticide with which the trophy had been preserved. The mannequin, mixed with the curious scent of naphthalene and urine, failed to entice the tiger. Seemingly confused with pungent odour of bug juice, he savored the tigress from outside and never entered the trap. Only once he approached the cage for a closer look and squirted on its bars, with his head resting upon the trap but the chemical smell was too strong for him to withstand.

For three days, the poor animal toyed with the idea of closing in to the mate and remained localized but the mannequin obviously remained stationary and unattainable. The tiger ate, slept and roared and tried to communicate with the tigress by repeatedly coming back to see her. He even rolled in the female urine and had several erections. Through binoculars we could guess its testosterone boiling high and it penis swollen to twice its normal dimensions. His drive to reproduce remained strong. But at the same time this 'tool creation and reverse engineering' of his mate by humans, kept him confused. What went on in his head was something only a cat psychologist might define better. However, the worst part was that none of the foresters could approach closer to him to risk a tranquilizer dart; and when people try to deal with predators without going near them, things don't happen easily.

The tiger finally became tired with the mannequin and started showing indifference and then as if in protest he started giving a long pass to the cage.

The rule book of wild animals' capture mentions that darting teams must accomplish their work by sunlight and no operations should be conducted during dark hours. It was only after sunset when the veterinarians moved away it came out of its hiding. It demonstrated its awareness of the operation being conducted to catch him. He roamed the area laid with various traps and nets that were set by a monkey catcher. In the extraordinary silence of winter nights, he would sniff the ladder from which the dart shooters climbed, observed the *machan* where they regularly sat and moved around the three cages. Despite the temptation of live bait and chunks of meat inside cages, he never stepped up even to their doors. He rather preferred to kill the tethered bait, which foresters provided him as a compulsion to keep him localized. He would chop the neck or leg that held rope and take away the kill.

Brander who regularly observed his tiger pet says, "They are animals of extraordinarily little intelligence. They possess very fixed habits and instincts and these serve them to get through life and deal with exigencies thereof… The cub although brought up with dogs, learned no dog habits and he was always a tiger, pure and simple, and acquired nothing except what developed out of his own nature." Perhaps Brander's pet was less intelligent and his experience about him does not give him the right to generalize the species as dumb. My experience tells that tigers are quick learners, and some of them also form habits and character that are made through learning and require reasoning. Unfortunately the first to excel in this trait are man-eaters because they interact with humans – a species more intelligent than what the normal tigers deal with. Interestingly in Lucknow Zoo, Krishna, the Kaanp Tanda man-eater and his partners Ipshita and Shishir, have learnt playing with a football. He has become so fond of it that he keeps the ball with him even when sleeping.

A day later we were again on tiger tracks when an iguana hurriedly crossed our path, followed by a chasing pariah dog. The speed of the lizard was terrific and the dog was unable to reach it. Perhaps the chase had been lasting for some time and the big creature not used to running long distances was tiring fast. It then turned for a straightforward fight. As the dog neared it turned again and used the whip of its tail on its face so fast from right and left that the dog was lashed across face

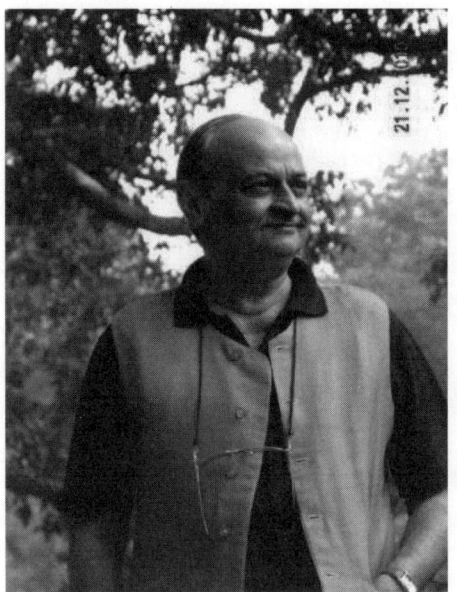

Ajay Kumar Mishra, I.A.S, former Chief Secretory of Jharkhand; A fearless tiger aficionado and a man of élan.

quite a few times. As the dog retreated at this attack, the lizard quickly slithered up a tree, managing to escape unimpeded.

Next evening my cousin Ajay Kumar Mishra, former Chief Secretary of Jharkhand, his son Gaurav and I reached the place and occupied the same *machan* which the foresters used during the day and vacated by evening. They had left a buffalo heifer tied to a peg. The exercise had helped localize the tiger so that he may be tranquilized at ease. By then the tiger had already lifted more than half a dozen calves from this place and he was in the habit of checking it regularly in the nights because so long their meals are guaranteed tigers give dime for the morrow. Laziness is their second nature and they have no objection to an existence which demands less effort.

For last two days, excessive machine activity in the area was going on but the tiger was not aware that a 3 feet wide and 12-feet deep trench had been dug encircling the spot where a fresh delectable invitation for him had rested. The encircling trench had been fully covered with grass sheets so that the ground appeared even at surface.

Langoors, being primarily herbivorous were plentiful in the area. As the sun dipped in band of pink clouds, a troop of these monkeys came to the place. They drank from the tube well pond and went up an *Amaltas* tree to take shelter for the night. Their silhouettes looked like so many gruesome spirits floating in a circle in a weird setting. They looked insecure, alert and cautious as they peeped here and there from their commanding position as if a predator was around.

Monkeys are like trained watchmen and are almost never known to render false alarms. They only call when the presence of the predator is confirmed and pinpointed. I have never seen or heard them joining the general volley of calls, which quite often proves false and adds to general confusion.

We sat for good long hours then as the chill begun to increase we abandoned the vigil and returned by midnight.

We only learnt the next day what an exciting story had unfolded after we left.

The tiger was very much around the *machan* since evening watching the heifer but had preferred to remain hidden. The *langoors* had already perceived its presence though they had yet not seen him. He came out of his hiding only when we had left and walking towards the heifer had tumbled down into the trench. Thereafter maintaining silence he made a great effort to free himself, scratching the trench walls with power and pulling down big chunks of earth from it. The extraordinary crescendo made by panicked monkeys at the sight of the predator was heard in the institute building as the guards on night duty wondered what had happened. They suspected that perhaps the tiger had been discovered but there were no whir of hideous growls from him.

Indeed keeping silent, the tiger stood on his hind legs and continued to scrape the wall, pulling down chunks of mud. As more and more mud fell on the ground, it provided the animal an ever-elevating platform from below that finally helped him earn his freedom and bolt away. The tiger was so panicked that he did not take any interest in the heifer and preferred to clear away from the place.

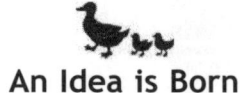

An Idea is Born

Because of much greater concern for human welfare that exists in all societies, usually wildlife gets eliminated if the conflict goes unresolved. For example, over last few centuries, most conflict prone wildlife species in India have suffered range constrictions of over 90%.
- Ullas Karanth

The tiger was the center of melodramatic news's. While some reporters admired his gracious behavior, the attitude of the general public was interesting. In the beginning the people wanted to get it eliminated but now things had changed drastically and the same people - even Lakshman whose buffalo and calf the tiger had killed - wanted it to live. The press was heavily critical of Forest Department's incompetence and a debate raged over the tiger's fate. A correspondent of Hindi daily *Amar Ujala* Ashutosh Mishra was candidly vocal, he wrote on 16 March, "Even Rahul Shukla is not brought in the affairs. It is like denying the champion fighter the right to enter the ring on the ground that he might get hurt."

The news revived the impetus of newly appointed Principal Chief Conservator of Forests JS Asthana. A friend of my friend Yogesh Kumar, Asthana invited me to discuss the matter at length and we began on a convivial note. "Four months have elapsed, great deals of funds have been spent and the result is nil," he said, reminding me of a meeting of Wildlife Advisory Board in 1996, in which I had suggested that a committee should be formed to write a manual for capturing large predators and their post-capture care. He told me with seriousness that due to the laxity of commitment, 2012 has arrived and the manual for handling darted animals is yet not set in writing. This way we are at a loss as how to proceed step by step when guidelines were missing.

But besides the absence of the modicum of statecraft, there are other equally serious problems that have brought the wildlife department to such a pass. There are structural and systematic issues, political compulsions, lack of practical policy making experience, and even intellectual capacity and lack of understanding the academia's suggestions, and a serious attention-deficit syndrome. All these have contributed to the shaping of problems of farm tigers as well as of their straying in distant lands.

My duties in the college were getting demanding so I expressed my inability to participate in action but conjured up a fresh blueprint for the operation with a request to include the name of Aftab Wali Khan in the team. The retired forester's association with me was well known to the present official. In the half-closed eyes of memories; many shiver-inducing days with him, huddled round the burning fires, had never marched out of the calendar.

Asthana relished the algorithm, sipped his coffee, stared into the cup as if it were a crystal ball and declared that the things will now really materialize.

In the meanwhile the state elections were over and a new government was formed in Uttar Pradesh by March 2012. In a pompous gesture, the new Forest Minister decided to tour Rahman Khera apparently to take stock of the efforts to capture the tiger. He arrived there followed by his staff, security guards, police, political followers, sycophants and hangers-on in 15 vehicles. The 50-plus entourage chased the tiger for the entire day, threw bricks, shouted and abused the animal, and the beleaguered, harassed beast moved from cover to cover to the joy of people.

Mary Taylor Young, the writer of *Guide to Colorado Mammals* believes that even just watching animals has an impact on them. Intrusion into their living space can expose them to predation, keep them from feeding or other essential activities, or cause them to leave their young. No photo or viewing opportunity is worth harassing or stressing wildlife. "In appreciating and watching them, we have a responsibility to protect and preserve the animals that share our state."

Tigers are disturbed by shock maneuvers and can easily turn on. Faulty actions are likely to lead to stressful interactions with humans and goad them into dangerous fury thereby making them a potential instrument of destruction. Such mischief-makers need to be educated that their method of dealing with a dangerous animal will only result in major increase of danger for rural people.

However when I questioned the minister who was from the same cadre of college teachers like me, his response was amazing: "People cannot enjoy wild life unless they can see it from close quarters". So this was his concept of entertainment, uncontrolled, intense wildlife tourism at the cost of animal's serenity.

The Capture & Relocation

"The immense longing not just to protect, but to rehabilitate the Earth".
- Laurens Van der Post

Soon temperatures began to rise and by the end of May, summers were quite acute. The grass cover had drastically reduced and the water puddles had become dry. The fields lay barren and the tiger had begun to seek water body for whole of the day.

Ashutosh Mishra, the journalist from *Amar Ujala* had taken to guiding the forest department through his reports. His contention was: "A predator must be vanquished at all costs." We would meet in the evening, discuss subtle gradations and next day his report would carry fresh advice for the foresters. One day we talked about the elephant ring method used by Maharaja of Nepal to shoot and trap big cats and next morning his paper carried all the guidelines point by point as how to proceed with the ring.

Maharaja Joodha Shumshere Jung Bahdur Rana of Nepal was a skilled hunter of great mammals. Olive Smythe of *One Thousand Miles on Elephants* fame tells about shoots in which big cats were shot inside the surrounding ring of elephants. It was no less magnificent to see the elephants' slow stately march through the swaying, crashing grasslands. With all the panoply and panache of unrestrained disbursements, over 500 of huge brutes moved through the river to surround the tiger, splashing the water along their heated sides to cool themselves. This sent huge waves dashing against the crumbling banks of rapid streams. A couple of elephants also served as mobile bars, their *howdahs* stocked with snacks and premium drinks including champagne and tonic water to rejuvenate the hunters who felt confident of realizing their pursuit pitching on the ponderous strength of huge creatures, as they heaved through the tangled brake, crushing everything in their relentless progress.

The circumference of the circle grew smaller as the elephants moved in, surrounding the grassland where the tiger was supposed to be lying, until ultimately all retreats were cut off. Then a staunch elephant, named Gaj Raj entered the ring with hunters sitting on the *howdah*. The ring would not let the tigers escape and the glimpses of one or more slinking forms were seen in the grass and undergrowth, when suddenly a tiger broke cover and charged with a roar to be met by shots from high powered cordite rifles or shouts or javelins if they dared to charge the ring. This generated a moment of climax as the tiger, often more than one, dashed here and there, backward and forward, determined to find an escape route, to a

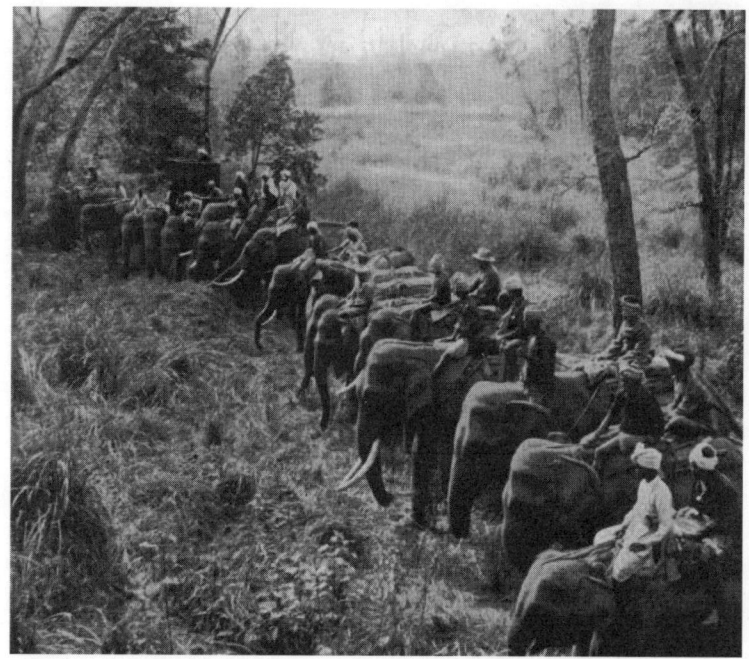

In the earlier 20th century, Maharana Jodha Shamsher Jung, the originator of organized hunting in Nepal, had started a ring system in which upto 500 elephants were employed in a shoot.

pandemonium of men shouting and panic stricken elephants trumpeting. The angry tiger with its all escape routes blocked inevitably charged the line of elephants and was met by a volley of shots as the hunters accomplished their job sanctimoniously, fostering an image of masculinity over sport killers.

Years later when the number of elephants declined and the mindless battues continued, the Maharaja initiated a ground-breaking innovation whereby the ring of elephants was complemented by long strips of cloth. The long white curtain like stretch prevented the escape of tigers from the ring; with their inborn suspicion of the unfamiliar, they did not willingly cross the white cloth line resulting in their ritualized destruction and phenomenal success of the hunt.

This system not only employed elephants in small numbers but also made it possible to operate several rings. Joodha Shumshere's mind-boggling hunting mortalities that ranged from episodic bag of 433 tigers in seven seasons or 120 in just one season of 68 days were enough a proof of the king's deadly innovation in waylaying the big-game; en extremely augmented success rate with much lesser efforts. But it was equally a maddening and dishonorable exhibition to manipulate an extreme beast, just to boost the ego of a single person. However, these true stories are no longer of our age and days; they belong to an epoch and regime that passed away more than half a century ago.

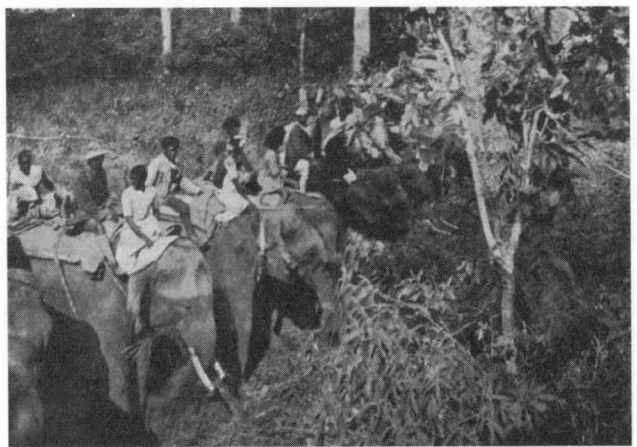

As soon the tigers were rounded up in the ring the ring converged upon them, slowly reducing in size.

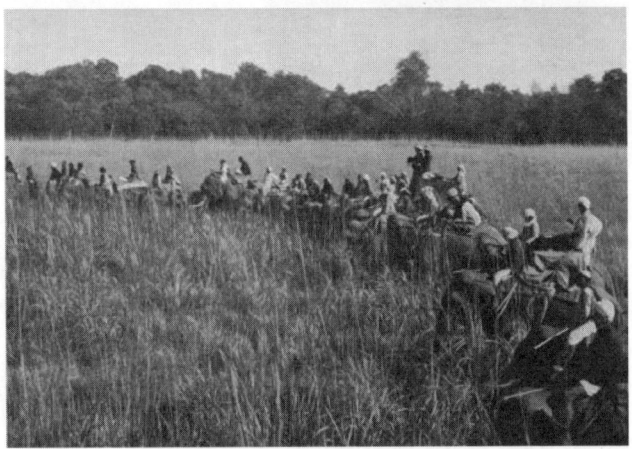

The elephants offered a living wall of flesh and muscle, standing shoulder to shoulder against the encircled tiger.

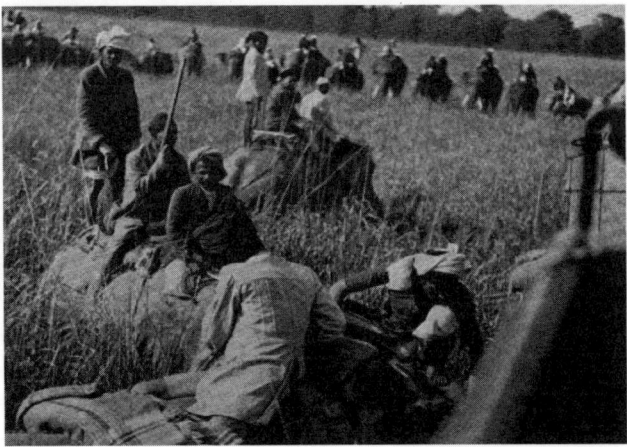

When the ring was complete some stout-hearted shikar elephants entered the ring to face the enraged predators.

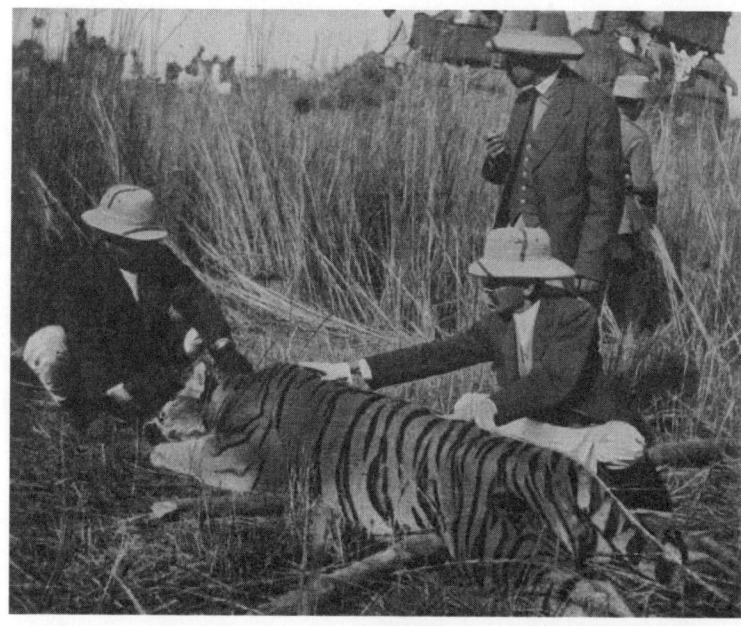

Genl. Bahadur (left) the first Nepalese Minister in England and Genl. Baber measuring a large man-eater which taped 10 feet 2 inches. (Shot by Elephant Ring Method)

❖

Both tiger and 'The Killer Ape' are strategists. Tiger is a hunter of first order and so is man. By this time the foresters had realized their mistakes. In last six operations whenever the tiger was cornered by elephants, all the retreats were not cut off, and in absence of proper stops, it had always managed to slip away.

On the morning of June 1, a message from a reconnaissance party arrived that the tiger was sighted at a crossing point. Hectic arrangements were made and the long-forgotten ring method was applied. Aftab introduced a two meter wide and hundred meter long strip of white cloth to contain the tiger within the circle and lead the beat. Everything went according to the plan. The tiger could easily jump over or rip through the flimsy cloth but it did not. Faced with unfamiliar white amidst the surrounding greenery, the naturally wary animal avoided the barrier and treaded its way cautiously towards the road, where it emerged out of the narrow exit. The zoo vet's gun went off with a crack as the godhead animal leaped forward, running a few paces before turning in surprise to search for the cause of momentary sharp pain as the drug laden dart pierced his skin with a measured dose of 5 milliliters of .CI-744.

After about five minutes as the sedation took effect the animal was found lying some 200 meters away. By a fortuitous chance it had avoided falling in a water pond. A bright red plump covered his thigh identifying the syringe and a giant owl, like a wheezing drone flew over it letting out a series of muffled hoots. The tiger was measured, weighed and blood samples were taken. After collaring it for monitoring, it was put in a cage and covered with a dark mattress. If not handled

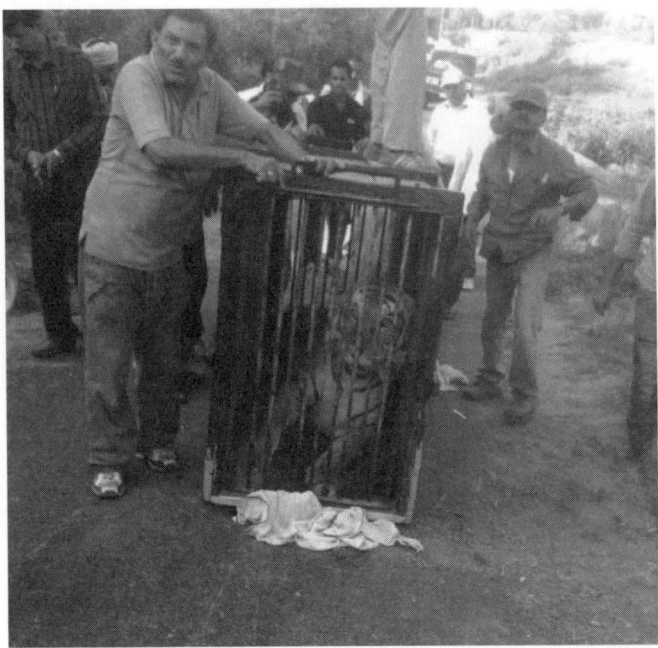

Author's old companion Aftab Wali Khan with the convival bachelor caught on 1st June, 2012 *(Photo credit : Chief Wildlife Wardon, UP)*

carefully the tigers may injure themselves by charging at the steel bars of the trap; the dark sheet prevents them seeing anything around and becoming aggressive when the drug automatically wears off, the recovery time of which might vary from two hours to four hours. In order to beat the heat, and keep its body cool since the drug makes the body temperature rise, the cage was half drenched in water.

There were a few uneasy moments for wildlife buffs as a section of officials that wished to earn cheap acclaim in the cocktail circle, felt the animal should be kept in the city zoo. The use of zoos as reservoir for problem animals is an old practice and though the space in the zoo was stuffed full but the prize catch was sure to attract massive footfalls.

Ipso facto, the imprisonment of an animal as superb as tiger is a crime. It may pander to the tastes of officials and mislead trans-national conservationist forums into believing that one more member of critically endangered species has been saved, but it is a misdeed to deprive Mother Nature of its magnificent creation and reduce into an atrophied and pale shadow of its natural self within the ghetto of zoo walls as its powers shrivel. The fact is no real wild tiger ever becomes reconciled to the restrictions of this new existence, which is truly a gateway to its destruction.

Fortuitously, good sense prevailed and the animal was shifted to Dudhwa, to be released inside the sanctuary. Though it is difficult to inject an outsider into the existing social system of tigers because resident tigers kill outsiders but on the basis of camera tracings and GPS locations, G. Ganesh the Deputy Director of the

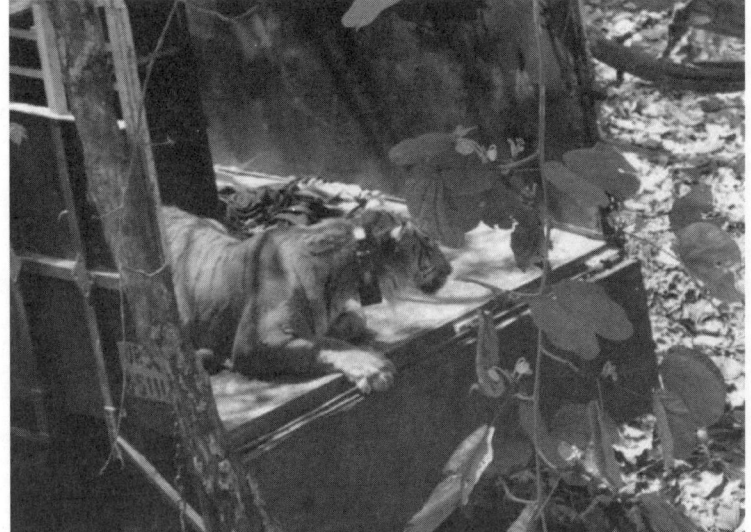

The radio colored Bachelor being released in Salukapur, Dudhwa, June 2- 2012.

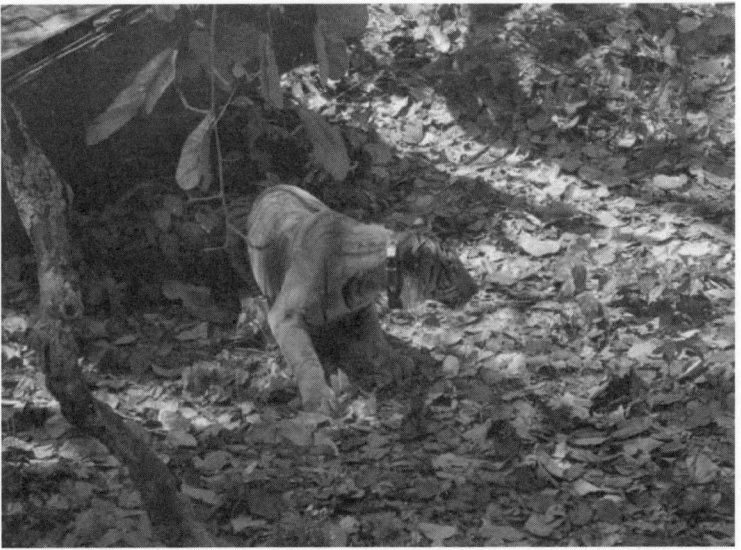

The translocated Bachelor finally seeks his freedom in the wilderness of Salukapur, Dudhwa National Park.

Park, had identified an area in Salukapur range which had no dominant male and marked it as apposite location for the tiger's rehabilitation. It may be mentioned that intraspecific antagonism towards an outsider causes social instability in big cat setups which is likely to lead to dismissal of either the introduced tiger or another individual for the local population often followed by increased rates of infanticides if the new comer triumphs. However, within 48 hours of its capture the tiger was successfully released there.

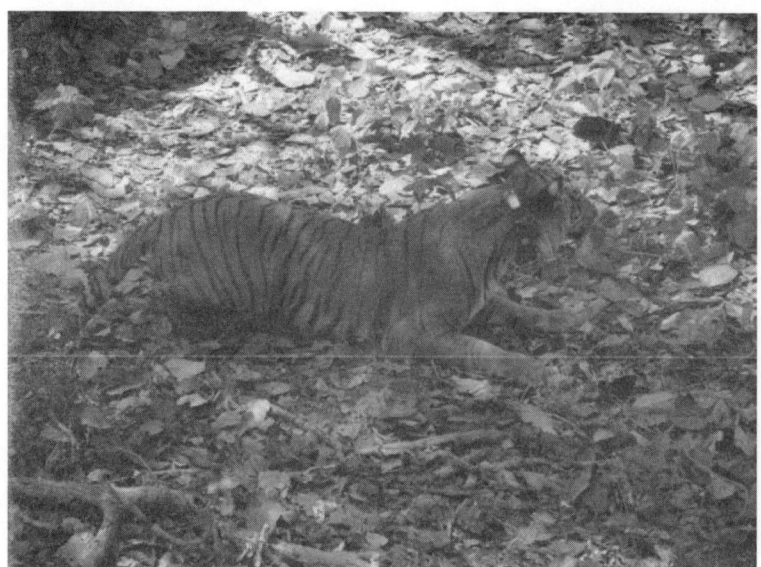

Enjoying freedom

This case is the first model of a stray tiger management in Lucknow that did not meet its nemesis at the hands of foresters but was successfully captured and relocated in the jungle. A free ranging animal that had never acknowledged humans as trespassers in his territory and which had managed to enjoy independence alongside man with his inhibitions and a large range, it was finally reintroduced to his own legitimate world of infinite freedom.

Some weeks later Dr Panday and I were roaming around the institute campus, when we neared a mango tree upon which the amiable fellow had regularly marked with his claws and sprayed his urine. It had left a deeply absorbed odour of his scent and urine that indeed helps the species to track each other. It was exactly fifty second day of his deportation from the institute and the pungent smell was still discernable on the tree. It reminded me of an old hunter's adage, "there is nothing more depressing than seeing a tree with scars healed over because the tiger that cleaned its paws against it is long gone."

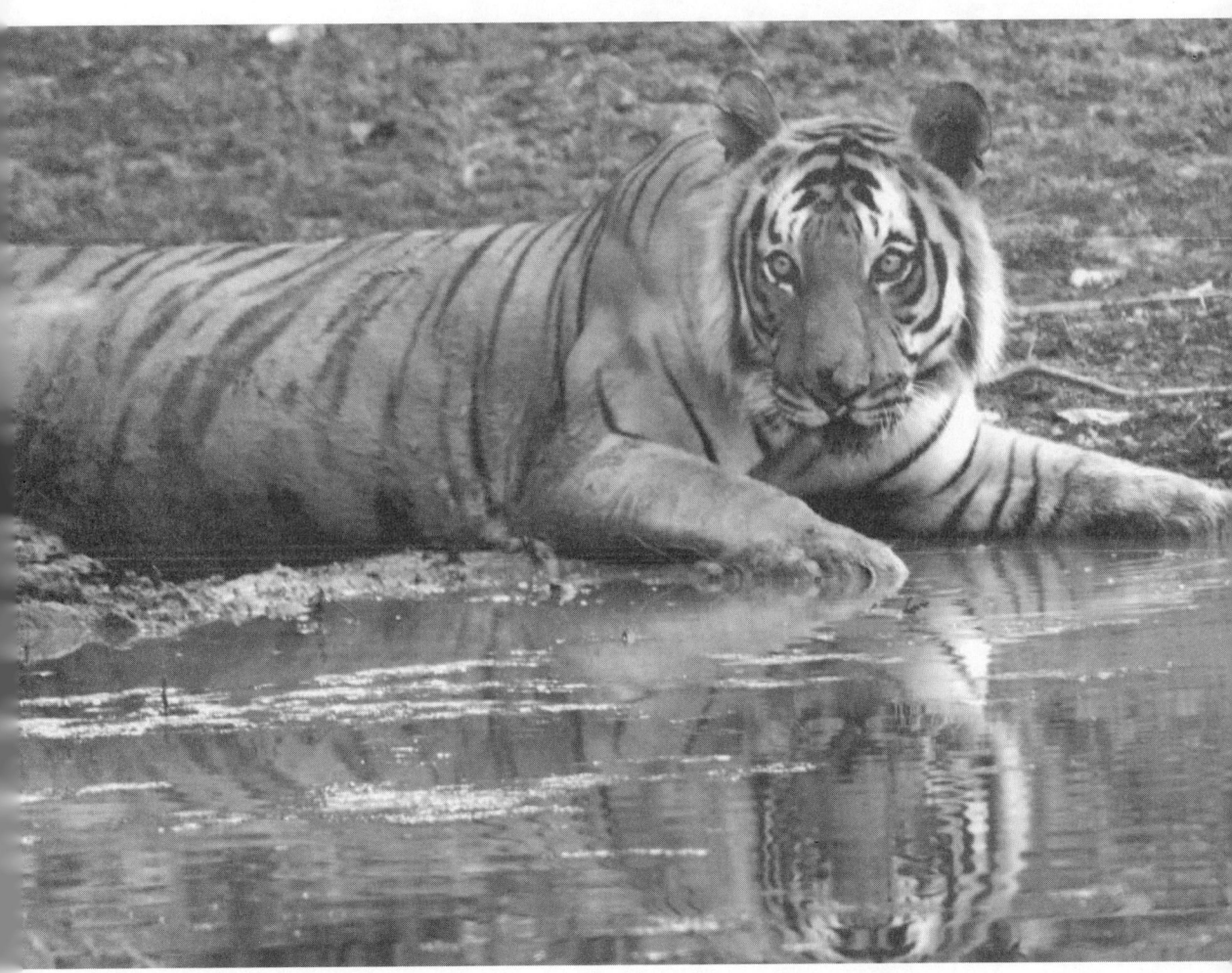

CHAPTER 10
OUT OF TOUCH WITH THE WILD :
A SCIENTIFIC REPORT ON KATRI
TIGRESS

Chapter 10

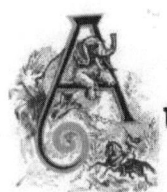

uthor's Note

At some point in 2012, possibly soon after the rains, a young tigress, having two cubs walks out of the jungles of Pilibhit district or perhaps its adjacent sugar fields. It then travels over 300 kilometres through heavily populated farmlands. She crosses the districts of Hardoi and Sitapur, reaching the small forest patch of Rahman Kheda in Lucknow, which is an hour's walk away from outer edge of the city, and then crossing over to Unnao district finally settles down near the Ganga river in a small forest of Katri. The small jungle falls on the border of two districts of Unnao and Kanpur and is closer to the Kanpur city. This tigress never turned aberrant; hence this report is a yardstick for determining that there is an abundance or overabundance of herds of feral cattle, including old timers, '*Chota-Shikar*' of prolific ungulate species like pig which definitely poses a serious problem to agriculturists.

Out of Touch with the Wild :
A Scientific Report on Katri Tigress

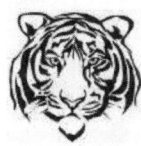

"Katri tigress is a gentle lady in true sense of word, if she is not diverted into unnatural ways by human dereliction."

- Shrivridhi Shukla to TOI

IN THE FIRST WEEK OF JUNE 2015, I WAS VISITING BALOO GHAT WITH MY daughter Shrivridhi and Vijay Kumar, then designated Additional Director General of Police (Arms Training Core of Uttar Pradesh Police.) As we alighted on the banks of Katri Jungle, we heard a cacophony of rhesus monkeys followed by the neighing of blue bulls. The snorting sounds carried far through the silence of evening. We went to investigate and came upon a bare stretch of sand extending to over 150 meters and surrounded by a running belt of reed and lemon grasses. A small herd of blue bulls containing five members, stood at the centre of the field. They were some hundred yards away and gazing at the 10 feet high grass. They soon huddled together as if facing some danger and started braying. They were aware of our presence but instead of giving any attention to us they seemed more attentive to some bigger danger. Clearly the tiger's hunt was in progress. Then I looked across them in a straight line that took me past the antelopes but there was nothing. Certainly the tigress was there and waiting for the blue bulls to approach within 20 yards of her but now her presence was detected through a waft of wind and the antelopes were restless. They did not run but rather stood rooted to the spot and continued neighing.

The drama continued for some five minutes then the blues bulls ran away. We walked up to the place where they had been looking. The sun was yet lambent and within a few minutes Vijay found out the marks of the tigress on the ground where she had been sitting and waiting. A micro search for more signs revealed a few hair of her body on the thick reed nails that had rubbed on her body closely when she had passed through them.

Later, as if tired of our presence, she decided to move from her hiding and crossed the dirt road before us. This was the first time I saw her in the evening lights, tucked amid grasses as good as amid reeds or sugarcane. The setting rays of the sun fell upon her and the fire of her eyes burned with awesome luster, reflecting the sun light with all its brilliance.

This was the stranded tigress of Katri island.

Mind you, this is no *shikaar* yarn by Jim Corbett or Kenneth Anderson but this is a report about the journey of a tigress through unfriendly terrain and her survival without causing any harm to human neighbours.

The Immigration Route

"Tigers possess many attitudes that increases their chances of surviving in altered landscapes as we must not loose sight of the evolutionary history of the species".
- Mel Sunquist, Tiger Biologist

The Tarai forests of Pilibhit district, falling to the west of Dudhwa National Park, are a part of similar environment. Outside the forest there is a large stretch of reed, *ikra* and tamarisk grasses, through which a large watercourse, made of many shallow intersecting streams, flows out. As it proceeds further it is joined by more *nalas* and rivulets, including two big rivers Garra and Khannaut, which transform it into a large river called Gomti, which crosses nine districts including Lucknow, finally merging into the Ganga. The grasslands along the origin of Gomti stretch up to many kilometers till they go across principal jungles and enter into farmlands. This is historical breeding grounds of tigers; a discerning habitat and a permanent source of fresh tiger populations to farmlands and jungles alike.

This is what Karanth explains: "Even if protected areas are designated for conservation of large carnivores, the wide ranging habits of carnivores and the dispersal needs of young adults can result in a spillover to these human dominated landscapes."

It is from this base that sometime in October 2012, a tigress with two half-grown cubs started on her journey towards the south. Moving along the course of Gomti river she walked into farmlands between Mahokpur range and stayed there for almost a year, where her cubs separated from her and the mother somehow walked on, breaking into the farmlands of Hardoi district. She was for the first time spotted by a group of herders when they were returning home. She followed their cattle, maintaining a fifty yard distance from the herd and tracked them for good two miles up to the edge of the village where she finally halted and stood watching the cattle enter the village.

In the meanwhile alarm was raised and a crowd gathered at the outskirts to see the animal. The charismatic mega fauna and its seeming ferociousness make it more attractive as a killer than a friendlier animal. For quite some time people had a grandstand view of her then as it happens some mischief-mongers raised the question of her possible return late in the night to prey upon their cattle. She was immediately half circled by some 200 people and chased away.

Then onwards the tigress' stressful existence started as she wandered disconcerted here and there. Harassed and bewildered in unknown lands, she crossed Pilibhit, Lakhimpur-Kheri, Hardoi, Sitapur, Lucknow and Unnao districts and finally reached Katri area, an outlying piece of forest near Kanpur city where she finally settled down.

Tigers inhabit any jungle of sufficient size which affords food, water and shade. Land use patterns of rural areas such as cultivation of certain crops or plantations help change the characteristics of the landscape and these changed landscapes act as habitats for the carnivores outside protected areas. Katri was such a kind of terrain that became her primary base in Unnao district. Its surrounding area consisted of villages, namely Satya Narayanpur, Nav Ghat and Ganga Ghat, there were stretches of National highways and a few patches of jungle that helped her free movement in the night. These served as halting stations where she could lay down and spend the day time sleeping in case she failed to reach her swampy base before the day broke and human activities started.

For an area so close to the big city of Kanpur, there is a relative local abundance of wildlife, especially herds of blue bulls and wild pigs. These supplemented the local cattle and buffalo baits as the tiger's primary prey base. Besides, the complex

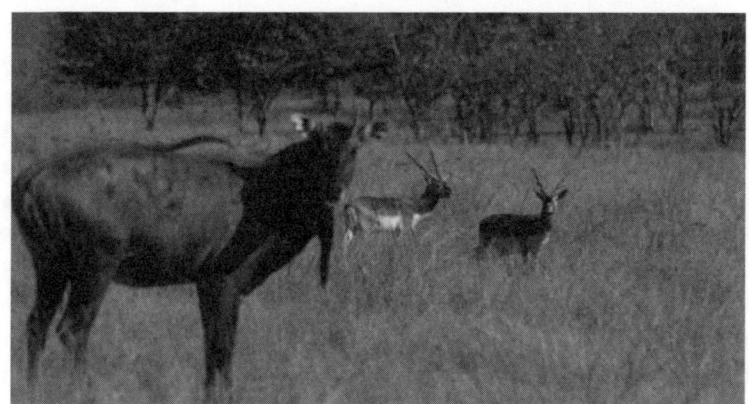

The route of Katri tigress carried plentiful of prey animals both wild and feral.

biota of Katri jungles' swampy ecosystem supported the tiger for good ten months, qualifying as a sample area on scientific scales to contain a large carnivore like a tiger. The heavily industrial area of Kanpur partly touches the parameters of futuristic Anthropocene age that scientists view as a period during which the human activity would cause dominant influence on climate and environment. It would be characterized by excessively dense concentrations of humans living in permanent settlements on a landscape that has been increasingly altered and degraded in order to support the growing human population, and where it will be difficult to define the stages of natural floral and faunal life.

Parenthetically in the neighbourhood, the holy land of Ganga river seems to present a quaternary period of Holocene, where wildlife is still a part of human cultural expression, and thus a hard combination of two different epochs that simultaneously exist side by side to come upon anywhere around world's mega cities.

It is not easier for people to overlook the apparent blessings of Mother Nature in trying to achieve balance even in its discrepancies. The tigress staying here presented an example as how unmolested, large carnivores develop their knowledge base to live near human habitations without confronting them. She stayed in this jungle for good ten months from October 2014 to August 2015, reflecting the better methods of governing its own existence, while continuously achieving greater level of coexistence with man than man himself knew. All through this phase she acquired education of self-preservation and perhaps for this reason she never chased or attacked any human being, save for occasional demonstrations. She also never behaved aberrantly despite excessive human incitement. It is the knack of the animal that it learns to live by the side of man without becoming a problem and it is the streak of man that he makes a problem of that presence.

However, her ten-month stay in Katri that acquired the monicker for her, vividly illustrates the need to study farmland behaviour of tigers in greater detail. The manner in which she carried on a daily routine without impairing humans, points to the fact that even in suspended and uncertain states of living, large cats indicate the ability for behavioral adaptations.

Tigers, being mercurial animals are entitled to freedom which is an undisputable component of their wildness. When they are free much of the activities they pursue in wilderness are identifiable and predictable to modern day scientists. But what they do in the inequitable freedom of human landscape is altered behavior. Territory maintenance and expression for recurring activities of mating are the instincts that comprise natural agenda for tigers that they pursue in the jungle. But in case of strayers there is no territory maintenance and mating is out of the question. Human pressure and constraints restrict them and don't allow them to follow even their normal movements.

Competition for prey resources and sometimes for prey itself becomes an intrusive problem with human neighbours. A tiger's biological requirement of being obligate meat-eater easily lands him in conflict with man and puts it continually on the run, seeking relief from one place to another and looking for sufficient space that is free from human molestation. Hiding and avoiding humans then becomes the most sensible path to achieve, whatever goals are deemed appropriate.

The requirements for a tiger's hiding wilderness that enable a straying tiger to work at his own level in an alien landscape, restrict his free behavioral pattern. It trims down to avoiding humans and manipulations for its own survival. This is despite the fact that there is plenty of food around.

During August 2015, when the monsoon was at its peak, the local streams came in spate. There was water everywhere with its level ever rising. The river Ganga swelled, flooding the Katri Island and the tigress was compelled to abandon its comfortable home. Tigers resort freely to swimming in a manner that denotes their familiarity with that element. But instead of crossing the Ganga and going further south she reasonably took a backward route and again set upon the course she had travelled to come here. It was this phase when on September 5, I butted again into the scene to follow her second part of journey.

Sadly this time her fortunes drastically changed. The carnivore that had managed to reach Katri almost undetected and incognito, thus without being resisted was spotted extensively everywhere she reached and was dealt with hard handedness by humans.

In rural landscape a tiger's life situation is different. George Scheller's estimate of an adult tiger's annual need for meat tells that "a tiger would be satisfied by some thirty of India's scrubby cattle." Obviously in the jungle killing and-eating of a standard prey takes a great deal of pressure off the professional predator. But in human landscape, a tiger kills more than this number because almost at every kill, they are by and large chased by men, especially when they bring down a livestock and often such kills are not even partly consumed because herders intervene.

I need hardly add that from whichever point she tried to secure food, she was hounded. She was even fired at by shotguns at two places though she escaped unscathed. But the distressing incidents kept her starved, and in trying to assuage her hunger, which became increasingly difficult to satisfy, her killing rate unnecessarily increased. Within six days, she had killed eight animals – one donkey, two buffalos, three cows and two goats, perhaps also killing some other forms of prey that I could not record. This made her life complicated but no doubt gave her an excellent understanding of the gradations of living along humans.

Tiger-trail - 400 kilometers

It is a well-known feature of animal behavior that further away from the centre of its territory an animal is forced to move, the more confidence it loses.

- Konrad Lorenz

Principal Chief Conservator of Forests/Chief Wildlife Warden of U.P, Dr. Rupak Day had employed Aftab Wali to monitor this tigress. The old friend kept me refurbished with every day development for many months as on weekends I also joined him every so often. This time my study area was no particular terrain but it was a long route of a straying predator, crossing some six districts, interspersed with developmental projects for irrigation, industry and mining, including railway tracks, metaled roads and three National Highways.

It is believed that there are some remote micro-ecological selective pressures, including obvious factors like drought, water logging, resource limitation or some kind of aggravation that compels a tiger to initially come into human settlements and it is the very same factor that again forces it to go back from there though apparently attributable to the change in seasons and competitive interactions with humans. Now if the tigress was returning to her *in situ* jungles then again it had to pass through this great track of more than 400-km inhabited by humans and a complex mosaic of various crop fields and patches of fallow land habitats, which could serve her as temporary halting stations amid households and townships dispersed across the landscape.

Throughout July the tigress moved on towards north, loitering here and there but keeping a constant pace of covering five to eight kilometers in northern direction. As I followed her I found that the habitat features of these sprawling farmlands, similar to that of Tarai could be safely divided into 3 major natural habitat strata made of tree plantations, moist grass swamps with water ponds and of grass meadows that served as *Charagah.* The other 2 were crop pattern habitat strata created by anthropogenic modifications, included maze and sugarcane crop areas besides other strata of vegetables, wheat, paddy and pulses, including mosaic of fruit plantations like, jack fruit, papaya, guava and banana that offered nutrition to ungulates, birds and primate populations.

In addition I came across, some of the spot light localities of green cover, numbering more than twenty and ranging from 20 to hundred acres in size, which the tigress had occupied during her passage. These were micro hot-spots of bio-diversity that also held rich carnivore diversity. There were four large-bodied species having a body mass up to 20kgs. On empirical scales, segregation of temporal and spatial aspects of the sympatric species environment, along niche dimensions simplifies partitioning of resources and facilitates co-existence of predators; accordingly there were middle order predators, scavengers cum group hunters like hyenas, jackals, rattles and wolves living with spatial heterogeneity. Since these are all potential carnivores they need more than one kilogram of meat every day.

Though meso-carnivore and hypo-carnivore like jackals and foxes can munch through a quantum produce of sugarcane in emergencies but their presence implied that natural food was there for all predators, in terms of species and body size and they were utilizing it in relation to biomass. I was aghast to see that over fifty million years of evolution of sympatric species which had attained specialist perfection was still existing over these farmlands with a complex interplay of extrinsic and intrinsic ecological equations, not yet subjected to absolute human vandalism. In addition, all these were populous places with an average human population density of above 300 people per sq. km (Government of India, 2015 census report).

Travelling this way the tigress continued through sugarcane and maze fields, utilizing suitable halting spots till incorrectly she killed some livestock. Consequently the human pressure escalated, compelling her to seek shelter elsewhere. Now as the tigress was constantly on the run, therefore in micro-ecological sense this conflict anywhere was of highly temporary and invariably of localized nature, which required no further management interventions than compensating the cattle owner.

This tigress was no competitor of man but the presence of livestock did impact the situation. This is a peculiar circumstance to which Katri tigress seems to have reconciled yet the most serious threat of human fatality by her remained prominent and the odds surely tilt in that direction when she was ruthlessly chased. During hunting years it was believed that unless the tiger had been wounded, it can scarcely be supposed to believe that it was being pursued. Probably it merely fears the unknown and unusual from man and recognizes the race as superior. Mostly cornered by mobs, sometimes quite unnecessarily because human-carnivore conflict in terms of livestock depredation is perhaps more common and thus the marooned animal had every reason to believe that she was being pursued. Moreover for simple villagers, chasing away any problem animal, whether feral cattle or a predator, that threatens their flora or livestock is the only practical option of its 'physical removal' from the place it has wrongly hit upon without lethal control.

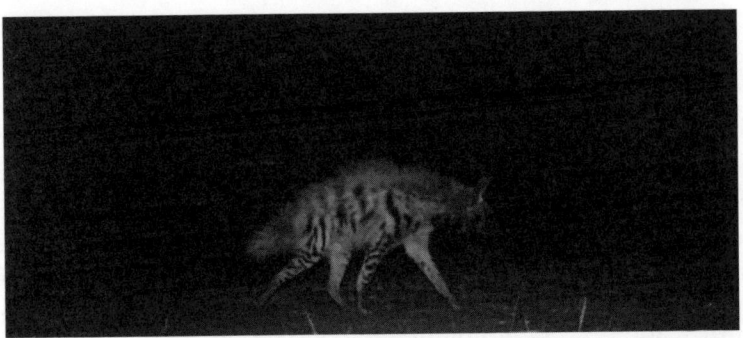

Hyenas are equally comfortable with grasslands and open farmlands. They occupy porcupine borrows to suit their needs and live on lesser lights of life including scavenging. *(Camera trap shot credit Maharashtra Forest Department)*

It is a nonviolent public method that has public acceptance in wildlife management including entertainment.

Excited behavior of villagers also spelled trouble for her and in some cases it reached the height of absurdity to the point of being suicidal. Tigers are rare animals and the news of their arrival inevitably produces great curiosity. During September 2015 the tigress reached Hardoi district again, coming through the same route that she had followed a year back to reach Kanpur. Here at Sandila and Bharavan area she killed a feral pig and a big crowd immediately surrounded her. But before she could eat she was chased away. Even in that excitement of escape, she deliberately avoided human beings, cutting her way zig-zag in full dash literally amid strong crowed of some 500 people. Though tigers are dangerous when feeding on their kills and just one slip is enough to give anybody a new look and make him spend the rest of his life on crutches, she didn't touch any onlooker.

It is easy to rationalize that it is just a short step from cattle-eating to man-eating, only one wrong move and a man-eater would be born. Within a fortnight she was chased no less than ten times by villagers. Considering the people's point of view, such impulsive acts are neither illegal nor immoral but rather justifiable because the horrors with which the activities of big cats are regarded are not irrational.

To say that no two 'straying' tiger observations are similar is nearly axiomatic. A case of an off track tigress comes to mind, which in 2010, Sanjay Pathak attempted to capture in sugar fields of Kheri and was later darted at Farrukhabad district. She had developed a habit of killing extra animals when on the run. That tigress had passed from Pihani of Hardoi district, where being chased by fun seekers she bounded across a grazing ground, and literally landed in the middle of a goat herd and immediately **st**arted destruction, boxing and slapping the goats, crushing their necks in jaws and tossing them high in the air. Of course she did this in a spate of anger. Unbelievably within thirty seconds of this energetic umbrage, she destroyed four goats, and then as the chasing crowd put her to flight, she plunged into a wheat field and disappeared, where she further killed a single mare and further on an oxen bull.

This certainly indicated not great hunger but great rage. Rendered wiser by the experience, a message went round natives "don't chase her or be prepared for the destruction of livestock."

In early October, graziers saw the Katri tigress dashing close by cattle herds to save herself from the chasing crowd. There was an unusual amount of shouting and screaming of people and the barking of pariah dogs sprinting along her, like a pack of wild dogs pursuing a tiger, when she jumped into Gomti with a great splash and swam across into another district. I recorded over a dozen incidents of her passing close to grazing herds of cattle but she never flashed any opportunistic attacks on them and never turned on the human crowd in a paroxysm of rage. Her patience with man is yet not short. She rather breaks away from the place and continued doing that.

Tigers are not designed to run like cheetahs. Their greatest weakness is their low endurance at speed. They can walk for days, but cannot take to any marathon. They are at their best in short bursts of speed within 150 to 200 meters, but a longer sprint tires them and instead of running further they turn back to fight. It is also observed that a stressed tiger will kill a beast out of a herd near which it is passing when being pursued, just as a hunted fox will snatch a fowl from the farmyard. But Katri tigress is recorded to have for couple of miles and though awfully tired and irritated she never turned on humans.

While I was at Jangaon village in Atauralla area of Hardoi, a native offered to take me to the tigress. He knew where she was resting after a dog's meal. Atul Kapoor a local correspondent of *Amar Ujala* and I immediately accompanied him. Close to the pond a flock of white egrets shimmered against the slate grey clouds. A little drizzle had just washed the emerald landscape that was resonant with plaintive calls of fish eagles, when we saw her abruptly get up and move towards a cane break. Her bulging stomach showed she was cat-napping post meal that we had interrupted. Near the spot we found her 'cologne scents' mixed with her urine and feces, called 'odour fields' in cat lexicon.

There nothing like ecological densities of prey in farmlands because farmland ecology of Gangatic planes is more or less similar with habitat strata and domination of feral cattle, the herds of which are embedded within larger landscape matrices but I must tell here that in hunting prone sites, I found considerable differences in wild prey densities. In principal Muslim areas blue bull were out while in Hindu areas wild boars were missing. This appeared attributable to different levels of hunting pressure.

Humayoopur and Dhobeya Ashram are smaller animal enclaves located inside remote farmlands. Being religious areas, developed by a Vaishanav Krishna devotee saint called Nepali Baba these were just about free from hunting pressure. Dhobeya Ashram had many gracefully posed mounds along Gomti River. As I monitored the tigress in this area with Atul Kapoor, I discovered a temporary shelter of tigress in

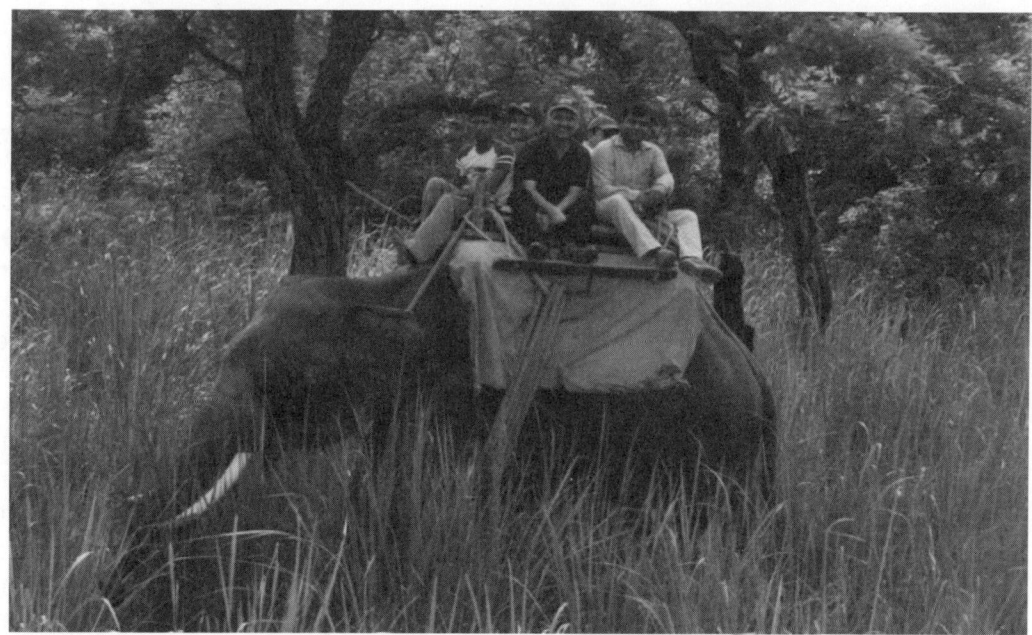

Sanjay Pathak, D.I.G, NTCA with his crew at Dudhwa, Deputy Director Mahavir and ArvindYadav IFS,
(Photo credit Vijay Kumar IPS, ADG Police U.P)

shallow cave which had been formed by licking of mineral salts by blue bulls, spotted deer and wild boar. It lay under the spread of a banyan tree, the roots of which grew on the sides of the mound and covered it from all around. She had stayed here for quite some time, satisfying her hunger on a large male peafowl; its brilliant feathers lay scattered on the floor. Then onwards I discovered her three kills in the vicinity of the cave, all of them were peafowls.

Moving in a closed environment of reed grass and sugar and finding kills was not devoid of risk but I got a first-hand opportunity to see the farmland wildlife of Hardoi district. Blue bulls rested in the open areas as monitor lizards scurried through canes and so did the peacocks and monkeys. At one point I came across the indication of a porcupine which had come grunting along with rattling quills upon the tigress and the latter had run away. Further on a pair of black bucks took to flight at our sight. I also learnt of a python pair inhabiting a pond and came across several flocks of red fowls and brown partridges residing in farmlands and small grass clumps.

By this time, monsoon was over and sugarcane had matured. Although there were many small, different habitat type spots all around but over preference to these, where cattle menace raged during daylight hours, she selected sugarcane plantations to spend her time resting. This showed that with the increased availability of sugarcane plantations, her habitat selectivity pattern had developed penchant for extremely dense grasses. Perhaps this helped her in effort to locate some wild prey as well as hiding it post meal.

Throughout this phase, using clues such as decomposition odour, locating innards and activities of scavengers, both birds and animals, I discovered over a score of large kills made by Katri tigress and studied them opportunistically. Since tigers' distribution has been dendritic, historically associated with watercourses and river basins, this tigress naturally stuck to Gomti's course. A large number of her kills were made in the river glitches, which held large scale of sugar plantations between Hardoi and Sitapur region where because of the loose sandy texture of the soil tracking was quite easy.

Lying inside dense crops of sugarcane and reed tangles, six animals, that I examined -4 nilgais', one antler chital and one feral oxen bull - had been caught from behind, disabled first by hamstringing and then instead of neck breaking the killer had crushed the windpipe and held it shut with its jaws, making the victim die of suffocation. Two were killed with throat bite and nape bite without neck breaking, while three killed through combined nape and throat bite without neck breaking and one seemingly by shock and loss of blood due to knee fracture and deep body punctures in stomach and back.

Over the length of my tiger observations I have repeatedly witnessed that most of the large kills, even moderate size kills, made inside tall crops had been by hamstringing. (It may sound funny but this pattern of killing is corroborated by Tarai natives and graziers who keep intersecting tigers.) The denser environment makes it difficult for a tiger to target the animal for a frontal attack and it finds easier to seize the prey from behind by grabbing its hind leg and pulling it down. This is because an animal with formidable horns and pronounced powers of resistance, such as blue bulls, would in some positions present obstacles to a seizure by the back of the neck. Though tigers ambush their prey in different types of covers but their killing style differs as per the size and behavior of the prey species. The pattern of attacks also showed that most were brought down inside the tall crop or within 5 meters of distance where the habitat feature was similar.

Though the tigress was not found near any kill but where she had hamstrung the prey, the prey was essentially large and the cover density was significantly higher where dragging of kill to a secure dining point was least needed. This again supported my claim that grasslands are more advantageous to the evolved hunting style of tigers and this factor makes the standard killers of large prey feel naturalized in sugar farms. Moreover hamstringing is a favourite method of matured tigers and it is also possible that their prey selection behavior is inspired by potential defenselessness of the prey to this specialized killing technique. It is so because any heavy-bodied and potentially dangerous animal, like a male blue bull or a stud bull, would be naturally helpless if one of its legs has gone completely sagging; for

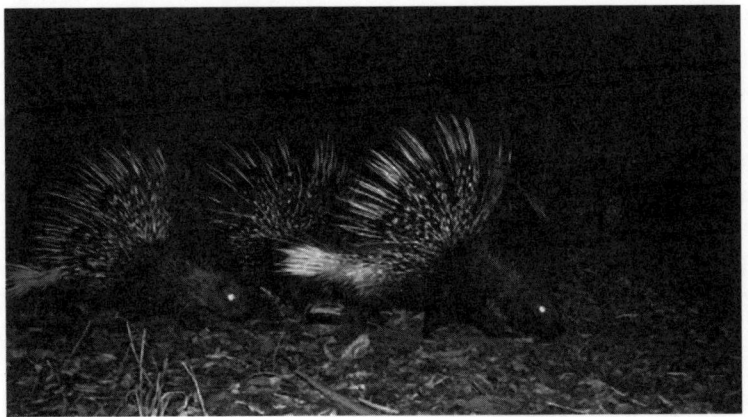

Porcupine adapts itself to any kind of country , moist or arid and inhabits both open land and forest. In Tarai they also shelter in sugarcane making regular runs through it. *(Photo credit : WCT)*

such animals are bitten by tigers at hock joints where canines puncturing of the bone and ligaments is thoroughly complete.

Col Fenton declares that while attacking camels, tigers invariably attack the legs while Captain Forsyth describes an instance in which a tiger seized the elephant's hind leg and worried him so severely that it died of terror induced heart-attack. It is the only instance he knew of a tiger killing an elephant.

It was for the first time that I expressed the possibility of the tigress getting back to home land. Scientists, who unveil the mystery of the cats' world, believe that the visual memory of cats is excellent and they are known to use it to find a way home at short distances in the area where they live. Some cats are also recorded using it for long distances. Newspaper reports begged a question from the foresters that when such great distances are involved, it seems implausible that even with extraordinary senses of smell and hearing, any cat would track down its native place it has left for long. But my argument was that the man-eating tigress of Moradabad had already shown that it can be achieved.

The ability of a cat to find its way home is called "PSI-traveling." Experts believe that cats either use the angle of the sunlight to find their way or that cats have magnetized cells in their brains that act as compasses and perhaps all cats, whether pets or wild have a sixth sense or some kind of psychic connection to their owners. In case of being away from places of their birth, they do navigate back. Sadly, no one knows it is indeed a psychic connection, and it's still not fully understood.

Predators when driven by hunger don't understand the laws of man. On one hand they are punished for not abiding with the diktats of the master race, which has at first itself dishonored all the laws of nature and subsequently created its own laws to control nature. On the other hand, human populations around tiger reserves are at much higher densities and the alpha killers like tigers have not progressed to the top of food chain to turn vegetarian. They will eat anything they can catch so a clash is a biologically inevitable consequence. Moreover, pressure induced hyper-activity in tigers easily makes them tired, and devoid of rest and sleep, they turn prone to conflict.

All told, this reminds me of famous Russian tiger catchers Averian Cherepnov and Vladimir Kurglov, who knew as how to capitalize on 'inability to run longer' weakness of heavy-bodied predators. They used to set their dogs free upon them in deep snow that would hold the panting predator at bay while the men advanced with long pronged tree branches and held it down. Then in a quick and carefully designed operation they would tie the tiger's head in a rope, tie its paws and put the gloves on them, quickly immobilizing it and packing it in a large bag. Kurglov is the only human being in the history of mankind who captured 41 tigers alive, grabbed many of them by ears and lived to tell the gauntlet of terrible hazards in his escapades. He did not let any of his henchmen handle the ears, for it is through them that he controlled the tiger's brain and body. He had told a researcher before his death in 2006 that "Ears are a tiger's steering wheel. You can turn off their teeth with the ears."

The title for most tiger catching in the heavyweight class unquestionably goes to this duo, but here the state foresters had none like Kurglov to go after a predator, weighing more than 300 pounds.

During months of December 2015 to June 2016, Katri was shunting back and forth between two districts of Hardoi and Sitapur, being constantly prevented by adverse human interference from reaching her in situ jungles. This made her kill more prey than needed for food because before she could eat she was chased away and this made her slaughter a fresh animal again. Small haphazard chases of predators by crowds do happen in nervous excitement when people fear them or go after them for sheer fun, but in the case of this unfortunate animal the extreme had already happened.

There were many recorded instances of fearlessness shown by herdsmen and even little herd-boys, in driving her away from their cattle, sometimes striking the fearsome beast with their staves. A herdsman riding his buffalo saw her being chased by a mob, he also threw his *lathi* swinging hitting her in legs, "As I got her, she lurched and accelerated her speed," he exclaimed in pompous triumph, muttering unprintables.

There is a marked difference between the existential situations for the strayed tigers that seek their living in far-off rural landscape, and the hardcore farm dwellers of Tarai. Tiger is a part of Tarai's consciousness which might be termed as traditional scientific consciousness. Particular tigers acquire a reputation for their behavior, such as boldness or timidity with the inhabitants of neighborhood over which they range, and to whom in course of time they become well known. Farmers, natives and tribals are long accustomed to living with them. They watch their behavior as ungulates get clues about carnivores. For example if a blue bull stops paying attention to them and looks in another direction, it means he is interested in

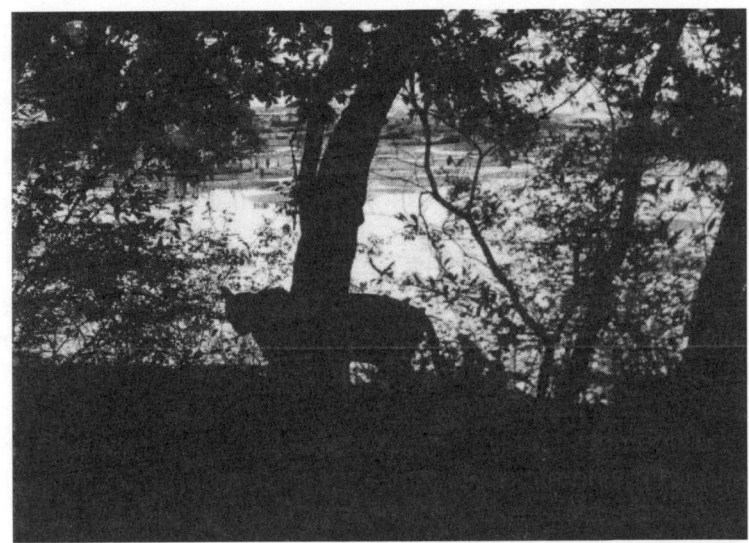

Katri tigress in the Kachaara of Gomtiriver, Hardoi district. *(Photo credit : Sanjay Singh, Director, Dudhwa National Park)*

something more threatening than man. This is how they learn and teach their children.

They don't disturb tigers nor show fear to their presence, for a predator can smell fear very well and anyone who shows fear is as good as gone. Through graziers and shepherds as well as firsthand participants in man-animal conflicts, they know the carnivore's possible locations, their sighting points and roughly about the size of their ranges. Sharing news helps them in prediction, prevention and staying out of the big predators' way.

A misplaced tiger on the run can break out anywhere, where people are not used to it. In fact many have never seen one before and this creates a strangely new situation. People don't know as how to deal with the mega fauna.

Use of dogs as guard animal is often useless in context of tigers. They do bark and warn their master about the presence of a carnivore but also attract the big carnivore as a prospective meal. Domesticated dogs and some breeds of animal husbandry like donkeys are known to counter-attack small carnivores, acting in a way that interrupts their predatory behavior. I was once shown an average-size leopard sitting away from a grazing donkey near Pathakpurva in Bahraich district that the graziers claimed had just been kicked at the jaw by the donkey. The poor leopard was actually nursing his jaw. Donkeys repel jackal and leopard attacks but there is no evidence that they can guard against wolves while guard dogs are vulnerable to leopards but can guard against wolves. The efficacy against tiger of any guard animals that can really counter attack and disrupt the predator's functioning has not been published by any scientist but for a few stray cases of counterattack by stud bulls that I related in my previous books.

When a large carnivore breaks out in an alien land there is no awareness among villagers about its strength and destructive ways but just an acute curiosity for its one glimpse. Often the naïve ways applied to handle the predator invite more danger. Villagers don't know what kind of serious trouble a resolute carnivore can cause if it goes uncharacteristic. An example is that of the Moradabad killer tigress, who on being disturbed had driven the entire village of Mithanpur on top of trees and held the natives of Hanspur hostage for days within their hutments with their doors closed and cut off from outside world.

In such situations, managing and coping with crisis is not easy but still we need scientific awareness about many aspects of tigers that can only be learnt when they are no longer inside their protected jungles yet they don't antagonize people at first. It is in this context that the inherent instincts of tiger's nature and human nature reveal themselves most starkly. We want to know how tigers fare in farmlands and what fundamentally designs their relationship to the environment to keep them alive.

Cats are too popular with people and sometimes this popularity generates outmoded fears and attitudes. Perhaps this factor has made Katri the most chased tigress I have ever known in history. However, throughout the investigation we kept wondering at her patience and endurance for not causing any human fatality.

In 1973, C. S. Holling introduced the word resilience into ecological literature as a way of helping understand the non-linear dynamics observed in ecosystems and in its actors. Ecological resilience, functional on both biotic and abiotic components of environment, is defined as the amount of disturbance that an ecosystem, as well as its living organisms, can withstand without changing self-organized processes and structures. Other authors consider resilience as a time of return to a stable state following a perturbation. A new term, adaptive cycles, is introduced to describe the process that modifies the resilience in life systems. This tigress offers an excellent opportunity to understand both the sides of resilience aspect.

The debate topics are hard; the subject makes for awfully interesting discussion for the media as well as for tiger buffs and foresters. Some inexorably justify tigresses' calm behavior while others question that for how long this goodness will last if the pressure remains constant. Fear in the psyche of people is bound to affect the long-term survival possibility of a wanderer in alien land. Much chasing can also become counterproductive for a carnivore might not tolerate excessive shifting and turn upon its chasers and then any unfortunate incident, such as a deliberate gunshot from a human supremacist, just for the inflation of his ego, would change the situation drastically.

Cory Meacham observes, "that which is wild is not controllable, nor is that which is controlled is truly wild. Moreover there are no wild tigers left; every area in which they now range 'wild' is plainly demarcated by surrounding human populations. The perimeters may lack metal bars but penalty subjected for transgressing the boundary is hard."

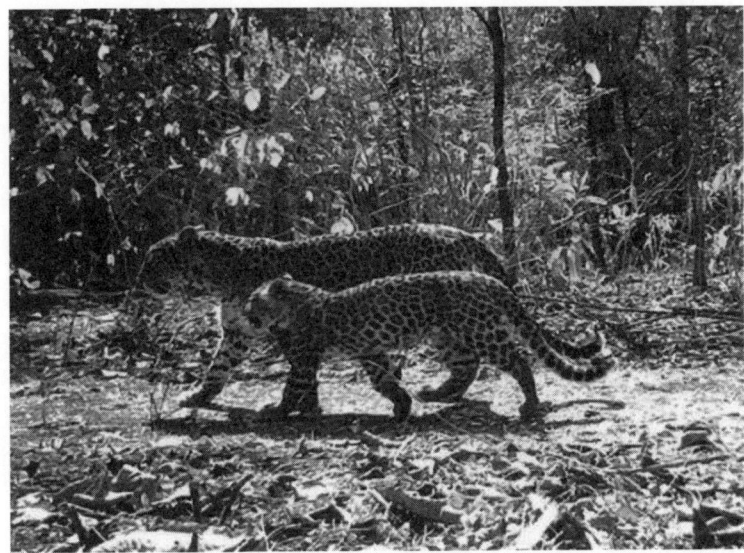

Leopard are perhaps more salitary than tigers. Here a mother with a female cub is seen taking her on the territorial patrolling *(Photo credit : WCT)*

Tigers have a superior ability to compete with humans and this creates problem. There is also much likelihood of some organized poaching operations taking place because most poaching is opportunistic and when people see a vulnerable animal in the farmland they see some hundreds of thousands of rupees or dollars moving unguarded, so they target the animal intentionally, cashing the advantage and turning the tiger into hard cash.

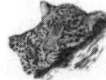

Abreast with a Spotted Ninja

"Should you fall for some of the trash that labels him as endangered, just remember that he is still the most widely distributed of the feline predators, and that for one reason; he is the very best at what he does".

- Peter Hathaway Chapstick

During mid-November, while my formative experience was building and delineations about behavioral traits of straying tigers under the period of maximum stress were shaping up, a leopard barged into the scene at Sariya village in Sitapur district. The five-year old leopard was spotted early morning in a field of *arhar* (a pulse variety) about five kilometers from Sidhauli township. The animal had certainly strayed from his area after walking by rivers and water bodies.

The news of leopard spread like wild fire. A team of forest officials was immediately sent as early as eight in the morning to the place where the leopard was resting inside a sugarcane field. By the time the rescue team arrived, there were thousands of people gathered at the place and the area was cordoned off. Controlling the crowd also meant seeking police help. The big cat was localized and tranquilized and brought to Lucknow Zoo hospital for examination. On being found medically fit it was later released on the fringes of Khutar forest area; falling three miles to the south of my ancestral village Larti. It was once my routine venturing ground, the old home of my favourite female leopard Spotty that I have described in my book "Leoprds in the Backyard".

It is interesting to mention that both a harassed leopard and a much seriously harassed tigress had been operating on the same ground. While the stripes had accounted for no human beings, the leopard within a few hours of his discovery had sharpened his offensive claws and injured three people in less than a minute. This makes the old hunters' adage stand unchallenged that "Tigers are killer of game and livestock and the leopard – a killer too –is not particular whether his object is beast or man." If disturbed, a normal leopard is statistically four times more likely to maul people than a tiger in a similar condition. Though confined to small reserves and in competition with tiger, they seemingly possess rich ability to adapt to any human pressure.

A fortnight after that, another male leopard was spotted in Imaliya Sultanpur village of the same area. In Sitapur and Hardoi, illegal sugarcane cultivation along Gomti makes it a paradise for both wild and feral boars. They persist in far larger numbers than farmers consider desirable. Their small groups congregate near water sites towards dawn and dusk and turn into large assemblies of over thirty, where they procure their varied food in a number of different ways. This naturally attracts the predatory killers, in which leopards figure at the top.

The natives saw the leopard being chased by a sounder of wild pigs. He had grabbed a piglet that had been left behind and its squeals had attracted the attention of the herd which had come charging and made the leopard run for its life. A week later the same four-year old male was found groaning in pain, with one forelimb caught in a pig trap. The animal was tranquilized and was found suffering from injuries in his right forelimb and a couple of serious scratches upon the stomach that I personally suspect were caused by boar tusks in his earlier confrontation with them. He was immediately shifted to Lucknow Zoo hospital for treatment, while a report was lodged at police station against the owner of sugarcane field for setting poaching traps.

Indeed tigers and leopards both like wild boar meat immensely but boars don't appreciate that much. Pigs that sport vicious curved tusks are particularly pugnacious adversaries to tackle. A large boar weighing over 250 pounds can easily disembowel a tiger if handled ineptly.

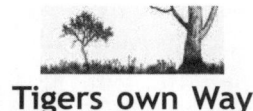

Tigers own Way

I believe there is no 'Indian Way' - or any other nation state way - of saving the tiger. There is only the tiger's own way.

- Ullas Karanth

Much of the information regarding Katri tigress is brutally time-sensitive. Since she is on the run and constantly changing her locations, hence situations are bound to change every day and many details would have changed before you end up reading this chapter. I have made every effort to supply the latest available information, and many aspects of her travel, presented here will retain their historical importance and value. Because some tiger aspects, though subjected to the vicissitudes of time are fantastically rare and only come out during jeopardy, need understanding.

A scientist Konrad Lorenz observes that the wild side of the domestic cats also allows them to keep their talents intact. This enables them to see the world like their ancestors had seen and their wild family members still do.

Cats can see the surface covered with an energy net made by geomagnetic fields coming from the ground. Zoologists believe that frogs, lizards and dolphins are equally capable or finding their way with the help of that net. Drop them anywhere, into some territory uncharted in their brain and some of them would reappear at their home.

Cats are sensitive to electromagnetism of the earth. And that they can efficiently use the pattern of the earth's electromagnetic and magnetic fields has been established by the discovery of tiny magnetic particles of metal on the 'wrists' of cats' fore and back paws. These particles, forming configurations can only be seen through a scanning electronic microscope and naturally respond to the earth's electromagnetic fields. But that's not all: researchers from the Natural History Museum in Stockholm have also discovered magnetic 'bracelets' on legs of cats and other animals that help them find a way back home easily.

It is believed that old cats are able to perform better in homing process. Perhaps as they age, more metal is deposited in these bracelets as well as their brain to develop this ability to return home when needed. This suggests that their wandering off from native places could very well be the result of human disturbance and chase.

It is difficult to encourage this grandiose dream because the human style of functioning easily topples nature's normal proceedings, where every computer model fails to predict and no sensible extrapolations are possible. But I am sure that since this tigress is aggressively on the back track and has already covered

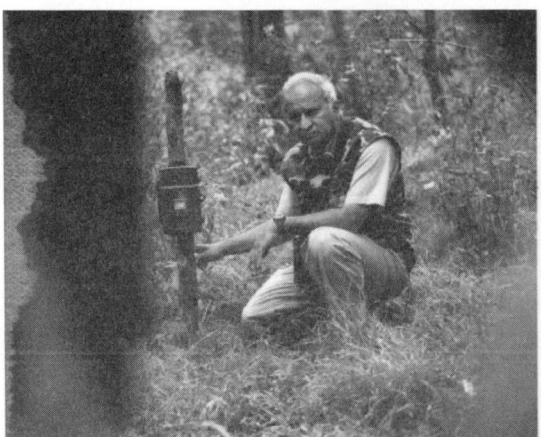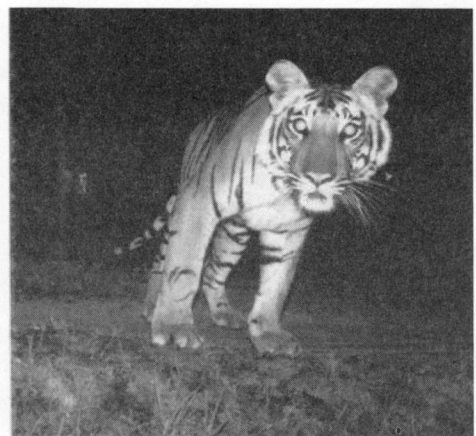

One of the world's foremost authorities on tigers, Dr. UllasKaranth is a senior conservation scientist and Director of the US-based Wildlife Conservation Society. He is known for introducing camera trap technique for wildlife census.

some two-thirds of that homing distance, the theory of PSI trailings offers striking evidence that cats can do it if left to themselves.

But unfortunately, not all cats with a strong bond with their home may survive long trips. It's a difficult and harsh world for a lost animal with a high mortality rate due to natural and anthropogenic causes, the odds of finding their home back hundreds of miles away are too high. Yet this tigress has shown an encouraging graph of navigating back.

Human operation easily complicates or overthrows any balancing act of nature. At any time, the route of the returning tigress might be diverted by human pressure. A mob of curious onlookers may disturb it for pleasure and she may be chased away to stranger places in opposite direction of her homeland.

Sticking to the banks of the Gomti river, inherently free from external control and of course wild in her nature, this tigress is not starving, sick or injured. It can go for a week or two without food if it has to, though there is no shortage of wild and feral prey in the area. If her fate is not tampered by humans tailing her such as she is not perforated, injured, eliminated by poisoning after consuming a dead buffalo or cow sprayed with insecticide or captured, and despite alternating between two districts back and forth in an endeavor to rationalize her existence in extremely disturbed conditions, this gives us hope that it can go back. Though circumstances are ripe for her to start killing humans, then eliminating her would clearly be preferred than trying to watch over her.

When all tiger stories are normally authored in the past, the journey of the Katri tigress shares the existing timeline. Still essentially wild in nature, she is a glaring example as how tigers are capable of exercising restraint even under extreme human pressures. Her return journey seems to create a new arc of survival and a

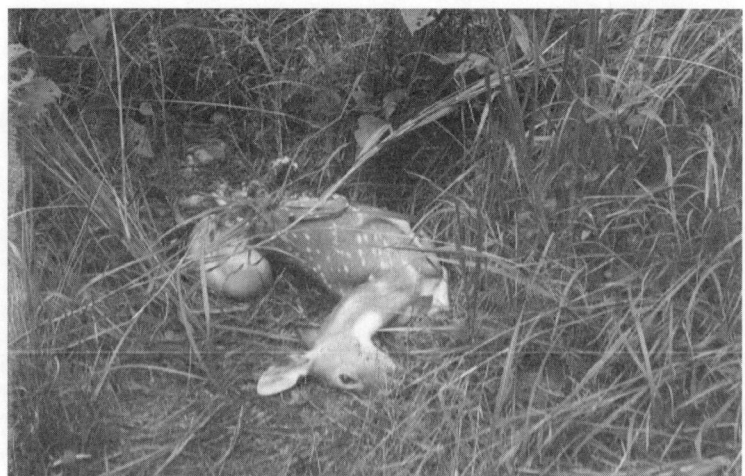

Jackals are master assasins. They take a heavy toll of deer life.

new model of bonds that essentially hold a wild tiger in relationship with its prime home and also to her capricious human neighbours, which indeed to her own nature are not broken. Every conservationist hopes for a peaceful resolution when she has already covered 250 plus kilometers without creating much pandemonium on her part. Shrivirddhi's spot-on words, "politically unprotected, she is truly a gentle lady in real sense of word", appear sorted out.

At the time of writing this chapter, her last location was recorded at Hasaiyapur village of Pihani Tehsil of Hardoi, on October 29, 2016. There she had killed three blue bulls and from there she was only 50 kilometers away from the Tarai-Arc landscape. If she finally manages to reach the safety of regular forests then the Katri tigress, after Moradabad's killer tigress, will stand as the foremost example of PSI trailing. She will be a unique animal that travelled some 600 kilometers inside the human zone, spent a good three years plus, including some 10 months near industrial city of Kanpur and then finally returned to her real holding grounds, the inviolate potential jungles, completely off limits to human traffic save for foresters and authorized tourists.

The thing is to never lose hope.

So let's keep our fingers crossed and see what happens.

Acknowledgements

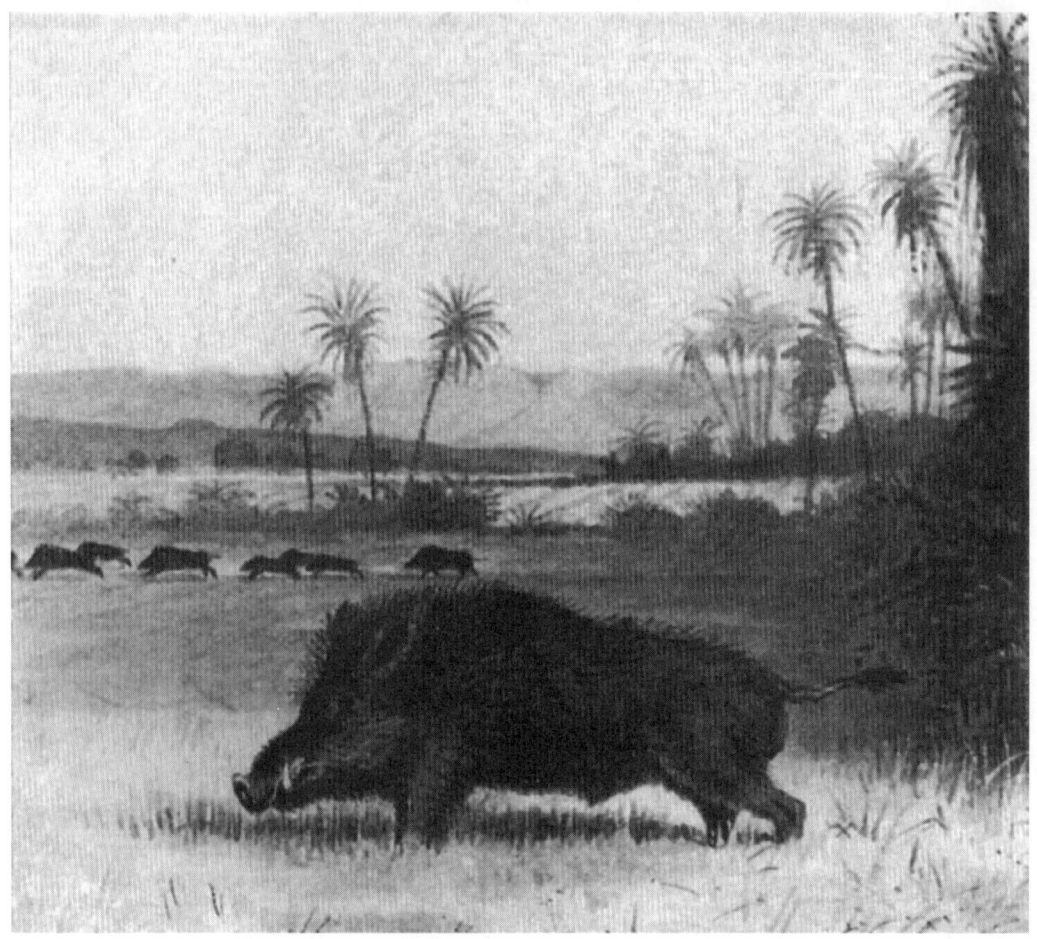

Just being in the Tarai farmlands, hearing if not seeing the tiger and conversing with the people of the old days gives me a new lease of life. Every time as I sit round the campfires, an old surge of thankfulness and joy overcomes me, over and over again. It makes me feel that I am away from the petty monotonies of urban existence and able to live the life I like. And this book is the outcome of those beautiful memories and those outstanding characters, aristocratic hunters, daring trackers, skilled gun-handlers and a hardened core of reformed poachers that can never walk out of calendar.

A very special thank is due to His Royal Highness, Dr Karan Singh, Maharaja of Jammu and Kashmir, a charming old world gentleman with most interesting shades of knowledge about Hinduism as well as of tigers. He not only showed a deep interest in my farmland wildlife research but remained concerned about the progress of my further investigations in this sphere and finally cared to write an informative introduction to this book. I feel indebted to his benign gesture.

Many of gracious people who helped me in this project are now no more but I cannot forget them. Foremost among them is Bharat Ratna Dr. APJ Kalam, who wrote the foreword of my introductory book on Sugarcane Tigers was in continuous correspondence with me about my second volume of the subject. I am in deep gratitude of Dr Kailash Sankhala who supported my idea of an emerging putative strain among these eco-type tigers and which needed to be protected from poachers for ultimate manifestation of that strain. My thanks are due to Late M Haider Mamman Khan, who gave me the opportunity to attend his tiger shoots with many personal accounts of the past, photographs and news clippings, including firsthand account of tiger shoots in farmlands.

I extend my heartfelt thanks to Late C. B. Singh, Chief Wildlife Warden of Uttar Pradesh, who invited me for a man-eater hunting expedition in trans-Sharda area thus generating a fresh opportunity for me to learn more about man-tiger conflict. I also thank the doyen of Dudhwa, Billy Arjan Singh who opposed my Cane Tiger theory tooth and nail, perhaps only to goad me more and more into this research. Finally late in life he observed that tigers do live in sugarcane farms and wondered why he himself had missed writing anything about this unique phenomenon in his books?

My grateful thanks are due to my cousin brother late Ajay Kumar Mishra, IAS, former Chief Secretary of Jharkhand, who accompanied me on my wildlife ventures including the chase of Rehman-Khera tiger on the outskirts of Lucknow. The best company in wilds, always ready to cover an extra mile for tiger, he not only encouraged me in writing this book but also generously helped me with anecdotes and opinions. I miss him at this moment.

Thanks to my brave gun bearers, the finest hunters of all, Chottey, Dilli, Phagunia and Bhajjenny, now no more and to trackers, Shri Pal, Neta, Shambho and Joginder, who still tirelessly cover miles with me, enduring pain and adventure while I continue to conduct this lengthy research on farmland wildlife.

My thanks are due to my old friends Yogesh Kumar, N. Ravi Shanker, Prabhas Kumar Jha, Jacob Thomas, Har Sharan Das, G.B. Pattanaik all IAS officers of Uttar Pradesh cadre, and Dev Raj Nagar, Balraj Bhalla, Ram Dev and Vijay Kumar all IPS officers of UP who occasionally joined my ventures and travelled the great vistas of Tarai with me.

Dr. R. L. Singh, former Director, Project Tiger, Government of India, Rupak De, Principal Chief Conservator of Forests, Uttar Pradesh, G.C. Mishra, former Field Director of Dhdhwa, Rashmi Kant Shukla, Shailesh Prashad, Uma Shanker Singh, Wung Longwa, presently all of them Principal Chief Conservators of Forests, stood by me as rock as I researched out hard facts about tigers in Tarai farmland. I feel grateful to all these well wishers.

My thanks are due to Dr Nirmala Singh, the principal of an intermediate college in Palia-Kalan, and her brother Dr P.N. Singh who helped me immensely in implementing my non-profit programme of 'Saving men from Tigers'. Rajesh Bharti, Mahesh Agarwal, Dev Kumar, Sardar Kuldeep Singh, Sukhdev Singh, Aman Singh and Pradhan of Kaanp Tanda, Ishwar Chand who joined the venture of public service by extending their helping hand to me in managing their local areas and also to Aparajita Shukla, my colleague in Christian College, who took pains to read and correct this manuscript.

Credit for photographs, lithographs, oil paintings and sketches produced in this book

The great Indian epic Mahabharat mentions of a famous character named Sanjay, who possessed a divine vision to see far-off events. This book contains the vision of some top photographers of wildlife. All of them are divine visionaries, whose celluloid and digital pictures show that there is a touch of divinity in free ranging animals and a special halo about them. That is why our ancestors regarded them as blood relatives, terrain guides and spiritual companions that connected us to the source of universal power and to our surrounding world.

These are:

- Yogesh Kumar, IAS
- Vijay Kumar, IPS, Additional Director General of Police, PAC, UP
- Sanjay Singh, IFS Field Director Dudhwa Tiger Reserve, UP
- Sanjay Pathak, IFS D.I.G, National Tiger Conservation Authority, New Delhi
- Sanjay Kumar IAS, District Magistrate of Allahabad, UP
- Pravein Rao, IFS, Principal Chief Conservator of Forests, UP
- Sanjay Narain, Owner of wildlife resort Dudhwa
- Sanjay Shah, artist contributor of wildlife sketches and monograms
- Sanjay Biswal, IFS, DFO South Kheri,
- Anurag Kumar, free lance wildlife photographer
- Mudit Gupta, Field Co-ordinator WWF, Kheri, Baharich and Pilibhit Districts
- Abhishek Verma, free lance wildlife photographer

My thanks are due to NTCA of the governement of India, WWF-India, Uttar Pradesh, Uttrakanad and Karnataka Forest Department, its foresters and dedicated field workers who helped me to profusely illustrate this book with their collection of photographs. My special gratitude to Maharashtra Forest department for providing me with data on wildlife living out side the protected areas. The data was collected over 27,970 camera trap days, making it the most rigorous camera trapping exercise ever carried out outside protected areas in India. The WCT team under supervision of Dr. Ullas Karanth and Vidya Atrayea also conducted several capacity-building workshops for the frontline forest staff so that they could conduct future assessments independently.

It is due their effort that this book reveals much about tigers and their transforming habitat of their prey. As a precaution, the photographs are not geo-tagged, which is to avoid getting undue attention to animals using specific areas.

Bibliography

Baker E. B, *Sport in Bengal*, London, 1888

Baldwin, J.A, *The Large and Small game of Bengal*, London, 1877

Baze W, *Tiger! Tiger!* London, 1957

Best, J.W, *Indian Shikar Notes*, London 1931

—*Forest Life in India*, London, 1935

Bindra, Prerna Singh, The King and I, Travels in Tigerland, Rupa &Co , New Delhi,2006,

Bolton, W, *Royal Chitwan National Park Management Plan*, Kathmandu, 1979

Brander A. A Dunbar, *Wild Animals of Central India*, London, 1923

Brown, J, Moray, *Shikar Sketches*, London, 1887

Burton R.G. *The Book of Tiger*, London, 1933

Campbell, Major Walter, *The old Forest Ranger*, London, 1843

Champion, F.W, *With a Camera in Tiger Land*,

—*The Jungle in Sunlight and Shadow*,

Corbett Jim, *Man-eaters of Kumaon*, New York and Bombay, 1944

The Temple Tiger, 1954

Jungle Lore, London, 1953

Tree Tops, London, 1955

Denial Johnson, Surgeon, *Indian Field Sports,* 1823,

Dockin, R, *The Selfish Gene*, Oxford University Press, 1976

Eardley Wilmot, S. *Forest Life and Sport in India*, London, 1910

Forsyth, J. *The Highlands of Central India*, London, 1872

Glasfurd A.I.R, *Rifle and Romance in the Indian Jungle*, London, 1905

Gordon Cumming, W, *Wild Men and Beasts*, Edinburgh, 1871

Hamilton, D. *Records of Sport in Southern India*, London, 1892

Hewett John, *Jungle Trails in North India*, London, 1938

Hanely, P. *Tiger Trails in Assam*, 1961

Hicks F.C. *Forty Years among Wild Animals in India*, Allahabad, 1910

Inglis James, *Tent Life in Tigerland*, London, 1888

Karanth Ullas, The *Science of Saving Tiger,* Universities Press, Hyderabad, 2001,

The Way of the Tiger, Centre for Wildlife Studies, Banglore.

Mac Dougal, Charls, *The Face of the Tiger*, London, 1977

Mishra Hemanta with Jim Ottaway JR, *Bones of the Tiger of Man Eating Tigers and Tiger Eating Men*

Mountfort, G, *Saving the Tiger*, London 1981

Patterson, J.H, *Man Eaters of Tasavo*, London, 1907

Perry, R. *The World of the Tiger*, London, 1974

Powel, A.N.W, *The Call of the Tiger*, 1957

Reader, J & Coze H, *Pyramids of Life*, London, 1977

Rice, W, *Tiger Shooting in India*, London, 1857

—Indian Game, 1884

Sanderson G.P, *Thirteen Years among the Wild Beasts of India*, London, 1887

Sankhala, K, *Tiger*, London, 1978

Schaller G.B, *The Deer and the Tiger*, Chicago, 1967

Shakespeare, H, *The Wild Sports of India*, London, 1860

Shukla, Rahul, *Killing Grounds*, Genesis Publications, Deryaganj Delhi, 1994

— *Leopards in the Backyard*, B.R. Publications Deryaganj Delhi, 2002

— *Tiger*, B.R. Publications, Deryaganj Delhi, 2008

— *Sugarcane Tiger; The phenomenon of wildlife in Tarai Farmlands*, IBDC, Deryaganj Delhi, *2013*,

Simpson, Frank.B, *Letters on Sport in Eastern Bengal*, London 1886

Singh Arjan, *Tiger Heaven*, London, 1973

——— *Tara the Tigress*, London, 1981

—— *The Legend of Maneater*, Delhi, 1999

Singh R. L, *Tara the Cocktail Tigress*, Allahabad, 2000

Stanley Breeden & Belinda Wright; *Through the Tigers Eyes*, California 1996

Storer J.H, *The Web of Life*, New York, 1953

Stephen Mills - Tiger. BBC Books Woodlands, London 2004

Thomas Pennant , A View of Hindoostan , two volumes, Printed by Henery Hughes, 1798

Thaper Valmik, *Secret Life of Tigers*, Oxford,

- *Tiger; the Predator*, London, 1986

Thomas Kuhn, *The Structure of Scientific Revolutions*,

Williamson, Thomas, *Oriental field Sports,* London, 1807

Wilson, E.O, *Sociobiology*, Harvard University Press, 1975

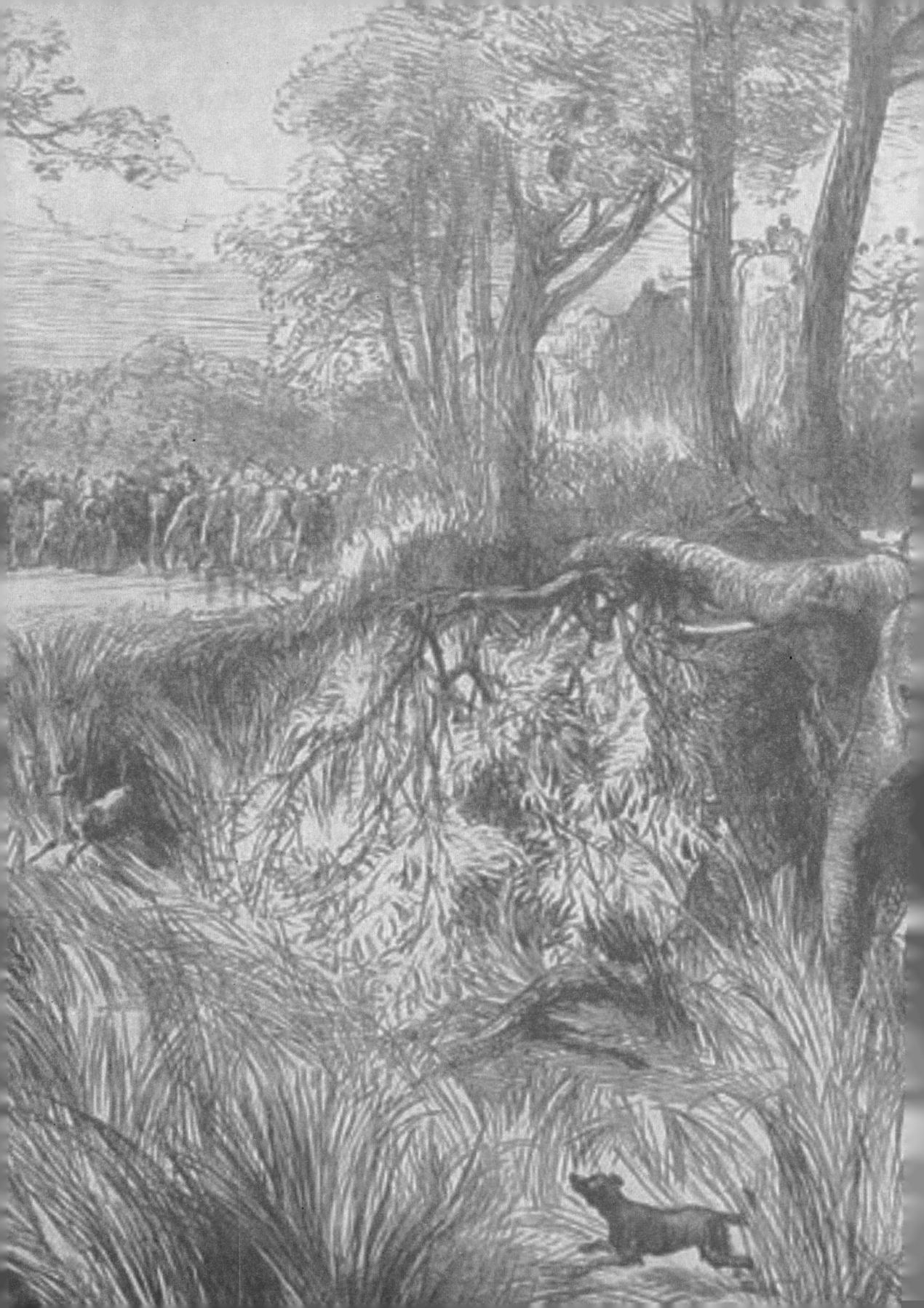